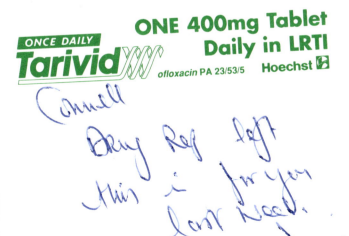
ONCE DAILY
Tarivid
ofloxacin PA 23/53/5

ONE 400mg Tablet
Daily in LRTI
Hoechst

Connell
Drug Rep left
this i for you
last week.

Epilepsy

Contents of Number 4

ISBN 0443 03915 1

You can place your order by contacting your local medical bookseller or the Sales Promotion Department, Robert Stevenson House, 1–3 Baxter's Place, Leith Walk, Edinburgh EH1 3AF, UK

Tel: (031) 556 2424; Telex: 727511 LONGMN G; Fax: (031) 558 1278

RECENT ADVANCES IN

Epilepsy

Edited by

T. A. Pedley MD

Professor and Vice-Chairman,
Department of Neurology,
College of Physicians and Surgeons of Columbia University;
Director, Columbia Comprehensive Epilepsy Center, New York, USA

B. S. Meldrum MA MB BChir PhD

Professor of Experimental Neurology,
Department of Neurology,
Institute of Psychiatry, London, UK

NUMBER FIVE

CHURCHILL LIVINGSTONE
EDINBURGH LONDON MELBOURNE NEW YORK AND TOKYO 1992

CHURCHILL LIVINGSTONE
Medical Division of Longman Group UK Limited

Distributed in the United States of America by Churchill
Livingstone Inc., 1560 Broadway, New York, N.Y.
10036, and by associated companies, branches and
representatives throughout the world.

First published 1992

ISBN 0-443-04494-6

ISSN 0 264 7400

British Library Cataloguing in Publication Data
A catalogue record for this book is available from the British
Library

Library of Congress Cataloguing in Publication Data
is available

Printed in Great Britain by Butler & Tanner Ltd, Frome and London

Preface

This issue, like its four predecessors, aims to provide authoritative reviews on a wide range of topics in the field of epilepsy. Criteria for selecting topics included not only timeliness and major recent progress, but also practical importance and lack of previous coverage in this series. Of the 14 chapters in this issue, 8 are devoted to fundamental mechanisms, pathophysiology and diagnosis of epilepsy, and 6 are concerned with treatment.

The first chapter shows how techniques of molecular biology can be applied to understanding the genetic basis of epilepsy. The properties of the various calcium channels in the nerve membrane and their possible roles in epileptogenesis and antiepileptic drug action are described in Chapter 2. The third chapter reviews the concept of cortical dysplasia, developing the view that pathological changes in focal epilepsy represent an intermediate developmental defect between lissencephaly and 'micro-dysgenesis'. Two chapters review new approaches to detection and analysis of EEG signals. Specific pathogenetic mechanisms for development of epilepsy are considered in three chapters. One assesses the role of prenatal and perinatal risk factors. Another discusses the contribution of craniocerebral trauma and emphasizes the crucial importance of preventive measures. The third chapter in this group reviews the growing problem of seizures associated with HIV infection. Next, the management of epilepsy is considered both in the larger medical context in which seizures may occur and from the point of view of the practitioner in the third world. Clinical data are presented for three novel antiepileptic drugs which may have a place in the future therapy of epilepsy. A final chapter reviews behavioural therapy of epilepsy.

Once again, we thank our distinguished contributors for providing concise and readable reviews and for conforming to editorial whims and deadlines. We hope that this issue will help to improve the lives of patients with epilepsy by providing guidance and stimulation to physicians, research workers and others in the field.

New York
London
1992

T.A.P.
B.S.M.

Contributors

D. Chadwick DM FRCP
Consultant Neurologist, Department of Neuroscience, Walton Hospital,
Liverpool, UK

Robert J. DeLorenzo MD PhD MPH
Professor and Chairman, Department of Neurology, Medical College
of Virginia, Virginia Commonwealth University, Richmond, Virginia, USA

John S. Ebersole MD
Professor, Department of Neurology, Yale University School of
Medicine, Connecticut, USA

Peter Fenwick MB BChir DPM FRCPsych
Consultant Neuropsychiatrist, Maudsley Hospital; Senior Lecturer,
Institute of Psychiatry, London, UK

Jean Gotman PhD
Associate Professor, Montreal Neurological Institute, Department of
Neurology and Neurosurgery, McGill University, Montreal, Quebec,
Canada

Ivan Janota MBBS FRCPath
Consultant and Honorary Senior Lecturer in Neuropathology, Department
of Neuropathology, Institute of Psychiatry, London, UK

N. A. Kshirsagar MD DClPh PhD DNB MNAMS
Associate Professor, Department of Pharmacology, Seth GS Medical
College, KEM Hospital, Bombay, India

Douglas R. Labar MD PhD
Director, Comprehensive Epilepsy Center, New York Hospital –
Cornell Medical Center, New York, USA

Jeffrey L. Noebels PhD MD
Director, Developmental Neurogenetics Laboratory, Department of
Neurology, Baylor College of Medicine, Houston, Texas, USA

Jonathan B. Perlin MD PhD
Department of Neurology and Department of Pharmacology and
Toxicology, Medical College of Virginia, Virginia Commonwealth
University, Richmond, Virginia, USA

Charles E. Polkey MD FRCS
Consultant Neurosurgeon, Maudsley Hospital and Bethlem Royal
Hospital, London, UK

Edward H. Reynolds MD FRCP
Consultant Neurologist, Maudsley and Kings College Hospitals,
London, UK

A. Richens PhD FRCP
Professor and Head, Department of Pharmacology and Therapeutics,
University of Wales College of Medicine, Cardiff, UK

Howard A. Ring BSc MRCPsych
Raymond Way Lecturer in Neuropsychiatry, Institute of Neurology,
London, UK

Mark L. Scheuer MD
Assistant Professor of Neurology, College of Physicians and Surgeons
of Columbia University, New York, USA

Pravina U. Shah MD(Gen Med) MD(Neurology)
Honorary Professor and Head, Department of Neurology, Seth GS
Medical College and KEM Hospital, Bombay; Consultant Neurologist,
Conwest Jain Hospital, Bombay, India

Sheila Wallace FRCPE
Consultant Paediatric Neurologist, University Hospital of Wales,
Cardiff, UK

L. James Willmore MD
Professor of Neurology, University of Texas Medical School, Houston,
Texas, USA

Contents

1

Molecular genetics and epilepsy

J. L. Noebels

You might think that a scientist who clones an unknown disease gene on the first attempt must be very smart. That would be like thinking that a man who enters a casino and wins at a slot machine on the first try is very smart.

R. Davis

INTRODUCTION

The human genome contains approximately 6 billion DNA bases, yet an alteration in only one is sufficient to cause disease. If these odds now seem commonplace to the modern gene hunter, consider that while an average gene extends about 2000 base pairs along the length of a chromosome, not all permutations in its coding sequence are equally deleterious. Furthermore, when the brain is the target tissue, a cascade of alternative gene-regulated homeostatic pathways mediating neuronal and synaptic plasticity may fully compensate for the gene error, even in the total absence of a functional gene product. Finally, consider the unique behaviour of the epileptic phenotype: although the molecular genetic lesion itself is fixed, its pathophysiological expression in the central nervous system is ephemeral. These inherent attributes make it clear why isolating and unravelling the cellular expression of epilepsy genes – a special subset of the genes that control the excitability of neural networks – present an unusually challenging goal for neurobiologists studying human genetic disorders at the molecular level.

Despite these unfavourable odds, recent advances in applying genetic strategies to define human neurological disorders are just beginning to direct attention to the promise these tools hold for similar gains in understanding the most common neurological affliction of all – seizures. The current excitement stems from the successful mapping of Duchenne muscular dystrophy to the X chromosome (Monaco et al 1987), hyperkalaemic periodic paralysis to chromosome 17 (Fontaine et al 1990), and neurofibromatoses nf1 to chromosome 17 and nf2 to chromosome 22 (Barker et al 1987, Rouleau et al 1987). Chromosomal markers for Huntington's disease on chromosome 4 (Gusella et al 1983) and myotonic dystrophy on chromosome 19 (Brunner et al 1989) give promise of finding the genes for these disorders in the near future.

In contrast with the unambiguous disease phenotypes initially selected for molecular genetic analysis, the epilepsies represent a heterogeneous group of disorders of neuronal excitability arising from inherited and acquired disturbances in neuronal bursting properties, connectivity and synaptic transmission. Although a hereditary predisposition is generally reported to contribute to 10–15% of epilepsy cases worldwide, these data account for only a small fraction of the larger category of prevailing cases considered to be idiopathic or cryptogenic (roughly 77% of all newly diagnosed cases) (Hauser & Hesdorffer 1990) in which genetic factors may also play a role in seizure susceptibility. Our understanding of the importance of genetic contributions will undoubtedly increase as: (1) medical and societal gains are made in preventable acquired aetiologies (trauma, stroke, infection and adverse birth history); (2) family histories are more carefully reported; (3) new insights emerge into the fundamental mechanisms most commonly disturbed in various epileptic phenotypes and the spontaneous mutation rate of major genes controlling those mechanisms; and (4) biochemical markers required for definitive ascertainment of the inherited lesions become available for molecular genetic diagnosis.

In this review, I will discuss several areas in which molecular genetic strategies are exerting an important influence on basic and clinical research in the epilepsies. These are: (1) mapping existing epilepsy genes from human pedigrees and delineating epilepsy syndromes; (2) identifying epilepsy genes in animal species and analysing basic gene mechanisms of epilepsy; and (3) defining novel candidate genes by examining the seizure-induced expression of neural genes.

SEARCHING FOR GENES OF COMMON DISEASES

It has been accepted dogma that common familial diseases with mixed clinical phenotypes lacking clear Mendelian patterns of inheritance are likely to be polygenic or multifactorial in origin, and unlikely to be controlled appreciably by alterations in a single gene. While this statement remains valid, it is now quite evident that buried within a wide variety of generic neurological diagnoses such as stroke, senile dementia of the Alzheimer type and epilepsy lie a proportion of cases that can be linked to specific chromosomal loci, for example genetic coagulopathies (Natowicz & Kelly 1987), the subset of Alzheimer's syndrome seen in trisomy chromosome 21 (St George-Hyslop et al 1987), and over 100 recessive disorders that include seizures as one phenotypic manifestation (McKusick 1990). Among the epilepsies, a wide variety of genetic and non-genetic phenocopies of various seizure patterns coexist, and it is only in elucidating their unique clinical and pathological features, rather than stressing their similarities, that we will achieve a full understanding of the basic mechanisms of epileptogenesis.

While a steady stream of new and complementary methods are being developed to compare and decipher gene sequences, the initial approach to human disease genes begins with the chance association of a marker phenotype with the inherited trait determined by linkage mapping. Two general strategies are employed. *Functional cloning* describes the path starting with the use of structural or functional information about the gene product. This usually implies the availability of a large amount of biological information about the natural history of the disease and the intervening cellular disturbances which can be used to generate a specific hypothesis based on the pathological expression of a candidate molecule. Examples of this approach have been the hypotheses that chloride ion channels were involved in cystic fibrosis (Rommens et al 1989), and sodium channels in hyperkalaemic periodic paralysis (Fontaine et al 1990).

The second strategy is termed *positional cloning*. When both the gene and its translated product are unknown, the approximate map position of the locus can be determined by linkage analysis relative to mapped anonymous chromosomal markers such as restriction fragment length polymorphisms and other internal repetitive DNA sequences (Nakamura et al 1987). A large number of evenly distributed chromosomal markers enhances the odds of tight linkage with the unknown gene error. Once the smaller DNA fragment containing the disease gene (and a large number of irrelevant sequences) has been cloned, several steps are useful in further pinpointing the boundary of the specific gene. These include interspecific comparisons to isolate evolutionary conservation of the gene sequence, and in vitro expression of mRNA transcripts. Finally, functional confirmation is needed that the gene and one of its alternative gene products actually causes the disease. This can be shown directly, either by verifying the presence of the mutation in a patient, or by introducing a copy of the wild-type gene into an experimental mutant genome to correct the defect. The latter proof was accomplished for the first time in the hypomyelinated, myelin basic protein deficient mutant mouse *shiverer*, where a syndrome of inherited tremor and seizures was averted by replacement of the defective gene (Readhead et al 1987).

Formal proof of the link between cloned gene and disease phenotype is crucial, even more so when the defective gene turns out to encode a protein end-product that was previously unknown, much less mapped. Unfortunately, implicit in the aforementioned transgenic approach is the constraint that definitive causal evidence in the form of a clear chain of pathological events triggered by the primary gene error is difficult to obtain in human nervous tissue. For practical purposes, then, the final elucidation of how human epilepsy gene mutations cause seizures at specific ages will need to be accomplished by indirect evaluation of the defective molecule in other animal model systems, and as a result the inferred mechanisms will be only as valid as the extent to which the model proves faithful to its human counterpart. The issue of incongruous clinical phenotypes across mutations in different species is a real, not theoretical, dilemma and has already arisen in other neuromuscular disorders, including the hypoxanthine phosphoribosyl transferase_ Lesch Nyhan mouse and the dystrophin_ mdx mouse, each entirely deficient in the gene product yet each lacking clinical symptomatology.

Practical limitations of gene mapping are minimized when: (1) the disease gene is highly penetrant; (2) the age of disease onset is known; and (3) the clinical phenotype is unambiguous (Leppart 1990, Anderson et al 1990). A high incidence of sporadic cases of a disease can also introduce difficulties, because it becomes unclear whether a high mutation rate or the presence of multifactorial causes are at play. For example, the increased spontaneous mutation rate in neurofibromatosis (50%, or about 100 times higher than the average gene) means that about one-half of the probands represent new cases with a negative family history. Altered severity of disease expression within the same family suggests the presence of modifier genes. Polygenic disorders pose a complex problem, but in principle should be amenable to the same strategy. All of the aforementioned difficulties are likely to be encountered in the search for epilepsy-related genes.

When linkage analysis is conclusive, a positive result demonstrates that the trait is genetic and provides the basis for definitive diagnosis and rational therapy. On the other hand, borderline results require appropriate scepticism, and access to original pedigrees and data by independent investigators is desirable. In particular, phenotypic markers such as electroencephalographic (EEG) findings and the clinical seizure history itself are susceptible to observer bias, and linkage based on these data should not be accepted without replication.

HUMAN GENE MAPPING STUDIES

Two distinct epilepsy syndromes have received detailed examination and tentative map locations have been assigned.

Juvenile myoclonic epilepsy (JME)

JME (Janz 1985) is a syndrome appearing in mid-adolescence characterized by a pattern of bilateral myoclonic jerks, generalized tonic–clonic seizures and, sometimes, absence seizures. Patients are neurologically normal, and both the myoclonus and other seizures respond to valproate. The EEG displays bilaterally symmetrical and synchronous 4–6 Hz multispike–wave complexes, with or without 2–3 Hz spike–wave complexes. In initial segregation and linkage studies in 28 families, lod scores of 3.05 were reported to the HLA and properdin (Bf) markers located on the short arm of chromosome 6 (Greenberg et al 1988). More recent analysis with additional pedigrees has yielded a lod score of 3.78 using an autosomal dominant model of inheritance with an assumed penetrance of 0.9, and a lod score of 3.05 with a recessive model assuming full penetrance (Delgado-Escueta 1990). While both linkage models yield scores exceeding the generally accepted significance level of 3, the apparent contradiction of the dual inheritance patterns has not yet been clarified. The inclusion and rejection criteria used for classifying affected individuals and the carrier status of family members have all been clearly enumerated (Delgado-Escueta 1990), and linkage of the JME phenotype assuming a dominant inheritance model has recently been independently confirmed using both serological (Weissbecker et al 1991) and restriction fragment length polymorphism (RFLP) (Durner et al 1990) markers for the HLA locus.

The major obstacles encountered in these pioneering studies were the uncertainties caused by phenotypic heterogeneity of the idiopathic generalized epilepsies, the lack of an obvious Mendelian pattern of inheritance, and the concern surrounding the carrier status of family members with non-specific EEG abnormalities and no clinical seizures. Overlapping variations in the age of onset and pattern of EEG discharge among the currently recognized clinical syndromes of idiopathic generalized-onset epilepsy present important nosological problems (Fig. 1.1). While some of these problems may not be fully resolvable, it seems likely that the determination of heritability of other subtypes of idiopathic generalized-onset epilepsy will yield to a systematic approach.

Benign familial neonatal convulsions (BFNC)

This syndrome, initially described by Rett & Teubel (1964), is a rare and benign form of neonatal seizures that can show autosomal dominant inheritance. Leppart et al (1989) screened DNA samples from over 47 family members in a four-generation American pedigree that included 19 members with historical evidence for the BFNC trait. Tests using nearly 100 DNA probes revealed that two markers on chromosome 20q – RMR6 and CMM6 – were transmitted along with the gene with a likelihood ratio of 450 000:1 favouring linkage. This analysis has been replicated in six French pedigrees of BFNC with the same probes used by Leppart, and an obligate recombinant in one of the families precluded significant linkage (Malafosse et al 1990). Using an additional RFLP marker for chromosome 20q13.3, however, a lod score of 2.93 was calculated, supporting a localization of the gene within this region. Other preliminary studies suggest the syndrome as currently defined may be clinically heterogeneous (Ryan & Wiznitzer 1990).

IDENTIFYING AND MAPPING MURINE EPILEPSY GENES

While the pathophysiological features of inherited epilepsy in various animal strains have been investigated for years, only in the last decade has

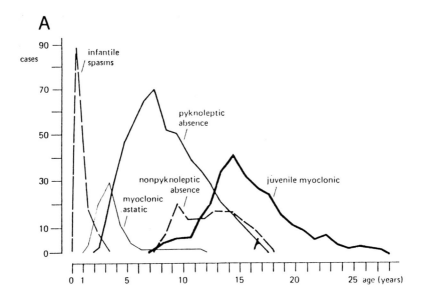

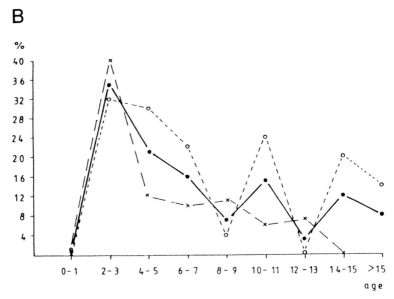

Fig. 1.1   Clinical heterogeneity of generalized epileptic phenotypes. **A** Temporal dispersion and overlapping ages of onset in various defined epilepsy syndromes. (From Janz et al 1989.) **B** Range of spike–wave EEG discharge frequencies in 302 siblings of probands with primary generalized epilepsy. x—x (boys), ○—○ (girls), ●—● (total). (From Doose & Baier 1989.)

there been a systematic search to identify the genes responsible (Noebels 1989, 1991). Phenotypic screening of single-locus mutations in inbred mouse strains offers a direct strategy to define new experimental models of epilepsy and to trace the developmental expression of the intervening cellular defects. Candidate mechanisms in mice are of major interest, because both gene sequence and chromosomal linkage homologies are highly conserved in mouse and humans (Womack 1987). Several important principles became immediately evident at the outset of the mutational analysis (Noebels 1979). The first was that single-locus gene mutations did indeed exist that could express chronic seizures, including the spike–wave seizure pattern, indicating that the membrane instabilities required to elicit this intermittent hyperexcitability phenotype can be transmitted as a recessive trait. The second principle was that more than one such genetic locus existed, because the spike–wave phenotype alone had been detected repeatedly in the survey of mapped spontaneous neurological mutants and currently includes five independent loci (Table 1.1). A third finding was that the gene defect could give rise to a reasonably precise cellular defect within the neuraxis representing the candidate destabilizing epileptogenic lesion. These conclusions represented more or less significant departures from previously held views. In the case of the spike–wave phenotype, there had been no prior indication from human studies (Doose & Baier 1989) that the general category of primary generalized spike–wave epilepsies could also contain a subset of lesions affecting neural hyperexcitability that follow a monogenic inheritance pattern, although this is consistent with newly emerging evidence (see above). The finding that the spike–wave phenotype in mice was under the non-exclusive control of several independent loci suggests not only that alternative conclusions over the exact modes of inheritance in man might not be contradictory, but also that the hereditary pattern and the intervening cellular pathology may both be reflections of the particular gene defect transmitted in the pedigree under study. Other experimental advantages of the mutant mice have been enumerated (Noebels 1985).

The first mapped epilepsy gene to be identified for the spike–wave seizure phenotype in the mouse was a mutation at the *tottering* locus on chromosome 8. This mutation results in a diffuse, gene-linked noradrenergic (NE) axon terminal hyperinnervation of the forebrain originating from locus coeruleus neurones and a generalized seizure disorder featuring brief, 6–7 per second cortical spike–wave EEG discharges associated with behavioural arrest (Noebels & Sidman 1979, Kaplan et al 1979, Levitt & Noebels 1981). The occurrence of the spontaneous neocortical epileptiform discharges increases in parallel with the postnatal development of cortical

Table 1.1 Mapped gene loci causing generalized spike–wave epilepsy in the mouse

Locus	Symbol	Chromosome	Mode
Lethargic	*lh*	2	Recessive
Tottering	*tg*	8	Recessive
Leaner	*tg^{la}*	8	Recessive
Ducky	*du*	9	Recessive
Mocha^{2j}	*mh^{2j}*	10	Recessive
Stargazer	*stg*	15	Recessive

noradrenergic innervation, and the onset of the seizure disorder in the adolescent mouse can be entirely prevented by selective denervation of the forebrain NE projection at birth (Noebels 1984). Although the molecular nature of the primary mutant defect remains unknown, these and other data (Noebels & Rutecki 1990) strongly suggest that in this genetic model central NE hyperinnervation facilitates the developmental expression of a specific pattern of synchronous cortical bursting. Recent intracellular recordings reveal that one mechanism underlying the hypernoradrenergic defect may be a reduction in the β-NE receptor-mediated membrane afterhyperpolarization (Fig. 1.2) (Helekar & Noebels 1991), a mechanism believed to contribute to epileptogenesis in other seizure models (Dichter & Ayala 1987).

By comparison, however, recent analysis of a newly described mutant, *stargazer* (Noebels et al 1990), which shares a far more severe but otherwise identical spike–wave seizure phenotype, shows no elevation of forebrain NE and neonatal NE terminal ablation has no effect on subsequent seizure expression (Qiao & Noebels 1991) (Fig. 1.3). These data suggest that the two genes act through independent intervening brain mechanisms to produce spike–wave epilepsy, and indicate that the severity of the clinical epileptic disorder can show a striking dependence on which of the specific genes associated with spike–wave discharges is inherited.

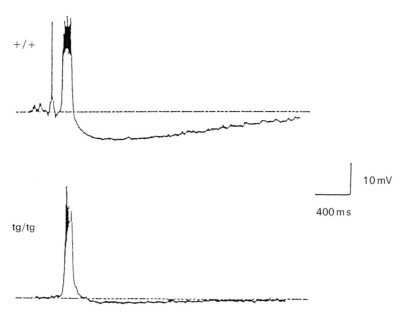

Fig. 1.2   A gene mutation for spike–wave seizures reduces NE-mediated afterhyperpolarization (AHP) in hippocampal neurons. Intracellular current clamp recordings from CA3 pyramidal neurons in wild-type ($+/+$) and tottering (tg/tg) mice reveal decreased AHP amplitude in the NE-hyperinnervated mutant cell following a paroxysmal depolarizing shift elicited by increased extracellular potassium ions. The defect is corrected in the presence of a β-adrenoreceptor blocker. (From Helekar & Noebels 1991.)

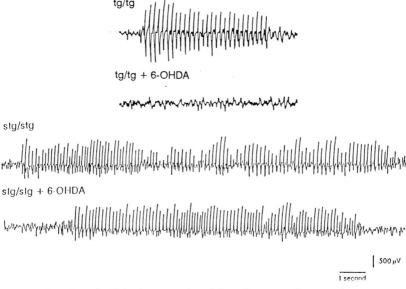

tg/tg

tg/tg + 6-OHDA

stg/stg

stg/stg + 6-OHDA

500 μV

1 second

Fig. 1.3   Genetic and cellular heterogeneity of the spike–wave phenotype in two mouse mutants. EEG tracings from two independent gene mutations, *tg/tg* (chromosome 8) and *stg/stg* (chromosome 15), reveal morphological similarity of the spontaneous cortical discharges phenotype, although the discharges are longer in duration and more frequent in the *stg* mutant. The onset of seizures in adolescence can be permanently prevented in *tg/tg* mutants by neonatal injections of 6-hydroxydopamine (6-OHDA), which reduce forebrain noradrenergic innervation (upper traces), while seizure expression in the *stg* mutants is entirely unaffected by noradrenergic lesions (lower traces). (Adapted from Noebels 1984 and Qiao & Noebels 1991.)

CANDIDATE GENES FOR EPILEPSY

Genes suggested by phenocopy experiments

A small group of genes that have a high probability for involvement in hereditary epilepsies can be nominated from the larger category of membrane-bound and intracellular molecules whose expression modulates excitability within neural circuits. The subset can be drawn at first approximation from the list of molecules where a hypothetical defect has been shown, in an experimental model, to precipitate seizures. While the initial impulse to consider defects in inhibitory mechanisms might logically direct attention to the genes encoding potassium and chloride channels and the receptors that gate them, it is worth noting that point mutations can result in kinetic or numerical changes in neuronal excitability molecules that alter function in a positive as well as a negative direction. Thus, a structural mutation that raises the affinity of an excitatory ligand for its receptor, or a regulatory mutation that increases the density of a specific voltage-dependent, burst-related cation channel, for example a sodium channel or the low threshold Ca^{2+} channel, are equally valid possibilities.

The locus encoding the $GABA_A$ receptor is a major candidate epilepsy gene since it represents the major inhibitory neurotransmitter receptor of the human brain and has long been implicated in mechanisms of epileptogenesis by phenocopy experiments that produce seizures following pharmacological blockade. The receptor contains α and β subunits, and several isoforms of these subunits have been cloned and mapped (human chromosomes 4, 5 and X) (Buckle et al 1989). The gene for the synthetic enzyme in the GABA pathway, glutamic acid decarboxylase, has been cloned from brain (Kaufman et al 1986), as has another related molecule in the pathway, the GABA transporter, designated GAT-1. GAT-1 possesses high affinity for GABA and exhibits pharmacological properties of the neuronal GABA transporter present in brain (Guastella et al 1990). These clones should enable molecular screening of human epilepsy pedigrees with the appropriate cDNA probe.

Genes encoding a variety of neuronal potassium channels are a second major generic candidate gene group. These channels play a key role in membrane repolarization, and blockade of one or more of the K^+ channel subtypes can initiate seizures. Over 30 different potassium channels have been characterized biophysically (Jan & Jan 1990). The number of parent genes is smaller, and the molecular diversity is ascribed in part to alternative splicing of the transcripts, heteromultimeric combinations of subunits, and post-translational modification of the channel polypeptide. The homologue of the *shaker* potassium channel gene has recently been cloned in human brain and mapped to the telomere of human chromosome 12p (Wilhelmsen et al 1990).

Seizure-induced genes

Important new evidence obtained from in situ molecular hybridization of cDNA probes to cerebral tissue has revealed that seizures induce both early and delayed changes in the pattern of neural gene expression (Morgan et al 1987, Gall & Isackson 1989) (Fig. 1.4). A list of gene transcripts whose

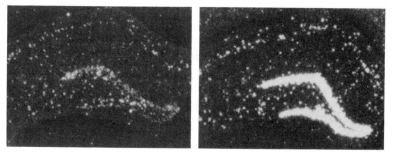

Fig. 1.4   Seizure-induced neural gene expression in hippocampus. Dark field autoradiograms of messenger RNA for nerve growth factor visualized by in situ hybridization in rat hippocampus in control (left) or 1 hour following a single seizure (right). Large increases were found in the stratum granulosum. (From Gall et al 1991.)

Table 1.2   Seizure-induced genes in hippocampus

mRNA	Latency	Duration	Cellular distribution	Ref.
Immediate early genes				
c-fos	Minutes	2 h	Diffuse increase	1, 2, 3, 5
c-jun	Minutes	2 h	Diffuse increase	3
junB	Minutes	2 h	Diffuse increase	3
NGF1A (zif/268)	Minutes	2 h	Diffuse increase	3, 5
Growth factors				
Nerve growth factor (NGF)	1 h	24 h	Selective increase	5
Brain-derived neurotrophic factor (BDNF)	1 h	6 h	Selective increase	5
Neurotrophin 3 (NT3)	1 h	12 h	Selective increase	5
Peptide neurotransmitters and enzymes				
Preproenkephalin	3 h	36 h	Selective increase	5
Preprodynorphin	3 h	24 h	Selective increase	5
NPY	6 h	10 h	Selective increase	5
Receptors				
Kainate	12 h	21 h	Selective decrease	4

(1) Morgan et al 1987; (2) White & Gall 1987; (3) Saffen et al 1988; (4) Gall et al 1990; (5) Gall et al 1991

abundance is significantly altered following seizures induced in different models is given in Table 1.2.

While the immediate significance of these gene transcription changes remains to be evaluated, the phenomenon may mediate long-term changes in excitability. A logical extension of this line of reasoning suggests the fundamental hypothesis that some epilepsy syndromes may arise, or change in character, along an alternative pathway of abnormal neural gene expression in the brain triggered by the first few seizure episodes. Alternatively, some may disappear for the same reason. If the premise can be accepted that a cascade of secondary neural plasticity involving rearrangements of neuronal membrane composition or synaptic circuitry is a basic mechanism in epileptogenesis, two critical predictions can be considered. The first is that a mutation in any of these loci could also be inherited as a primary defect; these seizure-inducible genes therefore comprise a plausible subset of candidate genes for epilepsy. The second is that it provides a rational basis for prevention or post hoc management of epilepsy by inducing compensatory changes in gene expression. Because new genes cannot be selectively substituted for old ones in the nervous system, advances in the molecular correction of inherited epilepsies may centre on strategies designed to alter the course and pattern of secondary cellular changes that themselves lead to sustained hyperexcitability. Single-locus murine mutations with highly reproducible patterns of early-onset epilepsy therefore provide valuable biological test systems, both for tracing the cellular pathogenesis of inherited seizure disorders and for future studies in the clinical management of epilepsy gene expression.

ACKNOWLEDGEMENTS

This work was supported by grants from the NIH, Blue Bird Circle Foundation for Pediatric Neurology, March of Dimes/Birth Defects Foundation, and a Pew Biomedical Scholars Award.

REFERENCES

Anderson V E, Hauser W A, Olafsson E, Rich S S 1990 Genetic aspects of the epilepsies. In: Sillanpaa M, Johannesson S I, Blennow G, Dam M (eds) Pediatric epilepsy. Wrightson Biomedical Publishing, London, pp 37–56

Barker D, Wright E, Nguyen K et al 1987 Gene for Recklinghausen neurofibromatosis is in the pericentromeric region of chromosome 17. Science 236: 1100–1102

Brunner H G, Smeets H, Lambermon H et al 1989 A multipoint linkage map around the locus for myotonic dystrophy on chromosome 19. Genomics 5: 589–565

Buckle V J, Fujita N, Ryder-Cook A S et al 1989 Chromosomal localization of GABA$_A$ receptor subunit genes: relationship to human genetic disease. Neuron 3: 647–654

Delgado-Escueta A V 1990 Gene mapping in primary generalized epilepsies. Epilepsia 31: S19–S29

Dichter M, Ayala G F 1987 Cellular mechanisms of epilepsy. Science 237: 157–164

Doose H, Baier W K 1989 Generalized spikes and waves. In: Beck-Mannegetta G, Janz D (eds) Genetics of the epilepsies. Springer-Verlag, Berlin, pp 95–103

Durner M, Sander T, Greenberg D A, Johnson K, Janz D 1990 Localization of idiopathic generalized epilepsy on chromosome 6p in families ascertained through juvenile myoclonic epilepsy patients. Epilepsia 31: 815

Fontaine B, Khurana T S, Hoffman E et al 1990 Hyperkalemic periodic paralysis and the adult muscle sodium channel alpha-subunit gene. Science 250: 1000–1002

Gall C, Isackson P J 1989 Limbic seizures increase neuronal production of messenger RNA for nerve growth factor. Science 245: 758–761

Gall C, Sumikawa K, Lynch G 1990 Levels of mRNA for a putative kainate receptor are affected by seizures. Proc Natl Acad Sci USA 87: 7643–7647

Gall C M, Lauterborn J, Bundman M, Murray K, Isackson P 1991 Seizures and the regulation of neurotrophic factor and neuropeptide gene expression in brain. In: Anderson E, Leppik I, Noebels J (eds) Genetic strategies in epilepsy research. Elsevier, Amsterdam

Greenberg D A, Delgado-Escueta A V, Widelitz H et al 1988 Juvenile myoclonic epilepsy (JME) may be linked to the Bf and HLA loci in human chromosome 6. Am J Med Genet 31: 185–192

Guastella J, Nelson H, Czyzyk L et al 1990 Cloning and expression of a rat brain GABA transporter. Science 249: 1303–1306

Gusella J, Wexler N, Conneally P et al 1983 A polymorphic DNA marker genetically linked to Huntington's disease. Nature 306: 234–238

Hauser W A, Hesdorffer D C 1990 Epilepsy: frequency, causes, and consequences. Demos.

Helekar S, Noebels J L 1991 Synchronous hippocampal bursting unmasks latent network excitability alterations in an epileptic gene mutation. Proc Natl Acad Sci USA 88: 4736–4740

Jan L Y, Jan Y N 1990 How might the diversity of potassium channels be generated? Trends Neurosci 13: 415–419

Janz D 1985 Epilepsy with impulsive petit mal (juvenile myoclonic epilepsy). Acta Neurol Scand 72: 449–459

Janz D, Durner M, Beck-Mannegetta G, Pantazis G 1989 Family studies on the genetics of juvenile myoclonic epilepsy (epilepsy with impulsive petit mal). In: Beck-Mannegetta G, Janz D (eds) Genetics of the epilepsies. Springer-Verlag, Berlin, pp 43–52

Kaplan B, Seyfried T N, Glaser G 1979 Spontaneous polyspike discharges in an epileptic mutant mouse (tottering). Exp Neurol 66: 577–586

Kaufman D, McGinnis J F, Krieger N R, Tobin A J 1986 Brain glutamate decarboxylase cloned in lambda-gt-11:fusion protein produces γ-aminobutyric acid. Science 232: 1138–1140

Leppart M F 1990 Gene mapping and other tools for discovery. Epilepsia 31: S11–S18

Leppart M, Anderson V, Quattlebaum T et al 1989 The gene for benign familial neonatal convulsions maps to human chromosome 20. Nature 337: 647–648

Levitt P, Noebels J L 1981 Mutant mouse tottering: selective increase of locus coeruleus axons in a defined single locus mutation. Proc Natl Acad Sci USA 78: 4630–4634

Malafosse A, Dulac O, Leboyer M, Schnittger S, Hansmann I, Mallet J 1990 Linkage studies of benign familial neonatal convulsions in six French families. Epilepsia 31: 816

McKusick V A 1990 Mendelian inheritance in man, 9th edn. Johns Hopkins Press, Baltimore

Monaco A, Bertelson C J, Colletti-Feener C, Kunkel L 1987 Localization and cloning of Xp21 deletion breakpoints involved in muscular dystrophy. Hum Genet 75: 321–327

Morgan J I, Cohen D R, Hempstead J L, Curran T 1987 Mapping patterns of c-fos expression in the central nervous system after seizure. Science 237: 192–197

Nakamura Y, Leppart M, O'Connel P et al 1987 Variable number of tandem repeat (VNTR) markers for human gene mapping. Science 235: 1616–1622

Natowicz M, Kelly R I 1987 Mendelian etiologies of stroke. Ann Neurol 22: 175–192

Noebels J L 1979 Analysis of inherited epilepsy using single locus mutations in mice. Fed Proc 38: 2405–2410

Noebels J L 1984 A single gene error in noradrenergic axon growth synchronizes central neurons. Nature 310: 409–411

Noebels J L 1985 Mutational analysis of the inherited epilepsies. In: Delgado-Escueta A V, Ward A A, Woodbury D M (eds) Basic mechanisms of the epilepsies: molecular and cellular approaches. Raven Press, New York

Noebels J L 1989 Experimental neurogenetics of the inherited epilepsies. In: Beck-Mannegetta G, Janz D (eds) Genetics of the epilepsies. Springer-Verlag, Berlin, pp 184–190

Noebels J L 1991 Mutational analysis of spike–wave epilepsy phenotypes. In: Anderson E, Leppik I, Noebels J (eds) Genetic strategies in epilepsy research. Elsevier, Amsterdam

Noebels J L, Rutecki P A 1990 Altered hippocampal network excitability in the hypernoradrenergic mutant mouse tottering. Brain Res 524: 225–230

Noebels J L, Sidman R L 1979 Inherited epilepsy: spike–wave and focal motor seizures in the mutant mouse tottering. Science 204: 1334–1336

Noebels J L, Qiao X, Bronson R T, Davisson M T 1990 Stargazer: a new neurological mutation in the mouse on chromosome 15 with prolonged cortical seizures. Epilepsy Res 7: 129–135

Qiao X, Noebels J L 1991 Genetic heterogeneity of inherited spike–wave epilepsy: two mutant gene loci with independent cerebral excitability defects. Brain Res (in press)

Readhead C, Popko B, Takahashi N et al 1987 Expression of a myelin basic protein gene in transgenic shiverer mice: correction of the dysmyelinating phenotype. Cell 48: 703–712

Rett A, Teubel R 1964 Wien Klin Wochenschr 76: 609–613

Rommens J M, Januzzi M C, Kerem B et al 1989 Identification of the cystic fibrosis gene, chromosome walking and jumping. Science 245: 1059–1065

Rouleau G, Wertelecki W, Haines J et al 1987 Genetic linkage of bilateral acoustic neurofibromatosis to a DNA marker on chromosome 22. Nature 329: 246–248

Ryan S G, Wiznitzer M 1990 Clinical heterogeneity in benign familial neonatal convulsions: a challenge for genetic analysis. Epilepsia 31: 817

Saffen D W, Cole A J, Worley P, Christy B A, Ryder K, Baraban J M 1988 Convulsant-induced increase in transcription factor messenger RNAs in rat brain. Proc Natl Acad Sci USA 85: 7795–7799

St George-Hyslop P H, Tanzi R E, Polinsky R J et al 1987 The genetic defect causing familial Alzheimer's disease maps on chromosome 21. Science 235: 885–890

Weissbecker K A, Durner M, Janz D et al 1991 Confirmation of linkage between the juvenile myoclonic epilepsy locus and the HLA region of chromosome 6. Am J Med Genet (in press)

White J D, Gall C M 1987 Differential regulation of neuropeptide and protooncogene mRNA content in the hippocampus following recurrent seizures. Mol Brain Res 3: 21–29

Wilhelmsen C, Tempel B, Gilliam C 1990 Cloning, mapping and sequencing of the human 'Shaker' gene family. Epilepsia 31: 819

Womack J E 1987 Comparative gene mapping: a valuable new tool for mammalian developmental studies. Dev. Genet 8: 281–293

2

Calcium and epilepsy

J. B. Perlin   R. J. DeLorenzo

INTRODUCTION

Calcium is a central biochemical component of neuronal function. The association of calcium with the coupling of excitation and neurotransmitter release has been appreciated for some time (Rubin 1972). More recently, there has been increasing recognition for the variety of functions subserved by calcium within the neurone. Calcium simultaneously acts as both an electrochemical agent exerting a depolarizing influence in the neurone as well as an agent of information transfer within the cell through its role as a major second messenger in neuronal signal transduction.

Calcium and calcium-dependent systems have been implicated in multiple aspects of the pathophysiology of epilepsy, and it is likely that many future strategies for the successful prevention of epilepsy as well as control of established seizure disorders will be based upon selective targeting and alteration of calcium systems. This chapter sequentially addresses: (1) mechanisms of calcium regulation and homeostasis in the neurone; (2) intracellular functions of calcium as they relate to normal neuronal function; (3) calcium and calcium-dependent systems which have been implicated in experimental models of altered neuronal excitability and seizures; and (4) the relevance of these findings to the clinical phenomena of epilepsy and its pharmacotherapy.

MECHANISMS OF CALCIUM REGULATION AND HOMEOSTASIS

Calcium homeostasis

Meticulous regulation of the intracellular ionic milieu is imperative for normal neuronal function. Extracellular Ca^{2+} concentrations are in the low-millimolar range. Through energy expenditure, which also generates internal negative transmembrane polarization, the level of calcium within cells is maintained at approximately 10^{-8} molar. Thus a substantial electrochemical gradient exists for movement of Ca^{2+} ions into neurones. Entrance of calcium into neurones occurs through both voltage-operated calcium channels as well as through receptor-operated channels. In addition, receptors which are not directly associated with ion-channel complexes can activate second messenger systems capable of releasing calcium from intracellular stores such as the endoplasmic reticulum.

Free intracellular calcium is regulated through a variety of mechanisms (Meyer 1989). Calcium-binding proteins such as calmodulin serve as principal intermediaries in calcium-activated signal transduction. Each calmodulin molecule binds up to four Ca^{2+} ions as flux concentrations of intracellular Ca^{2+} approach micromolar levels. Indeed, because calmodulin is so highly enriched (existing at cytosolic concentrations of $30-50\ \mu M$) it simultaneously serves, in effect, as a calcium sink (Kennedy 1989). Additional calcium-binding proteins including parvalbumin and calbindin are believed to buffer transient fluxes in calcium concentration and thereby indirectly modulate the activation of other Ca^{2+}-dependent processes.

In addition to being buffered by calcium-binding proteins, elevated cytosolic calcium is actively taken up into the endoplasmic reticulum through a Ca^{2+}-ATPase. An electrochemical gradient also drives mitochondrial uptake of calcium. However, mitochondrial Ca^{2+} buffering is probably more important during severe or pathological calcium loads. Mitochondria are a low-affinity, high-capacity system, and excessive mitochondrial accumulation of calcium may uncouple oxidative phosphorylation. Finally, there are active and secondarily active pumps on the cytoplasmic membrane which protect intracellular calcium levels. These include the Ca^{2+}-ATPase and the electrogenic Na^+-Ca^{2+} antiporter, respectively. Feedback for calcium homeostasis operates, in part, through the Ca^{2+} activation of calmodulin which increases the activity of the Ca^{2+}-ATPase (Kennedy 1989, Meyer 1989). Function of the Na^+-Ca^{2+} antiporter is dependent on maintenance of the transmembrane sodium gradient by Na^+/K^+-ATPase.

Excitatory amino acids and calcium

This past decade has witnessed a tremendous growth in information about excitatory amino acid (EAA) receptors. EAA systems constitute the majority of excitatory transmission in the vertebrate nervous system, and their relevance to the pathophysiology and potential pharmacological control of disorders of abnormally intense neuroexcitability is immediate. Collingridge & Lester (1989) have given a recent comprehensive review of EAA pharmacology. The present discussion will introduce EAA neurotransmitters and receptors only in the context of their contribution to the calcium flux.

The major EAA transmitters in the central nervous system (CNS) are glutamate and aspartate. Presently, five EAA receptors can be distinguished pharmacologically (Watkins et al 1990). These include the NMDA, AMPA and metabotropic receptors located postsynaptically and the kainate and L-AP4 receptors which may be situated presynaptically (see Fig. 2.1 caption for abbreviation definitions). Multiple isoforms of AMPA and kainate receptor subunits have been cloned, suggesting that an even greater number of glutamate receptor subtypes may exist, and that anatomical regions may be especially enriched in particular subspecies of the pharmacologically defined subtypes (Boulter et al 1990, Sommer et al 1990).

The NMDA subtype of glutamate receptors constitutes an important route for influx of extracellular Ca^{2+} and functions as a receptor-operated channel. The NMDA receptor–ionophore complex admits cations, predominantly calcium, when liganded by an appropriate agonist and simultaneous partial membrane depolarization has removed tonic blockade of the cation channel by Mg^{2+}.

In contrast, the metabotropic glutamate receptor generates a calcium flux through liberation of calcium from intracellular stores such as the endoplasmic reticulum. It is referred to as 'metabotropic', because activation of this receptor initiates a metabolic cascade in which phosphoinositol-bis-4,5-phosphate is cleaved to diacylglycerol (DAG) and inositol polyphosphates such as IP_3. AMPA receptors control a channel which conducts monovalent cations such as Na^+ (inward) and K^+ (outward) and are generally responsible for the fast component of excitatory postsynaptic potentials (EPSPs) in central excitatory pathways.

Except for their presynaptic location, kainate receptors are believed to be similar to AMPA receptors in that they control a monovalent cation channel. Less is known about L-AP4 receptors, which are speculated to act as autoreceptors inhibiting glutamate release when activated. NMDA and AMPA receptors are broadly distributed throughout the CNS: NMDA receptors, like kainate receptors, are highly enriched in the hippocampus (Watkins et al 1990).

Calcium channels

As already mentioned, one of the primary routes for entrance of extracellular calcium into the neurone is through voltage-operated calcium channels (VOCC). Presently, there are acknowledged to be at least three major types of VOCC. L-, N- and T-type Ca^{2+} channels share the property of activating (opening) and inactivating (closing) in a voltage-dependent manner. A complete survey of all distinguishing kinetic properties is beyond the scope of this chapter and excellent comprehensive reviews of VOCC in brain are available elsewhere (Hess 1990, Tsien et al 1988). Nevertheless, certain features of VOCC are pertinent to the present understanding of the role of calcium in seizures.

In the CNS most is known about L-type Ca^{2+} channels, which are sensitive to the dihydropyridine calcium channel blockers (e.g. nimodipine, nitrendepine) and are also strongly blocked by inorganic divalent cations such as Cd^{2+} and Co^{2+}. They are located postsynaptically, predominantly on the soma. L-type channels are opened by strong depolarizations (positive to approximately $-10\,\mathrm{mV}$), inactivate very slowly (approximately $\frac{1}{2}$ second), and have relatively large conductances ($25\,\mathrm{pS}$). L-type calcium channel activity is thought to be modulated by internal accumulation of Ca^{2+} ions as well as by cyclic AMP-dependent phosphorylation (Chad & Eckert 1986, Yue et al 1990).

Less is known about N-type channels, which are located presynaptically and may be important in neurotransmitter release in some neurones. Although sensitive to blockade by Cd^{2+}, N-type channels are resistant to dihydropyridines. Activated by slightly weaker depolarizations than L-type channels (positive to $-20\,\mathrm{mV}$), N-type channels have both a moderate inactivation rate ($\sim 65\,\mathrm{ms}$) and conductance ($\sim 13\,\mathrm{pS}$). Activity of N-type channels is inhibited in the presence of many neuroactive substances including acetylcholine, γ-aminobutyric acid (GABA), noradrenaline, opioids and 5-hydroxytryptamine (Hess 1990).

Finally, T-type Ca^{2+} channels are anatomically restricted post-developmentally and are associated with and may mediate intrinsic oscillatory activity in structures such as thalamus, pontine reticular formation and inferior olive (Coulter et al 1989). Interestingly, they are also found on hippocampal pyramidal cells (Tsien et al 1988). T-type currents are activated by weak depolarizations (positive to $-65\,\mathrm{mV}$), have relatively small conductances ($\sim 8\,\mathrm{pS}$) and inactivate rapidly ($\sim 35\,\mathrm{ms}$). They are blocked neither by dihydropyridines nor by the divalent cations which block N- and L-type channels.

INTRACELLULAR CALCIUM IN NEURONAL FUNCTION

Intracellular calcium-dependent systems

Calcium spikes, or transient elevations of intraneuronal calcium associated with depolarization and excitatory neurotransmission, initiate a plethora of calcium-dependent processes. In turn, these generally but not exclusively lead to activation of numerous enzymes including protein kinases, proteases, phosphodiesterases, phosphatases, phospholipases and regulatory proteins such as synapsin. Direct and indirect modulation of a number of Ca^{2+}-dependent ion channels also ensues. Some of the metabolic cascades initiated by the calcium flux are tightly regulated and rarely impinge on other calcium-activated pathways. Other cascades are comprised of less specific messengers creating the opportunity for substantial 'cross-talk' between signal transduction pathways. The ramifications of supranormal activation of these transduction cascades, especially those with less specific intermediaries, is determined by the particular physiological constituency of a given neurone.

Calcium/calmodulin-dependent kinase II and synapsin

The highly enriched cytosolic calcium-binding protein calmodulin (CaM) serves as an important intermediary in neuronal signal transduction. During calcium fluxes, calmodulin becomes activated as it binds Ca^{2+} ions. This endows CaM with messenger status, so that it may successively activate a variety of CaM-dependent processes. One of the most important is the activation of type II calcium/CaM-dependent kinase (CaM kinase II).

CaM kinase II has been implicated in the mediation of several second messenger effects of calcium in neurones, both pre- and postsynaptically. Reported roles include modulation of neurotransmitter release through vesicle–membrane interaction, synaptic function, cytoskeletal architecture and neuronal excitability (DeLorenzo 1981, 1986). In the forebrain, the CaM kinase II holoenzyme (M_r 460 000–654 000) generally exists as a heterologous dodecameric structure composed of 50-kDa α subunits and larger β, β' or β'' subunits of 60, 58 or 57 kDa, respectively. The stoichiometric ratio of α to β subunits has been variously determined as 8:2, 9:3 or 10:2, with the 9:3 ratio as the predominant form (Schulman 1988). The three isozymes of the β subunit are generated by alternative splicings of the β gene (Bennett & Kennedy 1987). The functional significance of the subunit isozymes or the various stoichiometries constituting different holoenzyme isoforms (and their potential alterations with increased neuronal excitability) remains unknown.

CaM kinase II is highly enriched in mammalian brain, constituting 0.8–1% of total brain protein. In regions such as hippocampus, which is important in learning and memory functions as well as in the development of seizures, CaM kinase II constitutes almost 2% of total protein weight. At the cellular level, CaM kinase II is concentrated at the synapse. Depending on the brain region, the α subunit of CaM kinase II constitutes 15–60% of the protein content of the postsynaptic density and is now known to be the major postsynaptic density protein (mPSDp) (Goldenring et al 1983).

Among the most prominent phosphoprotein substrates which the pleiotropic CaM kinase II phosphorylates are microtubule-associated protein II (MAP II) and synapsin I. The phosphorylation state of MAP II determines the extent of its polymerization. Presynaptic synapsin links neurotransmitter vesicles with the cytoskeleton. With depolarization, phosphorylation by CaM kinase II reduces the affinity of synapsin for neurotransmitter vesicles, consequently orienting neurotransmitter vesicles toward the membrane and improving the opportunity for vesicle–membrane fusion and the probability of neurotransmitter release (Llinas et al 1985).

Importantly, CaM kinase II is one of its own best substrates and undergoes autophosphorylation of its α and β subunits. The capacity for autophosphorylation endows CaM kinase II with an intrinsic mechanism for regulating its own enzymatic function. Initial autophosphorylation of CaM kinase II relieves its dependence on calcium and CaM for enzymatic activity. Subsequent autophosphorylation of the autonomous CaM kinase II produces inhibition of the kinase's enzymatic activity (Lou & Schulman 1987). Ultimately, this suggests an intrinsic mechanism for initial signal amplification followed by signal termination. As with other phosphoproteins, the phosphorylation state of CaM kinase II is also regulated by the activity of phosphatases. CaM kinase II from brain is enzymatically dephosphorylated in vitro by protein phosphatases I and IIa (Saitoh et al 1987).

Protein kinases C and phospholipase C

Protein kinase C (PKC) actually refers to a family of isoenzymes which are activated by the simultaneous stimulation of diacyglycerol (DAG) and elevated cytosolic Ca^{2+}. Inositol polyphosphates such as IP_3, which are independently capable of liberating Ca^{2+} from the endoplasmic reticulum, are simultaneously generated with DAG from the cleavage of phosphatidylinositol 4,5-bisphosphate (PIP_2) by phospholipase C (PLC). Many receptors, including the metabotropic glutamate and muscarinic cholinergic, are linked by a G-protein to a PLC isoform. Such receptors exert their effect following activation of this pathway (Huang 1989). In hippocampal pyramidal cells, PKC has been implicated in regulating conductances (Baraban et al 1985). PKC activation is also thought to increase the release of neurotransmitters, including glutamate (Malenka et al 1986).

Other calcium-dependent pathways

Calcium can also initiate activities of other protein kinases and phospholipases as well as those of phosphatases, proteases and the generation of cyclic nucleotides. For instance, subsequent to CaM activation, CaM-sensitive isoforms of adenylate cyclase can be activated. The ensuing rise in cyclic AMP (cAMP) leads to the activation of cAMP-dependent protein kinase (PKA). PKA has been implicated in the activation of L-type Ca^{2+} channels by phosphorylation. On the other hand, activated CaM also turns on the phosphatase calcineurin, which may be responsible for the desensitization or inactivation of L-type Ca^{2+} channels (Chad & Eckert 1986, Kennedy 1989). The Ca^{2+} flux can activate CaM-stimulated phosphodiesterase (PDE) which degrades cyclic nucleotides such as cAMP.

The activation of calpain, a calcium-dependent protease, may also occur with transient elevations of cytosolic Ca^{2+} (Huang 1989). One target for proteolysis by calpain is PKC. This process liberates the regulatory domain from the catalytic domain of the kinase which then constitutes the $Ca^{2+}/$ phospholipid-independent kinase, PKM. The functional significance of calpain activation and PKM liberation in neurones remains unclear. Phospholipase A_2 (PLA_2) activity also increases with increased intracellular Ca^{2+}. PLA_2 generates fatty acids including arachidonic acid which can subsequently be metabolized to prostaglandins and leukotrienes. Arachidonic acid and its metabolites have been shown to modulate a number of ion conductances. Arachidonic acid, specifically, could intensify EAA effects as it has been shown to inhibit uptake of glutamate by glial cells (Nicholls

& Attwell 1990). In addition to these metabolic events, regulation of a number of membrane ion channels has been shown to be Ca^{2+} dependent, including two types of K^+ channels which can modulate neuronal excitability (Marty 1989, Sombati et al 1988).

Finally, in addition to the aforementioned physiological effects and biochemical or post-translational modifications, Ca^{2+}-dependent processes may instigate a sequence of events which leads to the expression of 'immediate early genes' (IEG) and alterations in transcriptional and post-transcriptional programmes for gene regulation. As greater attention has hitherto been focused on this aspect of calcium function in the context of altered neuronal excitability or excitotoxicity, this facet of calcium action will be addressed below. Clearly though, initiation of processes of this sort suggests the capacity for Ca^{2+}-responsive long-term alterations in neural function and begs the investigation of their role in the ongoing adaptive mechanisms which constitute the basis of neuronal plasticity. (See Fig. 2.1 for an integrated summary of receptors, channels and calcium effector systems.)

CALCIUM SYSTEMS IN SEIZURE AND EPILEPSY

Interictal bursting, seizure, epilepsy and epileptogenesis

The present understanding of epilepsy derives from extrapolation from normal function as well as from experimental models and clinical investigation. These lines of inquiry establish calcium's importance in both the generation of interictal bursts (IB) and seizures and, especially, in the *induction* of epilepsy. It should be noted that there are practical and philosophical reasons for clearly distinguishing between seizures and epilepsy. At the minimum, it is recognized that not all stimuli which trigger a seizure produce epilepsy which is, by definition, a syndrome of recurrent seizures. Epilepsy implies a 'long-lasting' or permanent change in excitability (with a concomitant propensity toward seizure) and, thus, the *process* through which epilepsy has been induced is referred to as epileptogenesis (Dingledine et al 1990).

IB and seizures, in isolation and as a component of epilepsy, are characterized by abnormally intense, hypersynchronous discharges from populations of neurones. In the most general sense, these phenomena result from increased excitation or diminished inhibition which may be initiated by a variety of insults or functional aberrations. Given the manifold initiators as well as the diversity of neuronal architecture in which seizures or bursts can occur, a 'unified' theory of seizure disorders is unlikely, especially one which can encompass both focal (with which this chapter is chiefly concerned) and primary generalized disorders (Dichter 1987). Nevertheless, all of these phenomena must be expressed and executed through a variety of conserved calcium systems. In fact, it is in the context of localized enrichments of particular effectors of the calcium systems that intrinsic susceptibility to seizure disorders seems to arise.

Interictal discharges are the primary electrographic signature of increased excitability and arise from a population of neurones generating synchronous burst discharges. In an individual cell, a paroxysmal, high-voltage depolarization and superimposed fast and slow action potentials is termed the depolarizing shift (DS). Cellular depolarizing bursts are generally followed by an intense afterhyperpolarization. In a number of models, loss of this post-DS afterhyperpolarization signifies imminent transition from the interictal state to seizure activity (Dichter 1989).

Although they can be identified on the basis of their electrographic morphology, a conceptual distinction should also be drawn between interictal bursts (EEG 'spikes') and seizures. Even though the underlying mechanisms may be similar, the fundamental relationship between interictal phenomena and seizures remains unclear. Indeed, there are instances when interictal discharges seem actually to suppress ictal activity (Engle & Ackerman 1980). Several inhibitory processes converge functionally to create the post-DS afterhyperpolarization. Similarly, multiple mechanisms of excitation contribute to the DS. Excellent reviews of the cellular mechanisms and pathophysiology of epilepsy are available and should be consulted for further discussion (see Dichter 1989, Lothman 1990).

The influx of extracellular calcium

In a diversity of in vitro and in vivo models of seizure and epilepsy, extracellular Ca^{2+} declines prior to or during seizure onset. An increase in extracellular K^+ generally accompanies this process (Meyer 1989). As has been noted, the major conduits through which Ca^{2+} shifts from the extracellular space into the cell include the NMDA subtype of glutamate receptors and VOCC, especially of the L-type. Pumain & Heinemann (1985) measured the loss of calcium from the extracellular space of the rat cerebral cortex during stimulation by iontophoretic applications of the excitatory amino acid neurotransmitters, aspartate and glutamate. Blockade of calcium channels by the application of cobalt or manganese prevented loss of calcium from the extracellular environment. On the other hand, at doses and in anatomical regions where TTX, a sodium channel antagonist, blocked synaptic transmission, TTX did not block loss of extracellular calcium evoked by amino acid application. A conclusion drawn from this work was that loss of Ca^{2+} extracellularly could be accounted for by postsynaptic calcium uptake.

In some models the suggestion that seizures could be prevented by calcium entry blockers has been upheld. Indeed, seizures generated in mice by intracerebroventricular administration of the dihydropyridine calcium channel *agonist* BAY K-8644 are averted by pre-administration of similar calcium channel blockers (Shelton et al 1987). However, other investigators find that seizures evoked by intravenous administration of excitatory amino acid agonists are not prevented by VOCC antagonists (Meyer 1989). Collectively, these observations constitute evidence that calcium lost from the extracellular environment gains entrance into the cell largely through VOCC and the NMDA subtype of glutamate receptors. However, both of these avenues for calcium entrance are available only after partial membrane depolarization has occurred. Therefore, it has been postulated that at the canonical glutamatergic synapse the initial fast-component depolarization would be achieved by Na^+ influx through the cation channel associated with the AMPA receptor. Partial membrane depolarization would then relieve blockade of the NMDA receptor by Mg^+, and Ca^{2+} influx would then contribute to greater depolarization of the neurone and the late component of the EPSP (Dichter 1989). In turn, this would create the ideal situation for activation of L-type Ca^{2+} channels. Alternatively, experimental tetanic stimulation or interictal bursting of sufficiently high frequency might lead to summation of non-NMDA receptor-mediated EPSPs, rendering the membrane partially depolarized and thereby unblocking NMDA receptor-coupled channels.

Long-lasting alterations in neuronal excitability and epileptogenesis

The sequence of events described above is applicable both to the mechanisms which trigger interictal bursting and to those leading to seizures, as well as to processes believed to be involved in development of an enduring epileptic state. The process of epileptogenesis, however, implies a sustained alteration in neuronal excitability that persists beyond any seizure-like activity which may be initially generated. Recently, cellular mechanisms underlying induction of the hyperexcitable state have been increasingly characterized in the long-term potentiation (LTP) model of increased synaptic efficacy.

Hippocampal pathways, such as the Schaeffer collateral–commissural pathway in which LTP can be achieved by application of afferent tetanic stimulation, utilize EAA neurotransmitters. Non-potentiating EPSPs, generated from low-amplitude/low frequency stimulation in these pathways, can be blocked by non-selective EAA antagonists. On the other hand, the induction of LTP with appropriate and sufficient high-frequency ($>5 Hz$) stimulation, could be prevented by application of specific NMDA antagonists such as APV. After induction of LTP, however, APV did not block generation of the potentiated response (Collingridge et al 1983). This suggested that there were differences in the mechanisms responsible for the induction and maintenance of LTP. It must be noted that following induction of LTP by extremely intense stimulations, some potentiation of the NMDA component of the EPSP (possibly yielding increased Ca^{2+} influx) has also been observed (Bashir et al 1991).

After LTP had been established, potentiated responses could be depressed by CNQX, an antagonist of the AMPA receptor (Errington et al 1987). It was speculated that activation of the NMDA receptor during LTP led to positive modulation of a 'quisqualate' receptor (now more specifically identified as a glutamate receptor of the AMPA subtype). That calcium may be the essential second messenger in instigating a sequence of events leading to enhanced synaptic efficacy was strongly supported by the inability to establish LTP following intracellular injection of the Ca^{2+} chelator EGTA into the postsynaptic cell (Lynch et al 1983). Indeed, systematic investigation of Ca^{2+} target systems has revealed that at least two kinases, CaM kinase II and PKC, may be involved in the induction and maintenance phases of LTP, respectively (Reymann & Matthies 1989). Subsequent refinements in technique utilizing intracellular injections of increasingly selective kinase inhibitors implicate the postsynaptic involvement of both PKC and CaM kinase II in the induction of LTP, and the involvement of PKC, possibly presynaptically, in maintaining the potentiated response (Malinow et al 1989). Potentiation of a presynaptic process is in agreement with earlier observations of increased glutamate release (Errington et al 1987), and the recent reports by Tsien and Stevens which also suggest an increase in neurotransmitter release based on the technique of quantal analysis (see Barinaga 1990). Implication of either of these kinases presynaptically as a component of potentiation is possible on theoretical grounds as both have been shown to facilitate neurotransmitter release (DeLorenzo 1981, Llinas et al 1985, Baraban et al 1985).

Another mechanism for potentiating synaptic efficacy involves activation of the Ca^{2+}-dependent protease calpain. It has been proposed that occluded (AMPA) glutamate receptors could be exposed through proteolysis of a spectrin-like protein, fodrin, which is highly enriched in the dendritic cytoskeleton, freeing these putative receptors to participate in the potentiated synaptic response. Evidence for this was derived from inhibition of calpain activity by leu-peptin which, alternatively, also inhibits cleavage of the regulated form of PKC into the unregulated kinase, PKM (Staubli et al 1988). In another vein, an increase in IP_3, presumably generated by activation of the metabotropic receptor, has been observed with LTP too. Indeed, antagonism of the metabotropic receptor by D-AP4 (inactive at the presynaptic L-AP4 receptor) has been shown to block the late phase of LTP (Reymann & Matthies 1989).

Spatial resolution of calcium influx

Recently, technological advances in the optical imaging of ions have made sensitive and accurate spatially resolved measurements of intracellular Ca^{2+} concentrations possible. Interestingly, substantial regional variations in the amount of Ca^{2+} accumulation within the neurone have been observed. For example, orthodromic stimulation of hippocampal CA1 pyramidal cells led to Ca^{2+} accumulation in apical and basal dendrites, even in the presence of the NMDA receptor antagonist APV (Regehr et al 1989). This pattern of Ca^{2+} accumulation reflected the distribution of VOCC, and the calcium gradients were transient, persisting for less than 10 seconds.

In contrast, stimulation of hippocampal CA1 neurones by 1–3-second applications of glutamate or NMDA led to Ca^{2+} accumulation predominantly in apical dendrites. In this instance, however, regional calcium elevations were long-lasting and persisted for minutes at a time. With respect to possible mechanisms of synaptic potentiation underlying LTP, this long-lasting Ca^{2+} flux could be prevented by pretreatment with sphingosine, a confirmed protein kinase C inhibitor (Connor et al 1988). Consequently, in addition to the temporal constraints necessary for induction of altered neuronal excitability in LTP (i.e. stimulation at $>5\,Hz$), studies of this type imply that a spatial component is also likely.

Calcium, seizures and epilepsy in the intact brain

How are observations of altered neuronal excitability made in vitro related to seizures and epilepsy expressed in the intact brain? While it is debated whether or not LTP constitutes the cellular basis of kindling, the two models of increased excitability share many features, not the least important of which is a process of induction through which a long-duration state of increased excitability is achieved. Kindling, considered by some to be a model of complex partial seizures, describes a process in which the repeated administration of an initially subconvulsive stimulus ultimately elicits stereotyped electrographic discharges and behavioural seizures. Following induction of the kindled state, the change in neuronal excitability is permanent, and the kindled response persists for the life of the animal.

Studies of the sort utilized in the elucidation of mechanisms underlying LTP have been applied to kindling, and the results obtained have demonstrated major similarities. McNamara et al (1988) have shown that antagonism of the NMDA receptor by MK-801 (dizocilpine) retards the progression of the kindling process and the attainment of the fully kindled state. Furthermore, although NMDA receptor antagonists inhibit the kindling process and are thus 'antiepileptogenic', they only partially attenuate the established kindled response and function in this context as poor anticonvulsants.

It has also been recently demonstrated that activation of NMDA receptors mediates the loss of GABAergic inhibition as measured by paired-pulse depression of population spikes, an index of inhibitory efficacy (Kapur & Lothman 1990). In the rapid kindling model, MK-801 was not only observed to inhibit the lengthening of afterdischarges, but also to prevent the sustained decrease in paired-pulse inhibition which had been previously associated with highly selective antagonism of the $GABA_A$ receptor. The decrease in GABAergic inhibition was long-lasting and endured for at least 2 hours beyond the final seizure elicited. The sequence of events that ultimately couples activation of the NMDA receptor with altered GABA-mediated inhibition has not been established. Nevertheless, the conductance of hippocampal $GABA_A$ receptors is thought to be enhanced through phosphorylation by an as yet unspecified kinase and inhibited by a Ca^{2+}-dependent process such as the CaM-dependent phosphatase calcineurin (Stelzer et al 1988).

Another Ca^{2+}/CaM-dependent system which appears to be modulated in kindling is CaM kinase II. The initial finding that the most efficacious anticonvulsants (phenytoin, carbamazepine, diazepam) were among the best inhibitors of CaM kinase II activity in vitro propelled exploration of the possible involvement of this enzyme in models of altered neuronal excitability (DeLorenzo 1981, 1986). It has been reported that septal kindling leads to a permanent decrease in CaM kinase II activity from crude synaptic membranes (Wasterlain & Farber 1984). Historically, the lack of a selective CaM kinase II inhibitor suitable for in vivo applications has frustrated clarification of the relative importance of this protein kinase in either the kindling process or in the generation of established kindled seizures. Although data from the kindling model suggest that CaM kinase II is involved they do not establish a mechanism through which alterations in CaM kinase II activity might constitute either the basis of, or a response to, increased neuronal excitability. Teleologically, increased activity of CaM kinase II would not be unexpected given its capacity to increase neurotransmitter release. On the other hand, some investigators have postulated that CaM kinase II can lose its catalytic potential and adopt a structural function, perhaps modulating synaptic efficacy as it is physically poised to do through its enrichment as the major postsynaptic density protein (Goldenring et al 1983, Schulman 1988). One such example of postsynaptic potentiation includes the increased NMDA component of EPSPs which has been observed in dentate gyrus granule cells from kindled tissue (Mody et al 1988).

The loss of CaM kinase II activity has also been associated with experimental status epilepticus. Following 90 minutes of 'continuous' hippocampal stimulation (CHS) – a model which culminates in limbic status epilepticus – CaM kinase II activity was diminished (Perlin et al 1989). The decrement of activity was shown to correlate directly with the intensity and complexity of electrographic discharges observed during monitoring intervals in the stimulation protocol. Unlike the rapid kindling paradigm, the CHS model leads to significant cell death in the CA1 region of the hippocampus (Bertram et al 1990). It was unlikely that the decrease in enzymatic activity resulted from the early attrition of cells most highly enriched in CaM kinase II as concentrations of the kinase itself were unaffected. In this model of status epilepticus, it remains unclear whether loss of CaM kinase II activity relates to increased neuronal excitability (as with LTP and kindling) or excitotoxic processes which were likely to have already been initiated at the time of tissue sampling. In either case, loss of CaM kinase II activity could potentially degrade its capacity for autoregulation as well as the integrity of the signal transduction pathways it subserves.

Calcium and excitotoxicity

Although direct exploration of excitotoxicity in vivo has been difficult because of technical constraints, EAA or their analogues have been known to exert toxic effects on neurones for two decades. (See Dichter & Choi 1989 for an expert review of excitotoxicity.) Until recently, however, little was known about mechanisms underlying excitotoxic injury. Two components of excitotoxic damage have now been identified (Rothman & Olney 1987). First, sustained depolarization leads to massive influx of Na^+ ions. Coupled with the passive influx of Cl^- counterions, and amplified by the influx of additional cations, especially Ca^{2+}, this ionic shift leads to the osmotic influx of water and, ultimately, swelling and osmotic lysis. This process of osmotic damage is associated with immediate or 'early cell death'. The observed pattern of neuronal EAA damage has been described as 'dendrosomatotoxic', reflecting assumptions about the density of excitatory postsynaptic receptors (Rothman & Olney 1987, Dichter 1989).

The second component of excitotoxicity relates to the observation that the survival of neurones exposed to pharmacological levels of EAA could be markedly improved by limiting Ca^{2+} in the extracellular environment (Rothman & Olney 1987). The mechanisms through which Ca^{2+} loading produces late excitotoxicity or 'delayed cell death' are unclear. However, it has been speculated that given the plethora of Ca^{2+}-dependent pathways, profound changes ensue following cellular dysregulation initiated through disruption of normal calcium homeostasis. Kindled seizures generate strong but transient increases in cytoplasmic calcium (Kamphuis et al 1989a), and in experimental models of status epilepticus, as well as in surgically removed epileptic foci, Ca^{2+} accumulates not only in the cytoplasm but also in mitochondria (Meldrum 1986).

Calcium-binding proteins and calcium buffering

In vitro studies of excitotoxicity as well as reports of cell loss following status epilepticus or persistent experimental stimulation have revealed that not all neuronal populations are equally vulnerable to excitotoxic death especially delayed cell death. This phenomenon is thought to arise from a number of factors. Hippocampal pyramidal cells are notoriously prone to seizure discharge. Coincidentally, the hippocampus is highly enriched both in NMDA receptors (Collingridge & Lester 1989) and in CaM kinase II (Schulman 1988). Following sustained perforant path stimulation of the rat hippocampus, cell loss is substantially greater among cells apparently devoid of parvalbumin and endowed with relatively lower levels of calbindin (Sloviter 1989). Indeed, dentate gyrus cells identified as being devoid of calbindin or parvalbumin were protected from signs of deterioration during prolonged stimulation if BAPTA, a highly selective calcium chelator, was allowed to diffuse into the cytosol from an intracellular microelectrode (Scharfman & Schwartzkroin 1989).

Lack of the protective effect granted by calcium-binding proteins may play a role in possible long-term deficits in inhibitory function associated with epilepsy. In another study employing the kindling model, inhibitory interneurones which displayed co-localization of GABA and parvalbumin activity were spared relative to GABA-positive neurones which were devoid of parvalbumin activity (Kamphuis et al 1989b). There have also been reports that the Ca^{2+}-buffering capacity of surviving neurones may be impaired in experimental epilepsy. Dentate gyrus granule cells taken from kindled animals show subnormal levels of calbindin-like activity. Interestingly, Ca^{2+} currents in these cells inactivate more rapidly than in cells from control animals, and inactivation characteristics similar to those in controls could be restored by intracellular injection of BAPTA (Kohr et al 1990). Again, whether this constitutes a mechanism of, or a response to, increased excitability (or is simply epiphenomenal) is unclear. Nevertheless, in this or other situations in which the calcium-buffering capacity of the neurone is overwhelmed, the calcium signal may be 'shunted' into any accessible Ca^{2+}-responsive pathway.

Calcium-dependent ion channels exemplify another system that may be affected by the aberrant function of Ca^{2+}-regulated second messengers. In cultured spinal cord neurones, for example, injection of CaM kinase II resulted in the loss of the afterhyperpolarization that usually followed each spike. Conversely, injection of a monoclonal antibody against CaM kinase II suggested enhanced afterhyperpolarization (Sombati et al 1988). The loss of hyperpolarization could be mimicked by the application of apamin and charybdotoxin which block two Ca^{2+}-dependent K^+ channels, respectively. In addition to the possibility that these channels may be modulated by a phosphorylation event, it is plausible that in the context of Ca^{2+} flux and seizure initiation their dysregulation might constitute one component underlying the transition from interictal to ictal activity. On the other hand, the exaggerated expression of the normal contribution of these K^+ channels to repolarization is likely to be relevant to the regenerative nature of repetitive epileptiform discharges.

Calcium, seizures, epilepsy, the immediate early gene response, transcriptional and post-transcriptional gene regulation

In addition to calcium's function as a 'conventional' second messenger, contemporary research has increasingly recognized its role in the execution of immediate early gene (IEG) responses. It has become increasingly apparent that the physiological and, especially, the pathological stimulation of neurones can initiate cascades of events that culminate in the induction of transcription, message stabilization, translation or activation of gene products that, in turn, influence the transcriptional or post-transcriptional regulation of genes expressed in the course of normal neuronal function or adaptation. The ramifications for long-lasting changes or neuronal plasticity are profound (for expert reviews, see Morgan & Curran 1989, Dragunow et al 1989).

Many of the IEGs were initially described as proto-oncogenes owing to their identification in dysregulated neoplastic tissue. As a class, however, the protein products are better described as trans-acting elements which recognize motifs in the non-coding regions of genes through which they generally serve to promote or repress transcription. One such motif is the AP-1 site at which IEG members of the *fos*, *jun* and *fra* families exert their influence. In vitro, c-*fos* mRNA has been induced in PC12 pheochromocytoma cells by application of the L-type calcium channel agonist BAY K-8644 (Morgan & Curran 1989). In a variety of models of seizures (metrazol, picrotoxin, kainate) and epilepsy (kindling), c-*fos* message is transiently elevated following an ictal event particularly in the dentate gyrus and pyriform cortex. Interestingly, the NMDA channel blocker MK-801 inhibits the seizure-induced rise in c-*fos* (Labiner et al 1989). The potential connection between c-*fos* activity alone and plasticity is unclear. In the kindling model, c-*fos* levels are transiently elevated following seizures elicited during the kindling process as well as after the kindled response is fully established (Dragunow et al 1989).

An individual IEG does not exert an exclusively positive or negative influence on transcription. Interaction between various IEGs and the positional context of the recognition motifs in the genetic framework determines the direction of influence. For this reason, it is likely that alterations in neuronal gene expression affecting plasticity and epileptogenesis arise through the coordinated activity of several IEGs and other trans-acting elements. Indeed, in a variety of models of altered neuronal excitability, additional IEGs (including *zif/268*, c-*fos*, c-*jun*, *jun*-B) have also been induced (Dragunow et al 1989). Messages for at least two members of the heat-shock protein family (*HSP*-70 and *HSP*-84) were transiently increased after kindled seizures as well (Wong et al 1990). It must be cautioned, however, that the complete vocabulary and syntax for interaction between IEGs and other trans-acting elements is not currently understood.

Another family of trans-acting agents that influence gene expression are the cAMP response element binding proteins (CREBs) which modulate transcription by interacting with conserved recognition motifs known as cAMP response elements (CREs) (see Montminy et al 1990). As mentioned above, Ca^{2+} influx can initiate CaM-mediated metabolic cascades which culminate in increased production of cAMP and activation of PKA. Constitutively expressed CREBs are primarily activated through phosphorylation by PKA, and activation generally leads to increased transcription of CREB-inducible genes. Recently, CREBs have also been shown to be susceptible to phosphorylation and Ca^{2+}-activation by CAM kinase II (Sheng et al 1990). After PKA phosphorylation, CREB activity can be modestly increased through phosphorylation by PKC, a kinase whose activity is also stimulated in conjunction with a calcium flux. A number of genes coding for peptides appear to be regulated by CREBs (Montminy et al 1990). Some of these neuromodulators, especially somatostatin, have been implicated in seizure propagation (Perlin et al 1987).

We emphasize that the ultimate importance of IEGs, trans-acting elements, and post-translational regulatory mechanisms (including those which confer message stability) derives from their capacity to control gene expression in a fashion which can impart functional changes to a neurone's physiology. The manner in which the sustained accumulation of intracellular Ca^{2+} may initiate these mechanisms of neuronal reprogramming (including the sequela of excitotoxic injury) is under intense scrutiny in many laboratories, including our own. Calcium systems implicated in epileptogenesis and seizure generation are summarized in Figure 2.1.

CALCIUM, SEIZURE SUPPRESSANTS AND ANTIEPILEPTOGENIC DRUGS

Calcium is central to neuronal function, and many putative mechanisms of pathological neuronal excitability are calcium dependent. Thus, it is not surprising that present anticonvulsants are known or suspected to influence calcium systems either directly or indirectly (DeLorenzo 1988).

Ethosuximide and absence epilepsy

Evidence implicating calcium systems in absence epilepsy (as well as in the action of anticonvulsant drugs effective against this type of seizure) has been recently fortified. T-type calcium channels are associated with neuronal populations displaying intrinsic oscillatory activity including regions of the thalamus. These channels have also been implicated as having a role in some forms of primary generalized epilepsy. For example, characteristic spike and wave discharges associated with absence seizures are thought to be mediated by T-type currents of thalamocortical relay neurones (Coulter et al 1989). In support of this hypothesis, Coulter and his colleagues recently demonstrated that ethosuximide, an anticonvulsant effective mainly against typical absence seizures, blocked thalamic T-type calcium channels (Coulter et al 1990). Additional exploration of intracellular Ca^{2+}-dependent processes unique to the thalamus might help provide greater insight into mechanisms of primary generalized epilepsy and the role of calcium channel blockers as anticonvulsants.

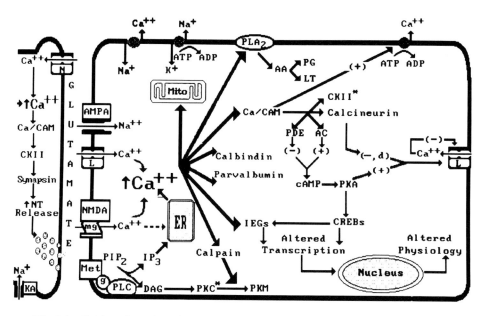

Fig. 2.1 Calcium-dependent signal transduction at the canonical glutamatergic synapse. Arrows indicate activation pathways and normal directions of ion flow. Putative pathways are indicated by dashed arrows. Upward arrows in the text indicate increases. Within pathways, '+' indicates increases or activation, '−' indicates decreases or inactivation, and 'd' indicates desensitization. '*' indicates kinases which also modulate activity of IEGs or trans-acting elements by phosphorylation (see text for details). The putative L-AP4 (L-2-amino-4-phosphonobutanoic acid) autoreceptor is not indicated. Components of this schematic are described in the text. In addition it should be noted that calcineurin has been implicated in both inactivation and desensitization of L-type calcium channels (Chad & Eckert 1986, Kennedy 1989). Additionally, it is speculated that non-IP$_3$-dependent (possibly calcium-activated) calcium release from the endoplasmic reticulum (ER) may occur (see Finch et al 1991, Harootunian et al 1991). Abbreviations: **AA**, arachdonic acid; **AC**, adenylate cyclase; **AMPA**, α-amino-3-hydroxy-5-methyl-4-isoxazolepropionic acid subtype of glutamate receptor; **Ca/CAM**, calmodulin (calcium-activated); **CKII**, type II calcium/calmodulin-dependent protein kinase; **CREB**, cAMP response element binding protein; **DAG**, diacylglycerol; **g**, G-protein complex; **IEG**, immediate early gene; **IP$_3$**, inositol 1,4,5-triphosphate; **KA**, kainate subtype glutamate receptor; **L**, L-type calcium channel; **LT**, leukotriene; **MET**, metabotropic subtype glutamate receptor; **mg**, magnesium (voltage-dependent blockade of NMDA receptor); **Mito**, mitochondria; **N**, N-type calcium channel; **NMDA**, N-methyl-D-aspartate subtype of glutamate receptor; **NT**, neurotransmitter; **PDE**, (cyclic nucleotide) phosphodiesterase; **PG**, prostaglandin; **PIP$_2$**, phosphatidylinositol 4,5-biphosphate; **PKC**, protein kinase C; **PKM**, protein kinase M; **PLA$_2$**, phospholipase A$_2$; **PLC**, phospholipase C.

Modulation of calcium channels

Because seizures can be elicited and inhibited by pharmacological modulation of calcium channels, calcium entry blockers of the dihydropyridine class, including nimodipine and nitrendepine, have been used as anticonvulsants in clinical trials, primarily in an adjunctive capacity. The novel 'selective' calcium entry blocker flunarizine is also currently in clinical trials. Although the mechanism of its anticonvulsant effect is still unclear, experimental data suggest that flunarizine will have clinical applications similar to phenytoin and carbamazepine (Porter 1989).

Modulating neuronal inhibition

Experimental paradigms (i.e. picrotoxin, metrazol, bicuculline) readily demonstrate that seizures can be initiated by antagonizing GABA-mediated inhibition. Other seizure models (e.g. kindling), in conjunction with NMDA receptor activation, lead to loss of GABA inhibition. Consequently, strategies directed toward improving inhibitory tone represent a proved and clinically useful strategy for indirectly antagonizing the electrochemical effect of intracellular calcium. In support of this concept, Uematsu et al (1990) recently demonstrated that the intracellular calcium flux associated with both an imminent seizure and the seizure itself could be reversed by intravenous administration of diazepam.

In addition to enhancing GABAergic function, supraclinical concentrations of barbiturates and benzodiazepines affect calcium systems directly. For example, barbiturates block N- and L-type calcium currents (Macdonald 1989).

Prevention of epilepsy – antiepileptogenic therapy

Phenytoin and carbamazepine are agents which retard development of potentiated neuronal responses in various models. Both block Na^+ channels in a use-dependent fashion (Porter 1989). Benzodiazepines have been implicated in blocking calcium effects mediated by CaM kinase II by diminishing vesicle–membrane interactions and neurotransmitter release and by inhibiting voltage-sensitive calcium uptake into synaptosomes (DeLorenzo 1986, 1988). Modulation of Ca^{2+} target systems by anticonvulsant compounds affords another level at which long-term neuronal excitability might be regulated.

EAA systems constitute the major component of excitatory neurotransmission and have been implicated in development of interictal bursting, seizures and epilepsy. It is not surprising, therefore, that EAA systems have been targeted as potential loci for modulating increased neuronal excitability. A novel approach to decreasing the effect of heightened EAA activity is exemplified by lamotrigine, a triazine derivative which has entered clinical trials as an investigational antiepileptic drug. Experimentally, lamotrigine reduces veratrine-induced glutamate release, and it may exert its effect through stabilization of neuronal membranes (Porter 1989; also see Ch. 12 for a discussion of lamotrigine).

Agents which modulate the activity of the NMDA receptor may also have the potential for modifying or preventing long-term changes in neuronal excitability. Examples include drugs such as APV, which competes at the NMDA site, and MK-801 (dizocilpine), which blocks the receptor-coupled cation channel. Based on experimental data which showed that it could block LTP and retard kindling, MK-801 was brought to clinical trials. Regrettably, MK-801 demonstrated only minimal success as an anticonvulsant drug, while it produced unacceptable behavioural and psychiatric side effects (Dichter 1989, Porter 1989). Nevertheless, given the strength of experimental evidence implicating NMDA receptors in epileptogenesis, the clinical investigation of agents which modulate alternate sites of the NMDA receptor complex continues.

CONCLUSIONS

Calcium systems are essential not only for triggering seizures, but also for the development of epilepsy. Each of the systems discussed in this chapter represents essential constituents necessary for the preservation of calcium homeostasis and maintenance of coordinated neuronal function. Simultaneously, they also constitute sites at which lesions can cause physiological aberrations which, in turn, result in neuronal hyperexcitability. Consequently, they predict potential points for pharmacological intervention. Present anticonvulsant therapy has exploited some of these opportunities. It is likely that future treatment strategies will employ knowledge of these mechanisms to address both the prevention of epilepsy in susceptible patient populations (such as following stroke or head injury) as well as the improved control of established seizure disorders. In addition to increased insight into the pathophysiological mechanisms of epilepsy, greater knowledge of the manifold roles of calcium as a central second messenger in neuronal signal transduction will broaden our understanding of physiological processes, including the cellular and molecular basis of neuronal plasticity.

REFERENCES

Baraban J M, Snyder S H, Alger B E 1985 Protein kinase C regulates ionic conductance in hippocampal pyramidal neurons: electrophysiological effect of phorbol esters. Proc Natl Acad Sci USA 82: 2538–2542
Barinaga M 1990 The tide of memory, turning. Science 248: 1603–1605
Bashir Z I, Alford S, Davies S N et al 1991 Long-term potentiation of NMDA receptor-mediated synaptic transmission in the hippocampus. Nature 349: 156–158
Bennett M K, Kennedy M B 1987 Deduced primary structure of the beta subunit of brain type II Ca^{2+}/calmodulin-dependent kinase as determined by molecular cloning. Proc Natl Acad Sci USA 84: 1794–1798
Bertram E H, Lothman E W, Lenn N J 1990 The hippocampus in experimental epilepsy: a morphometric analysis. Ann Neurol 27: 43–48
Boulter J, Hollmann M, O'Shea-Greenfield A et al 1990 Molecular cloning and functional expression of glutamate receptor subunit genes. Science 249: 1033–1037
Chad J E, Eckert R 1986 An enzymatic mechanism for calcium current inactivation in dialysed *Helix* neurones. J Physiol (London) 378: 31–51
Collingridge G L, Kehl S J, McLennan H 1983 The action of an *N*-methyl-aspartate antagonist on synaptic processes in the rat hippocampus. J Physiol London 334: 33–46
Collingridge G L, Lester R A J 1989 Excitatory amino acid receptors in the vertebrate central nervous system. Pharmacol Rev 40: 143–210

Conner J A, Wadman W J, Hockberger P E, Wong R K 1988 Sustained dendritic gradients of Ca^{2+} induced by excitatory amino acids in CA1 hippocampal neurons. Science 240: 649–653

Coulter D A, Huguenard J R, Prince D A 1989 Calcium currents in rat thalamocortical relay neurones: kinetic properties of the transient low-threshold current. J Physiol London 414: 587–604

Coulter D A, Huguenard J R, Prince D A 1990 Differential effects of petit mal anticonvulsants on thalamic neurones: calcium current reduction. Br J Pharmacol 100: 800–806

DeLorenzo R J 1981 The calmodulin hypothesis of neurotransmission. Cell Calcium 2: 365–385

DeLorenzo R J 1986 A molecular approach to the calcium signal in brain: relationship to synaptic modulation and seizure discharge. Adv Neurol 44: 435–464

DeLorenzo R J 1988 Mechanisms of action of anticonvulsant drugs. Epilepsia 29 (Suppl 2): S35–S47

Dichter M A 1989 Cellular mechanisms of epilepsy and potential new treatment strategies. Epilepsia 30 (Suppl 1): S3–S12

Dichter M A, Ayala G F 1987 Cellular mechanisms of epilepsy: a status report. Science 237: 157–164

Dichter M A, Choi D W 1989 Excitatory amino acid transmitters and neurotoxins. Curr Neurol 9: 1–26

Dichter M A, Herman C J, Selzer M 1972 Silent cells during interictal discharges and seizures in hippocampal penicillin foci: evidence for the role of extracellular K^+ in the transition from the interictal state to seizures. Brain Res 48: 173–183

Dingledine R, McBain C J, McNamera J O 1990 Excitatory amino acid receptors in epilepsy. Trends Pharmacol Sci 11: 334–338

Dragunow M, Currie R W, Faull R L M et al 1989 Immediate-early genes, kindling, and long-term potentiation. Neurosci Biobehav Rev 13: 301–313

Engle J, Ackerman R 1980 Interictal EEG spikes correlate with decreased, rather than increased, epileptogenicity in rats. Brain Res 190: 543–548

Errington M L, Lynch M A, Bliss T V P 1987 Long-term potentiation in the dentate gyrus: induction and increased glutamate release are blocked by D(−)aminophophonovalerate. Neuroscience 20: 279–284

Finch E A, Turner T J, Goldin S M 1991 Calcium as a coagonist of inositol 1,4,5-triphosphate-induced calcium release. Science 232: 443–446

Goldenring J R, McGuire J S, DeLorenzo R J 1983 Identification of the major postsynaptic density protein as homologous with the calmodulin-binding subunit of the calmodulin-dependent protein kinase. J Neurochem 42: 1077–1084

Harootunian A T, Kao J P Y, Paranjape S, Tsien R Y 1991 Generation of calcium oscillations in fibroblasts by positive feedback between calcium and IP_3. Science 251: 75–78

Hess P 1990 Calcium channels in vertebrate cells. Annu Rev Neurosci 13: 337–356

Huang K P 1989 The mechanism of protein kinase C activation. Trends Neurosci 12: 425–432

Kamphuis W, Huisman E, Wadman W J et al 1989a Transient increase of cytoplasmic calcium concentration in the rat hippocampus after kindling-induced seizures: an ultrastructural study with the oxalxte-pyro-antimonate technique. Neuroscience 29: 667–674

Kamphuis W, Huisman E, Wadman W J et al 1989b Kindling induced changes in parvalbumin immunoreactivity in rat hippocampus and its relation to long-term decrease in GABA-immunoreactivity. Brain Res 479: 23–34

Kapur J, Lothman E W 1990 NMDA receptor activation mediates the loss of gabaergic inhibition induced by recurrent seizures. Epilepsy Res 5: 103–111

Kennedy M B 1989 Regulation of neuronal function by calcium. Trends Neurosci 12: 417–420

Kohr G, Lambert C E, Mody I 1990 Inactivation of HVA calcium currents in granule cells following kindling-induced epilepsy: the Ca^{2+}-buffering role of calbindin-D_{28K}(CABP). Soc Neurosci Abstracts 16: 623

Labiner D M, Hosford D A, Cheolsu S, McNamara J O 1989 An N-methyl-D-aspartate channel blocker, MK-801, inhibits seizure-induced rise in c-*fos* mRNA in hippocampus of kindled rats. Epilepsia (Abstr F-3) 30: 697

Llinas R, McGuiness T L, Leonard C S et al 1985 Intraterminal injection of synapsin

I or calcium/calmodulin-dependent protein kinase alters neurotransmitter release at the squid giant axon. Proc Natl Acad Sci USA 82: 3035–3039

Lothman E 1990 The biochemical basis and pathophysiology of status epilepticus. Neurology 40 (Suppl 2): 13–23

Lou L L, Schulman H 1989 Distinct autophosphorylation sites sequentially produce autonomy and inhibition of the multifunctional Ca^{2+}/calmodulin-dependent protein kinase. J Neurosci 9: 2020–2032

Lynch G, Larson J, Kelso S et al 1983 Intracellular injections of EGTA block induction of hippocampal long-term potentiation. Nature 305: 719–723

Macdonald R L 1989 Antiepileptic drug action 1989. Epilepsia 30 (Suppl 1): S19–S28

Malenka R C, Madison D V, Nicoll R A 1986 Potentiation of synaptic transmission in the hippocampus by phorbol esters. Nature 321: 175–177

Malinow R, Schulman H, Tsien R W 1989 Inhibition of postsynaptic PKC or CaMKII blocks induction but not expression of LTP. Science 245: 862–866

Marty A 1989 The physiological role of calcium-dependent channels. Trends Neurosci 12: 420–424

McNamara J O, Russell R D, Rigsbee L C et al 1988 Anticonvulsant and epileptogenic actions of MK-801 in the kindling and electroshock models. Neuropharmacology 27: 563–588

Meldrum B S 1981 Metabolic effects of prolonged epileptic seizures and the causation of epileptic brain damage. In: Rose F C (ed) Metabolic disorders of the nervous system. Pitman, London, pp 175–187

Meldrum B S 1986 Cell damage in epilepsy and the role of calcium in cytotoxicity. Adv Neurol 44: 849–855

Meyer F B 1989 Calcium, neuronal hyperexcitability and ischemic injury. Brain Res Rev 14: 227–243

Mody I, Stanton P K, Heinemann U 1988 Activation of N-methyl-D-aspartate receptors parallels changes in cellular and synaptic properties of dentate gyrus granule cells after kindling. J Neurophysiol 59: 1033–1054

Montminy M R, Gonzalez G A, Yamamoto K K 1990 Regulation of cAMP-inducible genes by CREB. Trends Neurosci 13: 184–188

Morgan J I, Curran T 1989 Calcium and proto-oncogene involvement in the immediate-early response in the nervous system. Ann NY Acad Sci 568: 283–290

Nicholls D, Atwell D 1990 The release and uptake of excitatory amino acids. Trends Pharmacol Sci 11: 462–468

Perlin J B, Lothman E W, Geary W A II 1987 Somatostatin augments the spread of limbic seizures from the hippocampus. Neurology 21: 475–480

Perlin J B, Churn S B, Lothman E W et al 1989 Continuous hippocampal stimulation decreases calcium-dependent protein kinase II activity. Soc Neurosci Abstracts (Abstr 181.10) 15: 454

Porter R J 1989 Mechanisms of action of new antiepileptic drugs. Epilepsia 30 (Suppl 1): S29–S34

Pumain R, Heinemann U 1985 Stimulus- and amino acid-induced calcium and potassium changes in rat cortex. J Neurophysiol 53: 1–16

Regehr W G, Connor J A, Tank D W 1989 Optical imaging of calcium accumulation in hippocampal pyramidal cells during synaptic activation. Nature 341: 533–536

Reymann K G, Matthies H 1989 2-Amino-4-phosphobutyrate selectively eliminates late phases of long-term potentiation in rat hippocampus. Neurosci Lett 98: 166–171

Rothman S M, Olney J W 1987 Excitotoxicity and the NMDA receptor. Trends Neurosci 10: 301–304

Rubin R P 1972 The role of calcium in the release of neurotransmitter substances and hormones. Pharmacol Rev 22: 389–428

Saitoh Y, Yamamoto H, Fukanaga K et al 1987 Inactivation and reactivation of the multifunctional calmodulin-dependent protein kinase from brain by autophosphorylation and dephosphorylation: involvement of protein phosphatases from brain. J Neurochem 49: 1286–1292

Scheuer M L, Pedley T A 1990 The evaluation and treatment of seizures. N Engl J Med 323: 1468–1474

Scharfman H E, Schwartzkroin P A 1989 Protection of dentate hilar cells from prolonged stimulation by intracellular calcium chelation. Science 246: 257–260

Schulman H 1988 The multifunctional Ca^{2+}/calmodulin-dependent kinase. In: Greengard P, Robison G A (eds) Advances in phosphoprotein and second messenger research. Raven Press, New York, pp 39–112

Shelton R C, Grebb J A, Freed W J 1987 Induction of seizures in mice by intracerebroventricular administration of the calcium channel agonist Bay K 8644. Brain Res 402: 399–402

Sheng M, McFadden G, Greenberg M E 1990 Membrane depolarization and calcium induce c-Fos transcription via phosphorylation of transcription factor CREB. Neuron 4: 571–582

Sloviter R S 1989 Calcium-binding protein (calbindin-D_{28K}) and parvalbumin immunocytochemistry: localization in the rat hippocampus with specific reference to the selective vulnerability of hippocampal neurons to seizure activity. J Comp Neurol 280: 183–196

Sombati S, Forman R R, Attema B L et al 1988 Intracellular injection of CaM kinase II reduces spike afterhyperpolarizations in cultured spinal cord neurons. Soc Neurosci Abstracts (Abstr 438.13) 14: 1090

Sommer B, Keinanen K, Verdoorn T A et al 1990 Flip and flop: a cell-specific functional switch in glutamate-operated channels of the CNS. Science 249: 1580–1585

Staubli U, Larson J, Thibault O et al 1988 Chronic administration of a thiol-proteinase inhibitor blocks long-term potentiation of synaptic responses. Brain Res 444: 153–158

Stelzer A, Kay A R, Wong R K S 1988 $GABA_A$-receptor function is maintained by phosphorylation factors. Science 241: 339–341

Tsien R W, Lipscombe D, Madison D V et al 1988 Multiple types of neuronal calcium channels and their selective modulation. Trends Neurosci 11: 432–438

Uematsu D, Araki N, Greenberg J, Revich M 1990 Alterations in cytosolic free calcium in the cat cortex during bicuculline-induced epilepsy. Brain Res Bull 24: 285–288

Wasterlain C G, Farber D B 1984 Kindling alters the calcium/calmodulin-dependent phosphorylation of synaptic plasma membrane proteins in rat hippocampus. Proc Natl Acad Sci USA 81: 1253–1257

Watkins J C, Krogsgaard-Larsen, Honore T 1990 Structure–activity relationships in the development of excitatory amino acid agonist and competitive antagonists. Trends Pharmacol Sci 11: 25–33

Wong M L, Smith M A, Weiss S R B et al 1990 Induction of heat shock proteins in kindled brains. Soc Neurosci Abstracts (Abstr 138.10) 14: 309

Yue D T, Backyx P H, Imredy J P 1990 Calcium-sensitive inactivation in the gating of single calcium channels. Science 250: 1735–1738

Zorumski C F, Thio L L, Clark G D 1990 Blockade of desensitization augments quisqualate excitotoxicity in hippocampal neurons. Neuron 5: 61–66

3

Cortical dysplasia in epilepsy – a study of material from surgical resections for intractable epilepsy

I. Janota   C. E. Polkey

INTRODUCTION

In 1971 Taylor and his colleagues reported ten surgical cases under the title 'Focal dysplasia of the cerebral cortex in epilepsy' (Taylor et al 1971). The single localized lesions included congregations of large bizarre neurones and, in most cases, grotesque cells probably of glial origin in the depths of the cortex and the adjacent white matter. Most of the cases came from the late Murray Falconer at the Maudsley Hospital, with two from surgeons elsewhere. Similar cases continue to turn up at the Maudsley Hospital (Janota & Polkey 1985, 1986), and elsewhere, for example in Montreal (Andermann et al 1987) or Buffalo (Moreland et al 1988). Similar microscopic appearances are encountered in hemimegalencephaly and in a variety of developmental anomalies within the category of disorders of neuronal migration.

CLINICAL MATERIAL

We here summarize data obtained from surgical cases operated at the Maudsley Hospital and review the concept of 'cortical dysplasia'. The changes of cortical dysplasia were found in the cerebral cortex in 29 cases. These include 7 of the cases described by Taylor et al in 1971. Added to these are 4 cases from Murray Falconer's subsequent operative experience and a further 18 surgical cases, one of which was operated upon by Mr P. H. Schurr, the remainder by Mr C. E. Polkey.

These cases were found over a 35-year period between 1955 and 1990 and the clinical details are shown in Table 3.1. There are differences between the patients operated upon in the two periods 1955–1975 and 1980–1990; there were more extratemporal resections in the later group and the patients were younger when they came to surgery. All the patients presented with intractable drug-resistant epilepsy, and the object of the surgery was to improve the control of their epilepsy. They comprised 18 males and 11 females. Their fits started at a mean age of 7.8 years (range: birth to 40 years), and they came to operation aged between 2 and 49 years (mean age: 21 years). Eleven patients underwent temporal lobectomy, 9

Table 3.1   Clinical details

		1955–1975 (Falconer)	1980–1990 (Polkey[a])	Total
Number		11	18	29
Male/female		8/3	10/8	18/11
Age at onset	Mean	14.5	4	7.8
	Range	(3–40)	(0.1–27)	(0.1–40)
Age at operation	Mean	27.8	17.9	21
	Range	(16–49)	(4–47)	(4–49)
Temporal lobectomy		8	3	11
Frontal resection		2	7	9
Other resections		1	8	9

[a] One patient was operated by Mr P. H. Schurr.

frontal resections, and the others had brain resections from other regions and one had a hemispherectomy. Because they were selected from a group of patients investigated with the prospect of some kind of cerebral resection, they were subject to focal seizures usually appropriate to the area subsequently resected. Seven of the patients were also subject to generalized convulsive seizures and in three cases the generalized seizures were the main feature. The details of the patient's seizure type and the outcome of surgery are summarized in Table 3.2. There was significant neurological deficit in 8 patients prior to operation. The distribution between left and right hemispheres was roughly equal, 17 being left and 12 right.

The details of the neurophysiological findings are summarized in Table 3.3. Twenty-eight of the 29 patients had extensive scalp electroencephalography prior to surgery and sphenoidal recordings were also carried out in patients with temporal lobe problems. In one patient chronic subdural recordings were carried out prior to definitive resection to try to distinguish between a posterior frontal and central origin for the attacks.

A distinct focal electrical abnormality was seen in 17 patients, and additional bilateral abnormalities were seen in 3 of these 17 patients; widespread unilateral abnormalities were seen in a further 6 patients and

Table 3.2   Fit type and outcome

Operation	'Psychomotor' seizures	Other minor fits	Focal motor fits	Generalized seizures occurring regularly
Temporal lobectomy	7	2	0	2
Frontal resections	2	5	0	2
Other resections	0	5	1	3
Outcome:				
Worthwhile improvement	6	10	1	1
No improvement or worse	2	2	0	6

Table 3.3   Neurophysiological findings

Operation	Scalp EEG			ECoG	
	Unilateral lateralized	Unilateral widespread	Bilateral changes	Focal only	Widespread changes
Temporal lobectomy	8	1	2	8	3
Frontal resections[a]	6	1	1	6	2
Other resections[b]	3	4	2	4	4

[a] One patient had no neurophysiological tests.
[b] The patient who had the hemispherectomy did not have an ECoG.

bilateral abnormalities in the remaining 5 patients. Dr M. V. Driver, the clinical neurophysiologist who assessed many of the early cases, commented that there was no EEG pattern or waveform specific to cortical dysplasia; the EEG abnormalities related to a known or later discovered structural abnormality or corresponded to the 'focal' epilepsy.

At craniotomy 10 patients had clearly visible cortical abnormalities. In most cases acute electrocorticography (ECoG) confirmed the neurophysiological focus suggested by the extracranial recordings. In those cases where more widespread abnormalities were seen at ECoG the results of the resection were not as good. Such findings were found in 3 temporal resections, one frontal resection and 3 other resections. However, there were also four cases – one frontal resection and 3 extratemporal resections – where the result of the operation was bad even though there appeared to be a single focus at ECoG.

The details of the neuroradiological and neuropsychological investigations are shown in Table 3.4. Over half the patients were investigated in the period prior to the use of sophisticated methods of brain imaging. Eighteen of the 29 patients had computed tomography (CT) scans and the lesion was visible on only 4 scans. Seven of the 29 patients had magnetic resonance imaging (MRI) scans and 6 of these scans showed the lesion. Eleven patients had

Table 3.4   Radiology and psychometry

Operation	Brain imaging				Neuropsychometry		
	CT Done	Lesion	MRI Done	Lesion	Full-scale IQ Min.	Max.	Mean
Temporal lobectomy	3	0	0	0	64	126	93
Frontal resections	7	2	3	3	68	111	92
Other resections	8	2	4	3	60	104	78
Total	18/29	4/18	7/29	6/7	60	126	88

Note: the 11 patients investigated before modern brain imaging had either a lumbar AEG, which showed a dilated temporal horn in 4 of 11 examinations, or carotid angiograms; two were performed and one was abnormal.

Table 3.5   Results of surgery

Operation	Temporal lobectomy	Frontal resection	Other resection	Total
Number	11	9	9	29
Preoperative deficit	1	2	5	8
Postoperative deficit	4	0	7	11
Outcome – seizure control:				
Virtually fit free	8	5	1	14
Worthwhile improvement	1	1	3	5
Not improved or worse	2	3	5	10
Outcome – social status:				
Normal	9	4	3	16
Abnormal	1	5	6	12
Died	1	0	0	1

Mean follow-up 6 years, range 1–16 years.

lumbar air encephalograms which showed a dilated temporal horn in 4 of them. Two patients had carotid angiograms, one of which appeared to show diffuse swelling.

Detailed results of neuropsychological testing were available for 23 of the 29 patients; 3 others were described as subnormal and 3 others were not tested. There is a lower level of attainment in those patients undergoing resections from areas other than the temporal or frontal lobes and this reflects the larger, more widespread, lesions in these patients.

The results of surgery are shown in Table 3.5. The longest period of follow-up was 15 years and the mean was 6 years. The results do not differ from those seen in resective surgery as a whole and the results with temporal lobectomy are better than for other operations. The reasons for this are discussed below.

The final fate of the 29 patients is as follows: 13 are living normal adult lives; the remaining 7 adults are unemployed. Eight are children but only 2 are in normal education. One adult died, nine years after temporal lobectomy, from the ravages of his uncontrolled epilepsy. A post-mortem examination was not obtained.

PATHOLOGY

Methods

Since 1977 the specimens obtained by cerebral resection, i.e. from the last 18 cases in this series, have been examined in the Department of Neuropathology of the Institute of Psychiatry. In 5 of these 18 cases the abnormality was visible in the surgical specimen before it was sliced.

The fixed specimens were inspected, measured, sliced, photographed and usually weighed. Various abnormalities were felt and seen, usually an abnormally thick stretch of cortex, poorly demarcated from white matter. Blocks were embedded in paraffin wax, cut at 5 μm and 15 μm and stained with haematoxylin and eosin, with Luxol fast blue/Nissl and impregnated with silver according to Glees. Additional staining techniques, including immunohistochemical techniques, were employed. Some specimens were examined with electron microscopy.

Neuropathological findings

The details of the neuropathological findings in the recent 18 cases are shown in Table 3.6. The changes resemble what was described by Taylor et al (1971). However, some of the differences between our recent microscopic findings and theirs may be due to differences in processing. In two cases (Figs 3.1–3.3) there was an abnormally extensive smooth stretch of brain surface lacking any sulci. The abnormality, which included large nerve cells (Fig. 3.4) and glial cells (Fig. 3.5), often extended deep in the brain and was not confined to a single focus, sulcus or gyrus (Fig. 3.6). In some cases the abnormal area had not been completely resected. In the case where hemispherectomy was performed the large nerve cells deep in two temporal sulci were only found on microscopy. In retrospect, however, in that case the affected cortex was wider than normal and ill demarcated from the white matter. In that case, and in three others, only the large nerve cells were found. In one case abnormally large astrocytes in the white matter were the main feature. In one case, which has not been previously reported, a resection was made from the parietal region of a man aged 29 by Murray Falconer, who was convinced that the diagnosis

Table 3.6 Neuropathological findings in the last 18 cases

Biopsy number	Age	Sex	Site and type of resection	Pathological comments	Specimen weight (g)
137/80	25	F	Right frontal		33
71/81	1	M	Left frontal		Small
218/81	17	M	Left frontal		–
416/81	3	M	Left parietal	Lissencephaly	91
624/81	14	F	Right temporal lobectomy	Lissencephaly	46
B45/82	11	M	Left frontoparietal		101
B85/82	10	F	Right frontal		80
B644/83	15	F	Left frontoparietal		107
B812/85	36	M	Left frontocentral	Nerve cells only	14
B228/87	19	M	Right frontal (anterior)		123
B509/87	24	M	Right temporal lobectomy	Lissencephaly	39.4
B193/88	5	M	Left hemispherectomy	Nerve cells only	396
B318/88	23	M	Left temporal lobectomy	Glial cells only	51.7
B320/88	4	F	Right frontal		131.4
B369/88	15	M	Left frontal		82
B156/89	12	F	Right frontal	Nerve cells only	–
B466/89	19	F	Left frontal (central)		Small
B7/90	48	M	Right parietal (central)		Small

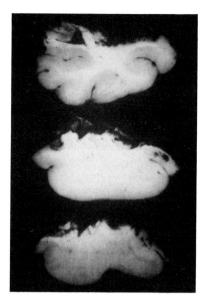

Fig. 3.1 Several slices from a fixed anterior lobectomy specimen, (624/81). Note the lack of sulci in the lower two slices and an abnormally wide gyrus above. The distinction between cortex and white matter is blurred. The temporal horn of the lateral ventricle is seen in the upper slice at the top left. Mildly magnified.

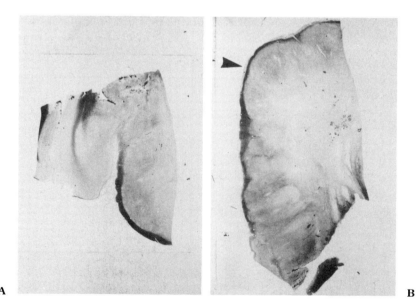

A B

Fig. 3.2 Two parts from a lissencephalic lesion (416/81). Note the superficial zone of myelinated fibres; more normal brain is seen on the left of **A**. The arrow in **B** indicates a thin pale leptomeningeal layer shown at higher magnification in Fig. 3.3.

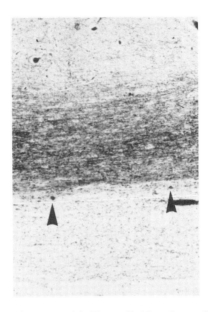

Fig. 3.3 Detail of the region arrowed in Fig. 3.2**B**. Note the myelinated nerve fibres deep to the surface and a pale glial zone in the leptomeninges that contains some nerve cells (arrows). (Luxol fast blue/Nissl, 160 × .)

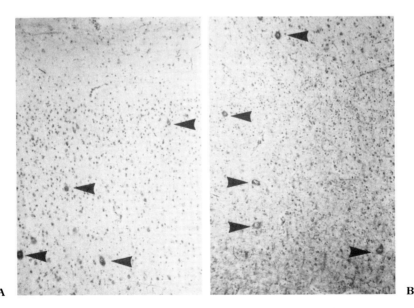

A   B

Fig. 3.4 Adjacent sections through the thick cortex from specimen B45/82. Note the sparsely scattered very large nerve cells. The leptomeningeal surface is at the top of **A** and white matter at the bottom of **B**. (Luxol fast blue/Nissl, 157 × .)

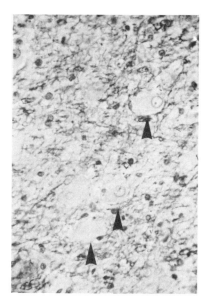

Fig. 3.5   Large ballooned astrocytes (arrows), amongst myelinated nerve fibres. (B37/80, Luxol fast blue/Nissl, 265 × .)

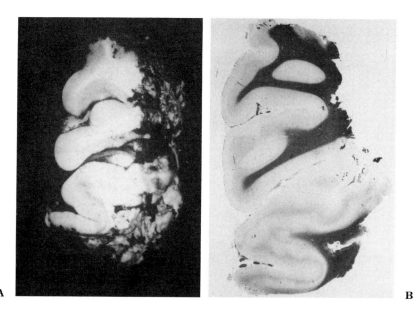

A   B

Fig. 3.6   A slice through the surgical specimen (B45/82) from the left frontoparietal region. Note the abnormal and thick cortex below. Mildly magnified. (**A** unstained; **B** section stained with Luxol fast blue/Nissl.)

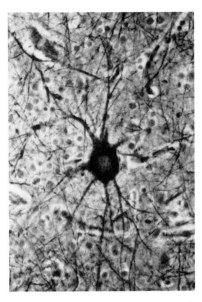

Fig. 3.7   An abnormally large nerve cell with several dendrites impregnated with silver. (B45/82, Glees/Bielschowsky, 265 × .)

was cortical dysplasia, but only a small patch of abnormally large astrocytes in the white matter was found and the cortex was normal. The patient was followed for nine years and remained virtually fit free. In several cases silver impregnation showed prominent numerous dendrites (Fig. 3.7), resembling the nerve cells in antegrade olivary hypertrophy. Electron microscopy in several cases did not show any synapses on the abnormal nerve cells but the material was not optimally fixed. The orientation of the large nerve cells was generally hard to establish; many appeared to be erratically arranged. The axons of some pointed in the appropriate direction. In one lesion with no gyri (partial lissencephaly) there must have been an element of inappropriate projection of at least some cortical nerve cells since there was a subpial layer of myelinated axons parallel to the meningeal surface (Figs 3.2 and 3.3). In that case there were also glial and neuronal elements in the meningeal surface – the so-called meningeal glioneuronal heterotopia (Friede 1989). The appearance and the position of the large glial cells varied. In some cases they were amongst the large nerve cells in the superficial 'cortical' zone, but often they predominated deep to the large nerve cells amongst myelinated axons. The staining of the perikarya of the large glial nerve cells with antisera to glial fibrillary acidic protein (GFAP) varied. Some of the perikarya were more and some less positive. Their processes, which appeared to be relatively sparse, were positive. In several instances the astrocytic nature of the cells was confirmed by electron microscopy; this occasionally showed more mitochondria than glial filaments in the perikarya, perhaps relating to the faint GFAP positivity. The large cells, neurones and astrocytes were recognized in smears when these were made at operation. There were other minor changes: subpial fibrillary gliosis (Chaslin's gliosis), loss of axons, gliosis deep to the cortex, calcific particles and corpora amylacea. These varied from case to case.

DISCUSSION

The lesion under discussion cannot be established from preoperative clinical studies. Taylor et al (1971) advance no clinical criteria for identifying the condition and this study, which includes a follow-up of some of their patients, does not resolve the matter. We would also agree that these patients are clinically distinct from those with tuberous sclerosis and other conditions, because of a lack of other lesions in the brain and elsewhere in the body.

Neurophysiologically a variety of abnormalities have been seen, none of which were diagnostic of the condition. Where the abnormalities were widespread, especially in the electrocorticogram, and where the resection was incomplete, whatever the reason, the results of surgery were unsatisfactory. This corresponds to the view of Rasmussen (1979) that if the results of a cerebral resection for epilepsy were unsatisfactory it was often because the resection was incomplete. He suggested that in such cases a further resection would improve the control of the epilepsy, but in most of these cases this would be impractical. In these cases, as in many other patients subjected to resective surgery, temporal lobectomy was more effective than other methods of resection in controlling the epilepsy. This is a reflection of the fact that temporal lobectomy involves each of the three mechanisms by which resective surgery may control epilepsy. These are: removal of the pathology; a considerable reduction in the potential epileptogenic mass; and a comprehensive neuronal disconnection.

The neuroradiological findings deserve some comment. This lesion, as we have already seen, has neither the vascular nor gross space-occupying properties necessary to demonstrate abnormalities prior to modern brain-imaging techniques. With the advent and then the improvement in CT and MRI imaging techniques, these lesions have become more obvious. Many of the smaller lesions, which are common in the surgical material, can be seen with MRI scanning, which also often suggests that the lesion is larger than it appears on CT scan.

In all our later cases the specimen contained normal brain. In two cases, for fear of producing an unacceptable neurological deficit, the resection was known to be incomplete.

Cortical dysplasia may be suspected on inspection of the specimen but histology is necessary to confirm the diagnosis. In contrast to the original series and Falconer's other four cases, which were all temporal lobectomies (Bruton 1988), in our cases cortical dysplasia is found more often in other parts of the brain than the temporal lobe (Table 3.6). This reflects to some extent different criteria for the selection of patients for operation. Some territories, which would have been avoided in the past, for example near the sensorimotor strip, have been explored albeit with modest resections and the use of multiple subpial transection (Morrell et al 1989).

The main microscopic features of cortical dysplasia are not unique to that condition. They are known in tuberous sclerosis, hemimegalencephaly, and are sometimes seen post-mortem in other brains, usually those of retarded and epileptic subjects. The distinction between tuberous sclerosis and cortical dysplasia has received much attention and has been discussed by Taylor et al (1971). Some regard the condition as a 'forme fruste' of tuberous sclerosis (Andermann et al 1987). There is an increasing interest in the relation of disorders of neuronal migration (Barth 1987) or of microdysgenesis (Hardiman et al 1988) to epilepsy. Our findings are of something more obvious than minor irregularities of the appearance of the cortex, or the presence of a few nerve cells in the white matter. Although we appreciate that these more subtle changes may be relevant to epilepsy our experience so far does not help to clarify the situation.

Similarity between cortical dysplasia and hemimegalencephaly has been stressed by a number of authors (King et al 1985, Harding 1987, personal communication, Robain et al 1988, Robain 1990, Norman et al 1990, personal communication). In hemimegalencephaly large abnormal nerve cells, similar to those seen in cortical dysplasia, are seen not only in the surface which can be recognized as cortex but also in the white matter. It has been suggested that cortical dysplasia and hemimegalencephaly may be linked with tuberous sclerosis or neurofibromatosis, in spite of the absence of the stigmata of these or other clinical conditions. Norman et al (1990) have recently studied a case of hemimegalencephaly and speculated that somatic mosaicism in the ventricular zone during embryonic life may be the explanation. They have suggested that DNA probes and chromosomal analysis might address this possibility and also any connection with tuberous sclerosis or neurofibromatosis. So far we have not done this.

The dearth of post-mortem reports and other evidence makes it difficult to assess the true incidence of cortical dysplasia or to know its true relationship to other malformations. Multiple cerebral lesions cannot be excluded on the basis of the surgical specimens but it is known that in tuberous sclerosis multiple lesions are often visible on scans. Why is there not more post-mortem evidence of cortical dysplasia? It is possible that there are some such appearances buried under the label of extensive cortical malformation, pachygyria or lissencephaly, or even that in tuberous sclerosis the histological sampling concentrated on the more typical tubers and the appearances of cortical dysplasia were missed. However, we have not encountered that appearance in brains categorized as tuberous sclerosis from patients ranging in age from birth to 60 years at death.

In our personal series of cortical resections for epilepsy we have encountered 18 cases in a total of 279 resections (6.5%) and in the Maudsley series overall it forms a similar proportion of the material. Not all series of cortical resections for intractable epilepsy published since Taylor's paper mention this lesion of cortical dysplasia and there may be a number of reasons for this. In some series the relevant material has not been examined. Thus Meyer et al (1986), describing 50 cases of temporal lobectomy in childhood, make sparse mention of the pathology in general because the medial temporal structures have been destroyed by suction and are therefore not available for examination. The lesion is also comparatively rare and will not be encountered unless the material from a substantial number of resections is available – say more than 50 in all. Jensen & Kliniken (1976), describing 74 temporal lobectomies from Denmark, note one specimen with cortical dysplasia and another with heterotopia. Recounting the experience in Oxford between 1957 and 1986 Ounstead and his colleagues describe the results of 65 resections in children with one case of cortical dysplasia in 54 temporal lobectomies and one further case in the frontal region in the remaining 11 operations, making an incidence of 3% (Ounstead et al 1987). Finally, the pathologist examining the material may classify the lesion of cortical dysplasia as something else. Mathieson (1975), in describing the Montreal material, notes 10 cases of tuberous sclerosis, or forme fruste thereof, in a total of 503 cases and some at least of these may be cortical dysplasia. Lieb et al (1981), describing 44 temporal lobectomies at UCLA, where the specimen is obtained using the 'en bloc' method, write of two examples of heterotopia. More recently Babb & Jann-Brown (1987) quote an incidence of 5.5% for heterotopia in material excised at UCLA.

The terminology in the field of cortical dysplasia is neither definitive nor ideal. Cortical dysplasia, as we have found it, is not confined to the cortex and the 'focus' can be rather large and so perhaps not focal. However, as abnormally large nerve cells in the cerebral mantle are a prominent feature, cortical dysplasia is a convenient term in our particular patients who have been selected for surgery. The occasional finding in some cases of only large nerve cells, or rarely predominantly large astrocytes, further complicates the question of terminology and of the origin of this condition.

For all these reasons it is difficult to interpret the findings of other workers but it seems likely that this lesion is present in 2–5% of specimens of cerebral cortex obtained by resection of such cortex for intractable epilepsy.

REFERENCES

Andermann F, Olivier A, Malanson D, Robitaille Y 1987 Epilepsy due to focal cortical dysplasia with macrogyria and the forme fruste of tuberous sclerosis: a study of 15 patients. In: Wolf P, Dam M, Janz D, Dreifuss F E (eds) Advances in epilepsy, Vol. 16. Raven Press, New York, pp 35–38
Babb T L, Jann Brown W 1987 Pathological findings in epilepsy. In: Engel J Jr (ed) Surgical

treatment of the epilepsies. Raven Press, New York, pp 511–540

Barth P G 1987 Disorders of neuronal migration. Can J Neurol Sci 14: 1–6

Bruton C J 1988 The neuropathology of temporal lobe epilepsy. Institute of Psychiatry, Maudsley Monographs No 31, Oxford University Press, Oxford

Friede R L 1989 Leptomeningeal glioneuronal heterotopia: developmental neuropathology, 2nd edn. Springer-Verlag, Vienna, pp 339–341

Hardiman O, Burke T, Phillips J, Murphy S, O'Moore B, Staunton H, Farrell M A 1988 Microdysgenesis in resected temporal cortex: incidence and clinical significance in focal epilepsy. Neurology 38: 1041–1047

Janota I, Polkey C E 1985 Focal dysplasia of the cerebral cortex in surgery for epilepsy. Neuropathol Appl Neurobiol 11: 325–326

Janota I, Polkey C E 1986 Focal dysplasia of the cerebral cortex in surgery for epilepsy. Abstracts of Xth International Congress of Neuropathology, Stockholm, No 161, p 83

Jensen I, Kliniken L 1976 Temporal lobe epilepsy and neuropathology: histological findings in resected temporal lobes correlated to surgical results and clinical aspects. Acta Neurol Scand 54: 391–414

King M, Stephenson J B B, Ziervogel M, Doyle D, Galbraith S 1985 Hemimegalencephaly: a case for hemispherectomy? Neuropediatrics 16: 46–55

Lieb J P, Engel J, Brown W J, Gervis A S, Crandall P H 1981 Neuropathological findings following temporal lobectomy related to surface and deep EEG patterns. Epilepsia 22: 539–549

Mathieson G 1975 Pathologic aspects of epilepsy with special reference to the surgical pathology of focal cerebral seizures. In: Purpura D P, Penry J K, Walter R D (eds) Advances in neurology, Vol. 8. Raven Press, New York, pp 107–138

Meyer F B, Marsh W R, Laws E R Jr, Sharborough F W 1986 Temporal lobectomy in children with epilepsy. J Neurosurg 64: 371–376

Moreland D B, Glasauer F E, Egnatchik J C, Heffner R R, Alker J J 1988 Focal cortical dysplasia. J Neurosurg 68: 487–490

Morrell F, Whisler W W, Bleck T P 1989 A new approach to the surgical treatment of focal epilepsy. J Neurosurg 70: 231–239

Ounstead C, Lindsay J, Richards P 1987 Developmental aspects of focal epilepsies of childhood treated by neurosurgery. In: Temporal lobe epilepsy 1948–1986: a biographical study. MacKeith Press, Oxford, pp 70–86

Rasmussen T 1979 Cortical epilepsy for medically refractory focal epilepsy: results, lessons, questions. In: Rasmussen T, Marino R (eds) Functional neurosurgery. Raven Press, New York, pp 253–269

Robain O 1990 Hemimegalencephaly. Communication to the European Neuropathology Group Meeting at Wallingford, June 1990

Robain O, Floquet C H, Heldt N, Rosenberg F 1988 Hemimegalencephaly: a clinicopathological study of four cases. Neuropathol Appl Neurobiol 14: 125–135

Taylor D C, Falconer M A, Bruton C J, Corsellis J A N 1971 Focal dysplasia of the cerebral cortex in epilepsy. J Neurol Neurosurg Psychiatry 34: 369–387

4

Equivalent dipole modelling – a new EEG method for localization of epileptogenic foci

J. S. Ebersole

INTRODUCTION

For six decades, electroencephalography (EEG) has been primarily a descriptive science, in which patterns of brain electrical potentials were characterized and correlated with clinical conditions. Although appropriate for young sciences, further progress requires that descriptive phases must be short lived. The EEG of epilepsy is a case in point. Epileptiform patterns have been described in great detail over the years. We now recognize many types of interictal and ictal activity associated with a variety of epileptic disorders. If, however, our understanding of epilepsy is to advance, we must go beyond simple description of the EEG waveforms and pursue the physiology and location of the underlying generators. Visual inspection and qualitative descriptions of EEG should be augmented if not replaced by quantitative measures.

Attempts to specify the location of epileptogenic foci have relied on several techniques: scalp EEG, behavioural seizure correlations, neuro-psychological testing, structural (CT and MRI) and functional (PET and SPECT) imaging. Most epileptologists would agree however, that intracranial EEG is the 'gold standard'. Nonetheless, intracranial recordings have limitations (Ajmone Marsan 1990) and associated morbidity. Therefore, there has been an increasing interest in developing better non-invasive localization techniques. Pre-surgical evaluations could be made more efficient, because intracranial EEG is often a rate-limiting factor in epilepsy surgery programmes. Potentially more patients could benefit from surgery with greater convenience and less morbidity. Among the non-invasive approaches under investigation, source localization and its precursor, voltage topography, applied to epileptiform EEG potentials look particularly promising.

This chapter is an introduction to equivalent dipole modelling of interictal EEG spikes. The discussion is directed to the clinical epileptologist and electroencephalographer. The mathematics of volume conduction of electrical potentials and of dipole localization methods are beyond the scope of this review but are readily available elsewhere (Wilson & Bayley 1950, Rush & Driscoll 1968, Brody et al 1973, Kavanagh et al 1978, Darcey et al 1980, Nunez 1981, Scherg & von Cramon 1986).

GENERATION OF EEG FIELDS

Neuronal excitation and inhibition are accompanied by current flow across membranes of affected cells. From these, secondary currents and a voltage potential field are generated in the extracellular space. The laminar organization of the cortex and the columnar arrangement of individual neurones, particularly pyramidal cells, provide a substrate for spatially coherent activity which can summate into macroscopic potential fields. Because scalp electrodes are relatively distant from the active neurones, cellular current sinks and sources can be approximated as dipoles and the corresponding potential fields as dipolar fields.

Because cortical neurones are arranged in parallel columns, dendritic fields are located above and below cell bodies. Regions of current sinks and sources are thus similarly positioned, and the resultant dipole fields have an orientation that is orthogonal to the plane of the cortical surface. In the case of an activated gyral crown, the field will be radial and the potential distribution on the scalp will reflect only one side of the dipole. If one side of a cortical sulcus is activated, the resultant dipolar field will be tangential and both the positive and negative fields reflecting both ends of the dipole will be evident on the scalp. In EEG terms, this would be called a 'horizontal dipole' field. In reality, a varying combination of radial and tangential dipoles contribute to the EEG.

The depth of a dipole determines the extent and gradient of the corresponding scalp voltage field. A small, superficial cortical generator will produce a voltage field that has relatively high amplitude, steep voltage gradients, and a relatively small area. Conversely, a small source that is deep within the brain produces a scalp voltage field that has relatively low amplitude, shallow voltage gradients, but a considerably larger extent. Superficial sources that are large in area can also produce a widespread voltage field, but the amplitude is relatively higher. Thus the location, orientation, size and shape of the generator region determine the topography of the voltage fields measurable at the scalp.

Evoked potentials or intrinsic potentials, such as epileptic spikes, are composed of waveforms which commonly alternate in polarity. Surface polarity depends upon the sequence in which cortical layers are activated (Ebersole & Chatt 1984). Sensory evoked potentials have a primary component that is surface positive due to an active current sink (negative) in the middle layers and a passive current source (positive) in superficial laminae. Epileptiform EEG spikes are usually surface negative secondary to active superficial laminar sinks and passive deep source. Subsequent reversals in sink–source locations produce scalp fields of alternating polarity.

LOCALIZATION OF EQUIVALENT DIPOLE SOURCES

Forty years ago electroencephalographers began to consider the physical relationship between electrical fields on the scalp and their underlying sources within the brain (Brazier 1949, Shaw & Roth 1955a, 1955b, Geisler & Gerstein 1961). The physical principles upon which dipole localization techniques are based, namely electric field theory applied to volume conduction, are substantially older having been developed by Helmholtz (1853) in the mid-nineteenth century. Nearly one hundred years later Wilson & Bayley (1950) developed a method for calculating the voltage field generated on a spherical volume conductor by a known dipole.

In simple terms, if the location, orientation and strength of a dipolar source within a spherical homogeneous conducting medium is known, one can predict the shape and magnitude of the potential field that is measurable on its surface. The answer to this type of problem has been called the 'forward solution', and it is unique. There is only one field that can be generated by a given dipole. Forward solutions can be used to test hypotheses directly, as will be discussed later.

However, the usual clinical problem is the opposite, namely trying to locate the intracerebral generator from the character of the scalp potential and its field. The answer to this is called the 'inverse solution' and, unfortunately, for any given voltage field there is no unique answer. Rather there are multiple possibilities, because fields of different sources in a volume conductor sum linearly (Helmholtz's principle of superposition). Accordingly, the field measured by a given electrode array may well be a composite from any number of different sources.

Certain assumptions are necessary to make the application of these principles to human EEG mathematically tractable. First, the brain is modelled as a sphere of uniform conducting material (Brody et al 1973). Concentric shells (two to four) can be added around this to imitate the skull and scalp (Rush & Driscoll 1968, Kavanagh et al 1978, Sidman et al 1978, Darcey et al 1980) (see Fig. 4.1). The brain and scalp are usually considered to be of equal resistivity with the intervening skull assigned a resistivity that is 80 times greater. The EEG field from which a solution is sought is considered to be dipolar in character, and the source of the field is modelled as a point-source dipole.

It is obvious that generators of scalp EEG potentials, such as spikes, are not point sources. They are comprised of large aggregates of neurones that probably extend over several square centimetres. However, the combined activity of such a generator region may be modelled effectively by a single dipole. That is to say, the field that would be produced by this 'equivalent dipole' is very similar to that of the real source. If the generator area is well localized, the equivalent dipole should reside close to its centre and have a similar orientation.

The most common form of source localization is the *instantaneous single dipole inverse solution*. This procedure takes voltage values from all electrodes at a given instant in time and searches, using iterative minimization techniques, for an equivalent dipole within the head that could generate such a field (Schneider 1972, Henderson et al 1975, Kavanagh et al 1978,

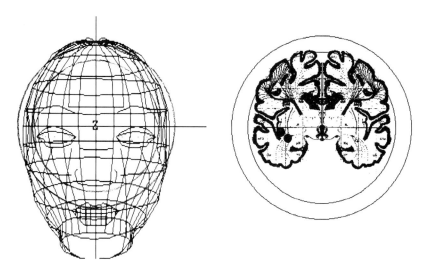

Fig. 4.1   Spherical shell models of brain and surface of scalp (represented as circles) superimposed upon diagrams of a head and brain (frontal cross-section at the level of anterior temporal lobe). Note that the spherical models only approximate true shape. Filled dots on brain cross-section correspond to locations of equivalent dipole sources depicted in Fig. 4.3.

Sidman et al 1978, Darcey et al 1980). In essence, localizing an equivalent dipole requires that the programme start at a given location in the model head, make repeated and progressively better estimates of dipole parameters that would be appropriate for the recorded potential field, calculate for each estimate the forward solution, and then determine how good that solution is. An error measure is computed, which is the sum of the squared differences between the actual field and that calculated from the most recent estimate. If the most recent estimate produces a larger error than the previous one, the direction of search is changed. The solution with the minimum sum of squared errors ('least squares') is considered to be the best one attainable. Search algorithms use a variety of techniques (Marquardt 1963, O'Neill 1971) to find an equivalent dipole quickly and at the same time avoid being trapped in a suboptimal local minimum of the errors criterion and missing the best solution.

Various factors can reduce source localization accuracy in addition to the assumptions of the model. EEG 'noise' which includes ongoing rhythms not associated with the potential of interest, can induce errors in localization of 5–10% of the head radius when it occurs at a level of 10–20% of the signal (Kavanagh et al 1978). It is essential, therefore, to model potentials possessing a high signal-to-noise ratio, such as 10:1 (Fender 1987). In the case of epileptiform spikes, this usually means that computer averaging of multiple individual spikes is required. Inaccuracy of electrode location by 1 cm from their specified positions (approximately a 5° error) will also produce localization errors of 5–10% (Kavanagh et al 1978). Measured electrode placement is a necessity. Normal variations in the thickness of the skull from the mean value used in the modelling process can cause errors of 7% for sources near the surface of the brain, while similar variations in scalp thickness about the norm may introduce errors of 3% of the head radius (Ary et al 1981).

Early applications of source localization techniques to brain activity were primarily limited to normal sensory evoked potentials. Investigations in this area have continued to be the major focus of dipole modelling in clinical neurophysiology. (For details, see the reviews of Vaughan 1974, Wood 1982, and Fender 1987.)

SPIKE VOLTAGE TOPOGRAPHY AND EQUIVALENT DIPOLE LOCALIZATION IN EPILEPSY

In studies of epilepsy, dipole localization techniques have been used to analyse focal spikes, such as the centro-temporal spikes of benign rolandic epilepsy of childhood (BREC) and the temporal lobe spikes of complex partial epilepsy. These seemed reasonable targets for early investigation, because the spike sources are more likely to be discrete and thus more modellable as a dipole than less localized forms of epileptiform discharge.

Benign rolandic epilepsy of childhood

In a review of EEGs from nearly 5000 children, Gregory & Wong (1990) noted that rolandic spikes were recorded in over 400 cases. These spikes could be divided into two major categories in terms of voltage topography. A classical 'horizontal dipole' distribution, i.e. with the negative maximum in the centro-temporal area and a concurrent positive maximum bifrontally, was observed in those patients with 'typical' BREC (Gregory & Wong 1984, 1990; Wong & Gregory 1988). These patients had few neurological deficits, were of normal intelligence, and were likely to have their seizures remit. A non-dipolar or complex voltage field characterized the spikes of another group of patients who were diagnosed as having 'atypical' BREC. They showed significantly more abnormality in motor and speech development and in school performance, and they usually had neurological abnormalities (Gregory & Wong 1985, 1990). Using only spatial characteristics of rolandic interictal spike foci analysed by a classification and regression trees (CART) strategy, these investigators were able to classify nearly 80% of patients correctly into one of the two clinical categories (Wong et al 1988).

In addition, spike data from these patients were submitted to dipole analysis using a single homogeneous sphere model with sequential instantaneous inverse solutions (Wong & Weinberg 1986). Equivalent dipoles for patients with typical BREC were localized to a cortical region just lateral to the C3 or C4 electrode sites within an area encompassing half an interelectrode distance. The consistency of equivalent dipoles over the course of the spike complex has also been examined (Wong 1990). A 'stability index' which quantified the fluctuations of source parameters (location, orientation and magnitude) was devised. Patients with typical BREC and spikes with dipolar fields tended to have more stable dipole solutions in general. Also, epochs of consistent dipole localization were observed in this group for a longer period of time after the primary spike, which often included later components of the spike complex waveform.

The physiological bases of these two different types of rolandic spikes are not known. One can speculate that the stable, dipolar BREC spikes arise from a consistent sequence of activation in discrete rolandic cortical areas, while perhaps the unstable and often complex atypical BREC spikes may reflect multifocal dysfunction with inconsistent spike-to-spike activation sequences across a broader area of cortex.

Complex partial epilepsy

We have applied similar quantitative EEG techniques to the study of interictal spikes in patients with complex partial seizures (Ebersole & Wade 1989a, 1989b, 1990a, 1990b, 1991, Wade & Ebersole 1989). Long-term EEG monitoring was usually necessary to record sufficient numbers of spikes on tape for off-line analysis. Individual spikes were visually identified on a video replay of the EEG. Voltage values from 19 electrode sites at 5-ms intervals were displayed concurrently as colour-coded topographic maps in order to assess the field of each spike. A mastoid electrode contralateral to the spike focus served as reference. Spikes were categorized according to their pattern of voltage topography and computer averaged within category in sums of 8–32. Bilateral, dependent discharges were not included in the analysis.

An expected mix of spike locations were observed despite the clinical categorization of these patients into one seizure type. Fifty spike foci of different location were recorded from 45 patients (Ebersole & Wade 1990b). The distribution of foci, determined by the electrode registering the negative spike maximum, was as follows: 24 (48%) frontal–temporal (F7, F8, F7–T3, F8–T4), 12 (24%) mid- to posterior temporal (T3–T5, T4–T6), 7 (14%) fronto–polar (FP1, FP2), 3 (6%) frontal (F3, F4), 4 (8%) occipital (O1, O2). The most common subcategory of spikes, fronto–temporal, has been subject to the most analysis to date.

Because equivalent dipole localization is a mathematical extension of voltage topography, the potential fields of temporal spikes first needed to be defined. Two patterns were observed repeatedly in the EEG of these patients. We arbitrarily designated them as Type 1 and Type 2 (Fig. 4.2). Attributes of Type 1 spike topography included negative fields that were sharply defined, had steep voltage gradients, were located inferolaterally, and were associated with distinct, contralateral positive fields in our recording arrangement. The addition of supplementary inferior temporal electrodes (F9, C9, M1 or F10, C10, M2), which were incorporated into

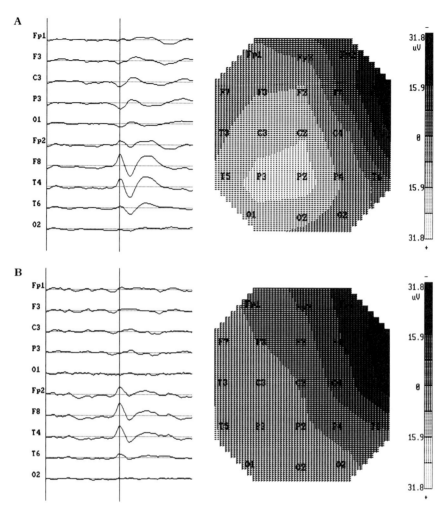

Fig. 4.2   Topographic representation of the scalp voltage field at the peak of averaged ($n = 8$): **A** right fronto–temporal spikes of Type 1 and **B** Type 2. An eight-level voltage scale (-32 to $+32\,\mu V$, dark to light) is shown on the right. EEG traces from selected electrodes are shown at left (1.28 s, common M1 reference, negative up). Cursor denotes time of the voltage map.

a laterally shifted, oblique topographic montage, provided a better view of the negative spike fields. Spikes with such a 'dipolar' field were the predominant type in the majority of patients with anterior temporal, mid-posterior temporal and occipital foci (54%, 62% and 60%, respectively). No patients with fronto–polar or frontal foci exhibited Type 1 spikes.

With Type 1 spikes, positive maxima were almost exclusively located in the hemisphere opposite that of negative maxima, and they usually occupied a parietal or fronto–central position. Negative and positive spike fields evolved in close temporal association, although in some patients one might lead or lag the other by 5–20 ms. Often the area of the positive field was larger than that of the negative field, and typically the voltage gradient across the positive field was more gradual. Although positive spike potentials could often be seen, on close examination of the raw EEG, at least in retrospect, the spike averaging process as well as the topographic display made them more evident.

Attributes of Type 2 spike topography included broad negative fields that extended to or beyond the midline, gradual voltage gradients, and less clear or no associated positive field. Only Type 2 spikes were seen in patients with fronto–polar and frontal foci. These spikes were also recorded from foci in other locations but less often than those of Type 1. It was possible to identify individual examples of both types of spikes by carefully searching the EEG in most patients, but there was usually a disproportionate (>80%) number of spikes corresponding to one topographic pattern. However, four patients had a nearly equal number of Type 1 and Type 2 spikes recorded from the same scalp region.

The characteristics which most distinguished the fields of Type 1 and 2 spikes, namely voltage gradients and dipolar pattern, were not dependent upon the choice of reference. We usually used a contralateral mastoid, because it was a distant site that was less likely to be active in the unilateral discharges we chose for analysis. Recalculating the spike fields to other reference electrodes or to an average reference only changed the absolute voltage values; the contours of the topographic landscape remained the same. Similarly, differences between the two spike types remained apparent after submitting the data to the 'source derivation' of Hjorth (1980).

Spike averages were also used as raw data for dipole localization. For single dipole modelling (three shells), instantaneous six-parameter solutions were obtained using a standard, least-squares minimization approach (Bio-Logic Dipole 1.3). We first examined the sources calculated for times around the peak of the primary spike component and specifically addressed the question of differentiating between patients with Type 1 and Type 2 fronto–temporal spike foci (Wade & Ebersole 1989, Ebersole & Wade 1990b).

In general, equivalent dipoles have been located in positions that are anatomically reasonable, i.e. within the brain lobe underlying the negative maxima. Incorporating data from inferior temporal electrodes, which contained a better representation of the negative field of temporal spikes, produced results that were more stable across the spike peak and appeared more plausible anatomically. Location (X, Y, Z) and orientation (azimuth, elevation) parameters of equivalent dipoles for Type 1 versus Type 2 spikes were compared across fronto–temporal foci from 24 patients. Dipole vector elevation was the only parameter mean that differed significantly in Type 1 versus Type 2 spikes (Fig. 4.3). Although there was variation from case to case, source locations were not statistically different between the two groups of patients. In nearly all cases, location of the equivalent dipoles, when transcribed to a standard brain atlas (Talairach & Tournoux 1988),

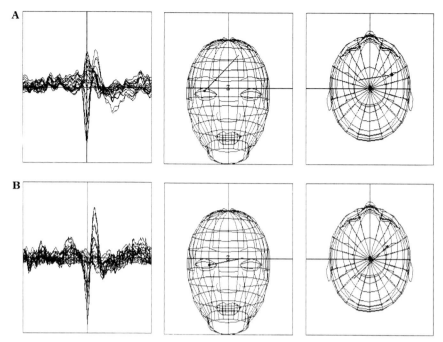

Fig. 4.3   Equivalent single dipoles calculated at the peak of averaged **A** Type 1 and **B** Type 2 fronto–temporal spikes. Source location is the dot at the beginning of the vector, which conveys orientation and magnitude parameters. Superimposed traces (21 channels) of the averaged spikes from which inverse solutions were obtained are shown at left. Cursor denotes time of dipole calculation. Note similar source location, but elevation of dipole vector, in Type 1 as compared to Type 2 spike.

appeared to be within a region approximating the temporal lobe (see Fig. 4.1). Calculated sources were usually deeper than the level of the temporal cortex, however.

INTERPRETATION OF SINGLE DIPOLE MODELS

It should not be surprising that equivalent dipoles are located deep to the cortex that is likely to be involved, because the solution is for a non-realistic point source. In general, dipole localization techniques are least accurate in depth determinations, because this estimation depends upon the size of the generator region. Single dipole solutions provide a reasonable approximation for superficial cortical sources if their diameter is smaller than 2 cm (Fender 1987, Scherg 1989). Activation of a larger area of cortex would produce a more diffuse scalp field that would model as a deeper equivalent dipole.

Additional anatomical considerations are also useful in trying to determine spike sources. Activation of both sides of a sulcus simultaneously would cause cancellation of the two opposing tangential fields, and only the radial component from the sulcus bottom would be evident. Because scalp-recordable EEG spikes probably require the activation of several square centimetres of cortex (Cooper et al 1969), tangential fields will often cancel one another allowing radial components to predominate. A simplification that is useful in field interpretation and dipole modelling is to treat scalp spike fields as if they arose principally from sources that are radial to the major outline of brain lobes. Both the temporal and frontal lobes have inferior as well as lateral surfaces. Therefore, fields tangential to the scalp can be generated even if individual sulci are disregarded.

When these ideas are incorporated into the interpretation of equivalent dipoles, one can conclude that the differences in source orientation for the two spike types does help to identify the involved brain regions. Extension of dipole vectors to intersect cortex lying more superficially would seem a reasonable approach toward achieving a better approximation of generator regions because it is likely that any location error is one of being too deep. This correction of the modelling would suggest that Type 2 spikes, with fields having a radial character, are generated from lateral temporal cortex, whereas Type 1 spikes, with dipolar fields suggesting a more tangential source, arise from inferior temporal cortex (see Fig. 4.1).

MULTIPLE DIPOLE MODELLING – BASIC CONSIDERATIONS

Although it is best to model a spike field first as a single dipole source, the question inevitably arises as to whether the generating neuronal aggregate is so dispersed or complex in structure that several dipoles will be needed to approximate it accurately. Techniques for multiple dipole localization are available; however, the added promise brings with it a new array of limitations, problems and traps for the unwary.

In order to define each dipole source, six parameters are required: three of location (X, Y, Z), two of orientation (elevation, azimuth) and one of magnitude. In a noise-free environment, at least one independent measurement is needed to determine each parameter. This means recording from at least six electrodes for each dipole in a source solution. However, clinical recordings are seldom noise free, and electrode placements are usually not where a given parameter can be determined best. Therefore, Fender (1987) has recommended that a safety factor of two be applied to electrode numbers. If, then, 12 electrodes are needed for each dipole, the 19–21 standard international 10–20 sites would barely suffice to characterize a two-dipole spike model. More electrodes would be better, but too many is not good either, because electrodes that are too close no longer provide independent measurements and noise becomes correlated among them. Fender (1987) has estimated that 40 electrodes equally spaced on the head would be an optimum number for source localization.

Solutions for the inverse problem become dramatically more numerous and therefore possibly misleading in the case of multiple dipoles. Because the measured voltage field is the sum of all contributing sources (again the principle of linear superposition), there are a multitude of two-dipole configurations that can produce the same field. Constraints need to be imposed to reduce the number of mathematical possibilities to a smaller manageable subset. The more restrictions that can be applied, the more likely that a reasonable solution can be found. This principle applies to single-dipole modelling as well, but it is essential for multiple-dipole efforts. The most straightforward constraints are biological. Dipole localization methods are physical ones that ignore anatomy and physiology. It it thus up to the investigator to use his medical knowledge to reduce possible solutions and to choose among those that are equally good mathematically.

A solution with two or more dipoles should be sought when a simpler model does not adequately explain the spike field mathematically or, as is more often the case, when there are other features in the data that suggest more than one source. A good mathematical fit can only be achieved with clean data; the dipole localization programme will otherwise attempt to model noise as well as the signal. A low signal-to-noise ratio will result in a high unexplained residual variance between the model and the data regardless of how accurate the model is.

A source that is well simulated by a single dipole should produce a field that varies over time only in intensity and polarity (Wood & Wolpaw 1982, Achim et al 1988). The brain does not move; therefore, an equivalent dipole for a spike from a discrete region also should not move. Changes in activity at the generator site will cause the scalp field to wax and wane in amplitude, and perhaps alternate in polarity, but apparent movement of a scalp field or asymmetrical changes in its shape means that other areas of brain are sequentially activated. In such a situation, more than one dipole may be needed to explain the spike field.

Similarly, all parts of a scalp field should evolve synchronously if there is only one source. This is particularly applicable to tangential fields where both negative and positive maxima are recorded. Both should peak simultaneously if they are generated by opposite ends of the same dipole. If one field leads or lags the other or changes shape independently of the other, more than one source is contributing to the field and a single-dipole model is no longer adequate.

MOVING DIPOLE ANALYSIS OF SPIKE FIELDS

Spatial analysis of spike fields over time can be performed by using the 'cartooning' feature of most topographic EEG instruments. Sequential instantaneous voltage maps are presented in rapid fashion to form a moving picture of the evolution of spike fields. Forty to 60 maps may be required to portray the dynamics of an entire spike complex when EEG sampling is done every 5 ms. However, the topographic voltage data within one instantaneous map can be synthesized into one equivalent dipole. The

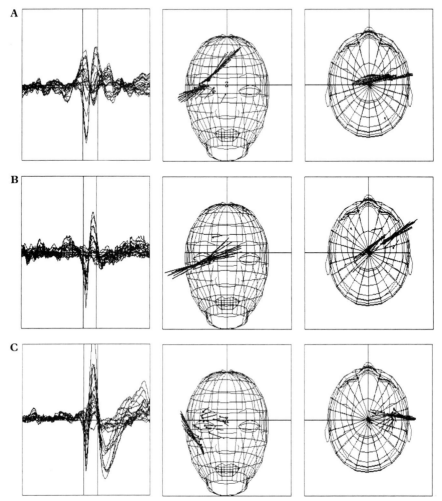

Fig. 4.4 Sequential, moving dipole solutions (instantaneous) during the spike and subsequent positive transient components of **A** a Type 1 and **B**, **C** two different Type 2 spike complexes. Note the consistency of sequential equivalent dipoles for each spike component, the closeness of the source locations for each component group, and their nearly opposite orientations in the top two examples. Sequential dipoles for **C** are unstable in position and orientation or unrealistic in location.

information in a series of maps can be reduced to one image which shows sequential instantaneous dipoles calculated for each time point. Considerable data compression is thus another advantage of dipole modelling. Any spatial instability of spike fields should be reflected as position and orientation variability in this 'moving dipole'.

When Type 1 spikes from patients in the present series were analysed in this fashion, stability in sequential dipole solutions for both the spike and the after-coming positive transient was uniformly evident (Fig. 4.4).

According to this test, multiple-dipole solutions would not be required. An analysis of Type 2 spikes showed marked variability among patients. Although two-thirds possessed stable dipole solutions for each spike component, the remaining third showed considerable instability (Fig. 4.4). Dipole location drift and vector rotation were evident during both waveforms, which suggested that a single-source model of the data was inadequate.

Noteworthy, but not as yet fully explained, was the unequal proportion of stable spike dipoles from different head regions. Essentially all the Type 2 foci in frontal, mid-posterior temporal and occipital areas were of the stable variety, whereas one-third of the fronto–temporal and nearly all of the fronto–polar equivalent dipoles were unstable. If this instability is related to multiple underlying generators, as we believe it is, our data suggest that multifocal cortical dysfunction is more common in these latter sites.

Sequential dipole analysis is less good than voltage map or simple waveform review, however, at discriminating field asynchrony. The evolution of negative and positive fields of Type 1 spikes was not synchronous in the majority of patients. Contralateral positive fields typically led or lagged the negative field to its peak by 5–15 ms. Despite apparently stable single-dipole solutions, temporal analysis demanded that Type 1 spikes be modelled with more than one source (Ebersole & Wade 1990a).

TWO-DIPOLE MODELLING OF TEMPORAL SPIKES

When we began to submit spike averages to two-dipole source modelling, it quickly became apparent that many instantaneous inverse solutions, although mathematically having low residual variance, were completely unrealistic in terms of anatomy and physiology. It was necessary to restrict the solution possibilities substantially. Such constraints are featured in a spatiotemporal technique called 'dipole source potential analysis'. This approach has been championed by Scherg and von Cramon, who have done considerable work in extracting multiple sources from evoked potentials (Scherg & von Cramon 1985a, 1985b, 1986, Scherg 1989). In essence, their method differs from instantaneous source solutions by postulating that dipoles, while fixed in location and orientation, vary in strength and polarity over time. Dipole fitting is based on an epoch of time, for example an entire spike complex or one of its components, and not just on one time point. Multiple temporal samples plus the fixed nature of the equivalent dipoles provide additional degrees of freedom for the calculations so that theoretically more than two dipoles can be extracted from standard 19-channel EEG data.

Fundamental to this approach is determining the source potential for each dipole in addition to its location. These source potentials (the activity of each generator expressed as a waveform) are obtained by a modification

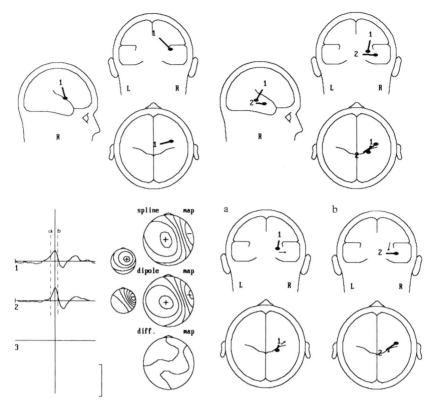

Fig. 4.5   One- and two-dipole models of a Type 1 spike (with a positive field lead) are shown at the top of the figure. The single equivalent dipole (top left) was calculated at the spike peak, whereas the two-dipole model (top right) was a spatiotemporal solution for a 100-ms epoch encompassing the spike. Source potentials for the two-dipole model are shown (bottom left) along with scalp voltage maps of the spike (spline), the two-dipole model (dipole), their difference (diff.), and each component dipole. Note in the source potentials that activity begins earlier in the mesial dipole (1). Dipole magnitude at cursor position 'a' is depicted in head model 'a' (bottom right). Both sources are active during the spike peak. Activity persists longer in lateral dipole (2). Dipole magnitude at cursor position 'b' is depicted in head model 'b' (bottom right).

of principal component analysis (Glaser & Ruchkin 1976) in which the restriction of orthogonality is not maintained. In deriving both the location and activity of putative sources, one can obtain the scalp voltage fields theoretically contributed by each dipole. Inspecting these fields can be very helpful in estimating the validity of a solution.

A particular advantage of a spatiotemporal modelling approach is the possibility of extracting sources whose activity overlap in time but are not entirely synchronous (Scherg & von Cramon 1986, Achim et al 1988). A clinically pertinent example would be a spike which originates in one brain region, propagates, and recruits another region. The ability to differentiate an original spike (one source) from a propagated spike (two sequential sources) would have definite utility.

This tactic has been used to analyse Type 1 spikes that show an asynchrony between negative and positive fields. Single equivalent dipoles can be obtained separately for those epochs during the spike complex in which one field is more prominent than the other. Modelling the interaction of these two sources over the course of the spike complex entails a gradual release of constraints on parameters of each dipole to obtain an optimal combined fit.

Figure 4.5 shows two equivalent sources obtained in this manner (BESA version 1.3) from a Type 1 frontal–temporal spike. Note that one dipole is more mesial and has an orientation that is vertex directed. Maps of the scalp voltage that would be generated by this source show a positive field near the midline. The second dipole is more lateral and has a nearly horizontal orientation. It would generate a lateral negative field during the spike. The theorized source potentials for each show that the mesial dipole is activated first and the lateral one later. The sum of fields produced by both dipoles approximates very closely the voltage topography of the Type 1 spike.

The residual variance of this two-dipole model is less than that of the best single-dipole model. This is not, however, the best mathematical solution that can be obtained. A better fit can be found by modelling with fewer constraints on dipole parameters, but the resultant equivalent dipole pairs are anatomically unrealistic. The illustrated solutions, on the other hand, make sense. Each dipole is orthogonal to a specific region of temporal cortex. If the source locations have a depth inaccuracy, as already discussed, the mesial dipole could represent a spike origin in the inferior mesial temporal cortex and the lateral dipole could represent a recruitment of lateral temporal cortex.

Similar analyses of Type 1 spikes with a positive field lag yielded a two-dipole model in which a lateral cortex source preceded a mesial source, suggesting propagation in the opposite direction. Type 2 spikes with stable fields could not be modelled better by two equivalent dipoles than by one. Satisfactory modelling of unstable Type 2 spike foci proved to be the most difficult to achieve. One-dipole solutions had high residual variances. In several instances of believable two-dipole solutions, the sources approximated different areas of lateral temporal or frontal cortex.

FORWARD DIPOLE MODELLING OF SPIKES

A completely hypothesis-driven approach to dipole localization can also be taken. Forward dipole modelling can determine how well source configurations, postulated by the investigator, fit the actual data. This technique is particularly useful when the goal is simply to discriminate between two or more source possibilities.

For example, one could develop a priori dipole models for fronto–temporal spikes with characteristics specific for certain source locations: inferior temporal, lateral temporal, temporal pole and frontal opercular cortex. By consulting a brain atlas or the patient's MRI, appropriate dipole location coordinates and orientations could be obtained. Having derived a set of dipole parameters for each hypothesis, the calculation of a forward solution would describe the scalp field generated by the test dipole(s) and determine the residual variance with the actual data. A dipole model with a distinctly better fit supports its associated hypothesis. New patient data could be screened quickly by a set of such models. In this case, classification of spikes into groups is the goal, not accuracy of dipole location. For some clinical work, differentiation rather than precise localization may be all that is necessary.

DIPOLE VALIDATION FROM SCALP AND INTRACRANIAL EEG

Although many equivalent dipoles appear to be reasonable explanations of recorded spike topography, validity can be sought from correlations with additional electrographic data. New scalp EEG evidence from the small group of patients who had a nearly equal number of Type 1 and 2 spikes from the same region lends credence to several hypotheses that arose from dipole modelling (Ebersole & Wade 1990a). If Type 2 spikes comes from sources on the lateral cortex convexity, and Type 1 spikes involve additional sources, subtracting a Type 2 spike from a Type 1 in the same patient should yield the field of the other source(s). When this was done, the remainder in all cases was a simple positive field with a maximum near the midline between FZ and PZ, which was remarkably similar to the scalp field of the more mesial source predicted by two-dipole analysis (see Fig. 4.5). That this positive spike potential was not merely a mathematical creation was confirmed by finding actual examples in a review of the raw EEGs of these patients.

Most convincing, however, has been the support given by intracranial electrode recordings in 8 of the 24 patients with fronto–temporal spikes (Ebersole & Wade 1989b, 1990a, 1991). Four patients had Type 1 spike foci and four had Type 2 foci. Consistent seizure onsets from mesial temporal structures were recorded in three patients, all of whom had Type 1 spike foci. Active spiking from the hippocampus and pre-hippocampus area was also observed in patients with Type 1 spike foci. These infero-mesial temporal spikes were frequently coupled temporally with more lateral cortical spikes that were recorded from both subdural and scalp electrodes.

Onset of seizures in three patients with Type 2 foci was localized to non-mesial or extratemporal regions. Hippocampal interictal spiking was less prominent, and often the potentials had the appearance of sharp waves. Scalp spikes that reflected independent discharges from lateral temporal and extratemporal cortex was a distinctive feature in patients with Type

2 spike foci. The remaining patient with Type 1 scalp spikes had seizures originating from both mesial and non-mesial temporal regions, and the other patient with Type 2 spikes had seizure onsets that were non-localizable.

Additional support for the proposed two-dipole origin of Type 1 spikes was obtained recently from intracranial recordings from a patient whose scalp EEG showed both Type 1 and positive midline spikes. Cross-averaging multiple intracranial sites to the positive scalp spike revealed synchronous activity only from the inferomesial temporal region. Typical Type 1 spikes were associated with inferomesial and lateral temporal discharge.

MAGNETOENCEPHALOGRAPHY (MEG) AND EEG DIPOLE LOCALIZATION

Although beyond the scope of this review, efforts to develop MEG into a useful tool for the evaluation of partial epilepsy deserve mention, because they parallel closely the EEG analyses discussed here (Barth et al 1984, Sato & Smith 1985, Rose et al 1987, Ricci et al 1987, Sutherling et al 1988, 1989). MEG measures extracranial magnetic fields produced mainly by intracellular electrical brain currents. These small magnetic fields are detected by a superconducting quantum interference device (SQUID), which is set perpendicular to the head. It 'sees' primarily magnetic fields coming out or going into the head, which are created by tangentially oriented dipoles.

MEG possesses certain theoretical advantages over EEG, namely that the scalp and skull are transparent to it. Thus, distortion of voltage fields by scalp and skull are not present, nor do they need to be taken into account for source modelling purposes. However, the procedure is technically more difficult, time consuming, and unavailable to most patients. Additionally, the devices are extremely expensive which likely further limits widespread use.

Source localization techniques are also used to analyse MEG data. In fact, dipole modelling of MEG interictal spikes preceded similar EEG analyses. Both iterative 'least-squares' approximations and more simple calculations based on the separation of the maxima have been used to estimate source locations (Sutherling et al 1988). Several investigators have compared MEG localization of spike foci to that obtained by intracranial EEG (Rose et al 1987, Ricci et al 1987, Sutherling et al 1988), and the results have been comparable. The ability of MEG to define deep epileptic foci, such as those in the mesial temporal region, is still controversial (Rose et al 1987, Sutherling et al 1989), but spike propagation has been demonstrated between magnetic sources localized to inferior and lateral temporal cortex (Sutherling et al 1989).

EEG and MEG dipole localization of spikes have not been systematically compared in the same patients. However, in a recent study of artificial dipoles created by stimulation through depth electrodes, EEG and MEG source solutions were nearly comparable (Cohen et al 1990). The average localization error for MEG was larger than expected (8 mm), while that for EEG was better than expected (10 mm), based upon theoretical considerations and previous data (Smith et al 1985).

Most investigators believe that MEG and EEG are complementary in terms of characterizing current dipoles such as a spike focus. The special sensitivity of MEG to tangential and not radial sources can clarify ambiguities in EEG fields and identify the more likely of competing hypotheses. However, given EEG's ability to record both radial and tangential fields simultaneously from many channels over both hemispheres, and given the ease with which it is performed, it is reasonable to begin any quest for intracerebral spike generators with EEG voltage topography and dipole localization.

FUTURE OF DIPOLE MODELLING IN EPILEPSY

The future appears bright for EEG voltage topography and dipole localization. The application of these techniques to the evaluation of epilepsy is only in its infancy. Already multiple directions for further investigation are apparent, and a host of ideas for improving data acquisition and analysis are being developed.

To take full advantage of the power of these techniques, spatial sampling of the EEG will need to be increased from the customary 19–21 scalp electrodes to 32–40. Likewise, temporal sampling rates should be increased from the present EEG monitoring standard of 200 Hz to 400–800 Hz or more. The former will provide a more accurate description of spike fields to be modelled; the latter will allow easier extraction of multiple sources whose activity is only slightly asynchronous.

More sophisticated, multiple-dipole models with a variety of modifiable constraints will by necessity be developed. Anatomical realism will be increasingly incorporated into source localization programmes. The spherical head of homogeneous material will be replaced by realistically shaped models containing pertinent brain anatomy. MRI data from an individual patient will be incorporated into head/brain models used with that patient's data. The location and orientation of all cortical areas will be specifiable, and source solutions will be restricted to those configurations that are anatomically correct.

Dipole modelling of extended, rather than point, sources will be increasingly utilized. Source depth versus source size/shape equivalences will be available so that a solution can be tailored to the cortical anatomy in the region of an equivalent dipole. Increased accuracy might also be achieved by adding intracranial data to the scalp EEG. Correction factors to take into consideration the location and recording characteristics of the intracranial electrodes will need to be developed.

Intracranial EEG data will also be increasingly analysed by a combination of quantitative techniques. Subdural grid recordings, in which there are often multiple interacting radial and tangential sources, are particularly difficult to interpret by visual inspection. Voltage topography and dipole modelling will prove to be very useful.

EEG source localization will also be applied to a broadening range of electrographic phenomena. Among the more important are seizures. Types or stages of seizures in which the rhythms are composed of distinct potentials may be amenable to traditional dipole analysis. Waveforms early in an ictal discharge may be generated by sources discrete enough to be modelled as one or more dipoles, whereas potentials late in a seizure are probably too diffuse. In some cases, seizure propagation may be approachable by these techniques. Early investigations have already shown that a modification of dipole localization methodology that accepts spectral rather than voltage data can characterize the source of EEG rhythms, instead of transients (Lehmann & Michel 1990).

CONCLUSION

The era of descriptive EEG is ending. We can no longer afford simply to use pattern recognition as the exclusive basis of analysis. An untapped wealth of information is contained in these bioelectric signals. Voltage topography and source modelling are two new techniques available to the clinical investigator to mine these riches, both for the benefit of patients and for science.

What really can be expected of these techniques, in terms of clinical utility, is an important question. It is true that the validity and accuracy of source localization depends upon the degree ot which dipole models can depict reality. However, even if localization is imprecise, dipole modelling may have considerable use if the technique can discriminate among clinically important categories of disease.

Improved pre-surgical evaluation of patients with medically uncontrolled focal epilepsy will probably be the most immediate benefit provided by these new methods of EEG analysis. Spike voltage topography and source localization will add significantly to other non-invasive measures. More patients will be able to have surgery without intracranial monitoring, and those patients who still require it will be more accurately identified.

REFERENCES

Achim A, Richer F, Saint-Hilaire J M 1988 Methods for separating temporally overlapping sources of neuro-electric data. Brain Topography 1: 22–28
Ajmone-Marsan C 1990 Chronic intracranial recording and electrocorticography. In: Daly D D, Pedley T A (eds) Current practice of clinical electroencephalography, 2nd edn. Raven Press, New York, pp 535–560
Ary J P, Klein S A, Fender D H 1981 Location of sources of evoked scalp potentials: corrections for skull and scalp thicknesses. IEEE Trans Biomed Eng 28: 447–452
Barth D S, Sutherling W, Engel J, Beatty J 1984 Neuromagnetic evidence of spatially

distributed sources underlying epileptiform spikes in the human brain. Science 223: 293–296

Brazier M A B 1949 The electrical fields at the surface of the head during sleep. Electroencephalogr Clin Neurophysiol 1: 195–204

Brody D A, Terry F H, Ideker R E 1973 Eccentric dipole in a spherical medium: generalized expression for surface potentials. IEEE Trans Biomed Eng 20: 141–143

Cohen D, Cuffin B N et al 1990 MEG versus EEG localization test using implanted sources in the human brain. Ann Neurol 28: 811–817

Cooper R, Winter A L, Crow H J, Walter W G 1969 Comparison of subcortical, cortical, and scalp activity using chronically indwelling electrodes in man. Electroencephalogr Clin Neurophysiol 18: 217–228

Cuffin B N, Cohen D et al 1991 Tests of EEG localization accuracy using implanted sources in the human brain. Ann Neurol 29: 132–138

Darcey T M, Ary J P, Fender D H 1980 Methods for the localization of electrical sources in the human brain. In: Kornhuber H H, Deecke L (eds) Motivation, motor, and sensory processes of the brain: progress in brain research. Elsevier, Amsterdam, pp 128–134

Ebersole J S, Chatt A B 1984 Laminar interactions during neocortical epileptogenesis. Brain Res 298: 253–271

Ebersole J S, Wade P B 1989a Intracranial EEG validation of spike topography and dipole modelling in the presurgical localization of epileptic foci. Epilepsia 30: 696

Ebersole J S, Wade P B 1989b Temporal spikes are not all the same: a topographic EEG analysis in surgical candidates. Neurology 39 (Suppl 1): 299

Ebersole J S, Wade P B 1990a Spike voltage topography and equivalent dipole localization in complex partial epilepsy. Brain Topography 3: 21–34

Ebersole J S, Wade P B 1990b Intracranial EEG validation of single versus dual dipolar sources for temporal spikes in presurgical candidates. Epilepsia 31: 621

Ebersole J S, Wade P B 1991 Spike voltage topography identifies two types of fronto-temporal epileptic foci. Neurology (in press)

Fender D H 1987 Source localization of brain electrical activity. In: Gevins A S, Remond A (eds) Methods of analysis of brain electrical and magnetic signals. Elsevier, Amsterdam, pp 355–403

Geisler C D, Gerstein G L 1961 The surface EEG in relation to its sources. Electroencephalogr Clin Neurophysiol 13: 927–934

Glaser E M, Ruchkin D S 1976 Principles of neurobiological signals analysis. Academic Press, New York

Gregory D L, Wong P K H 1984 Topographical analysis of the centrotemporal discharges in benign rolandic epilepsy of childhood. Epilepsia 25: 705–711

Gregory D, Wong P K H 1985 Centrotemporal spike focus: the clinical signficance of a dipole field. Electroencephalogr Clin Neurophysiol 61: S183

Gregory D, Wong P K H 1990 The clinical relevance of a dipole field in rolandic spikes. Epilepsia 31: 621–622

Helmholtz H 1853 Uber einige Gesetze der Vertheilung elektrischer Strome in korperlichen Leitern, mit Anwendung auf die thierischelektrischen Versuche. Ann Phys Chem 29: 211–233, 353–377

Henderson C J, Butler S R, Glass A 1975 The localization of equivalent dipoles of EEG sources by the application of electrical field theory. Electroencephalogr Clin Neurophysiol 39: 117–130

Hjorth B 1980 Source derivation simplifies topographical EEG interpretation. Am J EEG Tech 20: 121–132

Kavanagh R N, Darcey T M, Lehmann D, Fender D H 1978 Evaluation of methods for three-dimensional localization of electrical sources in the human brain. IEEE Trans Biomed Eng BME 25: 421–429

Lehmann D, Michel C M 1989 Intracerebral dipole sources of EEG FFT power maps. Brain Topography 2: 155–164

Maier J, Dagnelie H, Spekreijse H, van Dijk B W 1987 Principle components analysis for source localization of VEPs in man. Vision Res 27: 165–177

Marquardt D W 1963 An algorithm of least-squares estimation of non-linear parameters. J Soc Industr Appl Math 11: 431–441

Nunez P L 1981 Electrical fields of the brain. Oxford University Press, New York

O'Neill R 1971 Function minimization using a simplex method. Appl Statist 20: 338–345

Ricci G B, Romani G L, Salustri C et al 1987 Study of focal epilepsy by multichannel neuromagnetic measurements. Electroencephalogr Clin Neurophysiol 66: 457–466

Rose D F, Sato S, Smith P D et al 1987 Localization of magnetic interictal discharges in temporal lobe epilepsy. Ann Neurol 22: 348–354

Rush S, Driscoll D A 1968 Current distribution in the brain from surface electrodes. Anaesth Analgesia Current Res 47: 717–723

Sato S, Smith P D 1985 Magnetoencephalography. J Clin Neurophysiol 2: 173–192

Scherg M 1989 Fundamentals of dipole source potential analysis. In: Hoke M, Grandori F, Romani G L (eds) Auditory evoked magnetic fields and potentials: advances in audiology. Karger, Basel, pp 40–69

Scherg M, von Cramon D 1985a Two bilateral sources of the late AEP as identified by a spatio-temporal dipole model. Electroencephalogr Clin Neurophysiol 62: 32–44

Scherg M, von Cramon D 1985b A new interpretation of the generators of BAEP waves I–V: results of a spatio-temporal dipole model. Electroencephalogr Clin Neurophysiol 62: 290–299

Scherg M, von Cramon D 1986 Evoked dipole source potentials of the human auditory cortex. Electroencephalogr Clin Neurophysiol 65: 344–360

Schneider M R 1972 A multistage process for computing virtual dipolar sources of EEG discharges from surface information. IEEE Trans Biomed Eng BME 19: 1–12

Shaw J C, Roth M 1955a Potential distribution analysis. II. A theoretical consideration of its significance in terms of electric field theory. Electroencephalogr Clin Neurophysiol 7: 285–292

Shaw J C, Roth M 1955b Potential distribution analysis. I. A new technique for the analysis of electrophysiological phenomena. Electroencephalogr Clin Neurophysiol 7: 273–284

Sidman R D, Giambalvo V, Allison T, Bergey P 1978 A method for localization of sources of human cerebral potentials evoked by sensory stimuli. Sens Processes 2: 116–129

Smith D B, Sidman R D, Flanigin H, Henke J, Labiner D 1985 A reliable method for localizing deep intracranial sources of the EEG. Neurology 35: 1702–1707

Sutherling W W, Barth D S 1989 Neocortical propagation in temporal lobe spike foci on magnetoencephalography and electroencephalography. Ann Neurol 25: 373–381

Sutherling W W, Crandall P H, Cahan L D, Barth D S 1988 The magnetic field of epileptic spikes agrees with intracranial localizations in complex partial epilepsy. Neurology 38: 778–786

Talairach J, Tournoux P 1988 Co-planar stereotaxic atlas of the human brain. Thieme, New York

Vaughan H G 1974 The analysis of scalp-recorded brain potentials. In: Thompson R F, Patterson M M (eds) Bioelectric recording techniques: B. Electroencephalography and human brain potentials. Academic Press, New York, pp 157–207

Wade P B, Ebersole J S 1989 Spike voltage topography and equivalent dipole localization: new noninvasive adjuncts to presurgical evaluation in complex partial epilepsy. Epilepsia 30: 696

Wilson F N, Bayley R H 1950 The electric field of an eccentric dipole in a homogeneous spherical conducting medium. Circulation 1: 84–92

Wong P K H 1989 Stability of source estimates in rolandic spikes. Brain Topography 2: 31–36

Wong P K H, Gregory D 1988 Dipole fields in rolandic discharges. Am J EEG Technol 28: 243–250

Wong P K H, Weinberg H 1986 Source estimation of scalp EEG focus. In: Pfurtscheller G, Lopes da Silva F (eds) Functional brain imaging. Hans Huber, Toronto, pp 89–95

Wong P K H, Gregory D, Farrell K 1985 Comparison of spike topography in typical and atypical benign rolandic epilepsy of childhood. Electroencephalogr Clin Neurophysiol 61: S47

Wong P K H, Bencivenga R, Gregory D 1988 Statistical classification of spikes in benign rolandic epilepsy. Brain Topography 1: 123–129

Wood C C 1982 Applications of dipole localization methods to source identification of human evoked potentials. Ann NY Acad Sci 388: 139–155

Wood C C, Wolpaw J R 1982 Scalp distribution of human auditory evoked potentials. II. Evidence for overlapping sources and involvement of auditory cortex. Electroencephalogr Clin Neurophysiol 54: 25–38

5

Automated detection and analysis of seizures and spikes in the EEG

J. Gotman

INTRODUCTION

When evaluating epileptic patients, documentation of ictal and interictal EEG patterns is often important, but this becomes essential when considering epilepsy surgery. Such documentation can be obtained with long-term monitoring during which the EEG and the patient's behaviour are observed and recorded continuously. Thus, all spikes and seizures are recorded and electroclinical correlations can be performed. In order to characterize a complicated seizure problem properly, which often involves multiple seizure types, it may be necessary to monitor a patient for two to three weeks. The simplest method is to record the EEG continuously on paper using a standard EEG machine and to observe the patient or record the patient's behaviour on videotape. The role of computer analysis during long-term monitoring, particularly using automatic detection methods, can be best understood by considering the pitfalls associated with this basic 'continuous paper–videotape' recording procedure:

1. Recording the EEG on paper during many days requires a large quantity of paper and ink. It also requires the presence of a full-time technologist, because a simple paper jam or ink problem could ruin a whole monitoring session. If only spikes and seizures are of interest, then 95–99% of the recording is not useful. I will discuss below whether computers can be programmed to detect this small fraction of interesting EEG and leave out uninteresting parts, thus solving a problem which has both economical and ecological implications.

2. The EEG recorded on paper cannot be manipulated after it has been recorded: gains, montages and filter settings cannot be altered. The EEG cannot be quantified with techniques such as spectral analysis or visualized as topographic maps. An advantage of computer-based automatic detection methods is that the EEG is recorded digitally and is thus immediately available for such manipulations.

3. Archiving represents a major difficulty when large amounts of paper are recorded. Automatic detection methods greatly reduce the amount of EEG that is recorded and thus facilitate archiving. The digitally recorded EEG can be archived on optical disc, providing easy access to archived data.

I will discuss the promise as well as the difficulties of automatic detection methods; the easy review and manipulations that are made possible by digital recording; and present techniques for analysing spike and seizure discharges. I will discuss the detection of spikes and seizures separately because the different patterns require different approaches to detection. Furthermore, missed detections have different implications in the two instances. On the other hand, detection of spike and seizure discharges share common problems: detection of both are difficult, and existing methods are far from perfect despite the large computing power of modern equipment. For more information, readers can also consult several reviews of automatic event detection in epilepsy and applications of computer methods to the analysis of the EEG in epilepsy that have been published in the last few years (Frost 1985, Gotman 1985a, 1985b, 1986, Ktonas 1987, Wieser 1987).

AUTOMATIC SEIZURE DETECTION

Although considerably more work has been done on spike detection, I will discuss seizure detection first because it is the more important in clinical practice. One might wonder what is the use of automatic seizure detection, because seizures are behavioural events that can be noted by an observer or the patient. In fact, however, patients are not aware of many of their seizures, and observers cannot be constantly watching every patient. So-called 'subclinical' seizures are also important in evaluation. Automatic seizure detection is thus helpful in detecting all seizures, whether or not associated with clinical manifestations. After presenting the methods and their performance, I will discuss the clinical context in which they are best implemented.

Seizure recognition from EEG data alone is a difficult problem, because seizures are primarily behavioural events and not electroencephalographic events of consistent and specific morphology. A large proportion of seizures have clear EEG accompaniments but some do not, or they have mild and non-specific changes (Ajmone Marsan 1984). The computer receives information only about the EEG, and therefore it is reasonable to expect it to detect only seizures having clear and unambiguous EEG features. Even with this caveat, the problem remains a difficult one because seizure activity can consist of a variety of morphologies. Unlike spikes, which have a relatively well-defined morphology, seizures can include patterns such as low-amplitude desynchronized activity; polyspike activity; rhythmic waves occurring with a wide range of frequencies; or spike and waves (Blume et al 1984). In extracranial recordings, seizures are often obscured by EMG, movement and eye-blink artefacts. From the perspective of signal processing, the problem is therefore complex. This may be one reason why so few publications deal with automatic seizure recognition, the one exception being detection of 3-s spike–wave bursts which is one of the few seizure patterns of well-defined morphology.

Methods of seizure detection

Prior et al (1973) described the use of a cerebral function monitor to identify generalized tonic–clonic seizures. These would be recognized on the monitor's record as a large increase followed by a major decrease in EEG voltage (the postictal depression) and by accompanying intense EMG activity. Lockard et al (1980) found that similar convulsive seizures with major changes could also be identified in monkeys with experimental epilepsy by a characteristic pattern on slow paper tracings (0.25 mm/s). Ives et al (1974) described a method in which 16 channels of EEG were added, bandpass filtered and subjected to amplitude discrimination. This technique detected widespread, intense seizure discharges but was otherwise quite insensitive. Babb et al (1974) implemented an electronic circuit for detecting seizures in recordings made from intracerebral electrodes. A seizure was recognized when a rapid succession of large-amplitude spikes, lasting at least 5 s, occurred. None of the above methods were formally evaluated.

Gotman (1982) presented a computer method which attempted to recognize a wide variety of seizure patterns. This method selected patterns that represented possible seizure activity for later definitive examination by traditional visual inspection. The method was therefore designed to be as sensitive as possible. False detections, as long as they were not extremely frequent, were not detrimental. Observation of numerous seizures led to the conclusion that most seizures, at some time during their development, included activity that was *paroxysmal* compared to the background (the paroxysm could consist of increased voltage or a sudden increase in frequency); *rhythmic* (with frequencies varying from 3 to 20 c/s); and relatively *sustained* in duration (lasting several seconds).

It was possible to obtain measurements of these characteristics by first breaking down the EEG into half-waves (Gotman & Gloor 1976) and then measuring, for each 2-s epoch, the average amplitude of the half-waves relative to that of the background (indicating whether an epoch was paroxysmal); the average duration of the half-waves (indicating frequency); and the coefficient of variation of half-wave duration (indicating the regularity of duration, or rhythmicity). The background was defined as indicated in Fig. 5.1, and included some time before and some time after the epoch of interest. Comparing voltage, frequency and rhythmicity measurements of the background to those of the detected epoch allowed a decision tree to be formulated for detecting seizure activity. Detections could be triggered by rhythmic activity of large amplitude (Fig. 5.2) or by a sudden increase in frequency (Fig. 5.3). It is often not realized that it is unnecessary to detect the *onset* of a seizure. A detection occurring at any

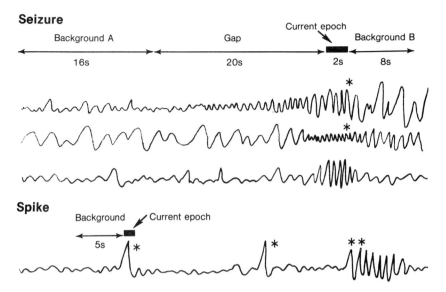

Fig. 5.1 Definition of the concept of 'background' for the purpose of seizure and spike detection. For seizure detection a relatively long background is used, including before and after the epoch under investigation, thus preventing the detection of short events. For spike detection, the background is much shorter. A * indicates detection.

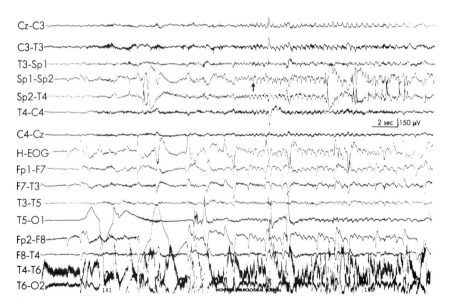

Fig. 5.2 Example of a seizure automatically detected because of its rhythmic discharge of paroxysmal amplitude. The alarm button was not pressed by the patient or an observer. The seizure was detected despite a large amount of artefact and not a very large amplitude. (From Gotman 1990.)

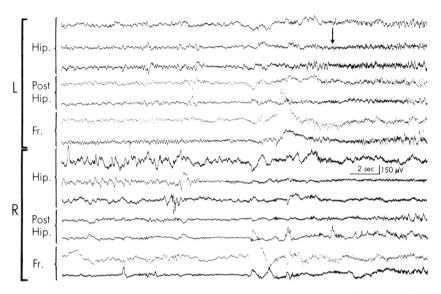

Fig. 5.3   Example of seizure automatically detected because of a rhythmic discharge of high frequency compared to the frequency of the background. Note that the amplitude of the discharge was not larger than that of the background. The alarm button was not pressed. (From Gotman 1990.)

time during the course of the seizure is sufficient, because the computer can hold in memory the preceding 2 or 3 minutes of EEG, thus ensuring that EEG immediately before and at seizure onset is preserved.

Validation of seizure detection methods

Evaluating the performance of automatic detection methods is difficult because results may depend more on the selection of EEGs included in the evaluation set than on the detection method itself. For instance, a spike detection method may perform well when the patient is resting with eyes closed, perform less well when eye blinks are present and fail completely with EMG and movement artefacts. To give a fair impression of performance, what type of EEG should be included in the evaluation? The person selecting the EEG segments is often subjective, and this can bias results.

In evaluating our seizure detection method, we made all efforts to avoid bias in data selection (Gotman 1990). EEGs were recorded from 293 *consecutive* monitoring sessions from 49 patients. Monitoring was performed in the absence of an EEG technologist. All EEGs were included irrespective of patterns present and technical quality. Electrode problems and other technical difficulties were frequent, but all EEGs were retained. Most patients were above 10 years of age and had medically refractory epilepsy; all were being considered for surgical treatment. The average recording duration was 18.1 hours, ranging from 12 to 23 hours. The method was

Table 5.1 Percentage of seizure recordings that were triggered by both the alarm button and the automatic seizure detection (1st line) or by only one of them (2nd and 3rd lines). Total number of seizures is $86 + 59 + 99 = 234$

Seizure	Alarm	Automatic detection	N	$\%$
Yes	Yes	Yes	86	35
Yes	Yes	No	59	24
Yes	No	Yes	99	41

293 recordings; 49 patients; average duration of recording 18.1 hours; total duration of recordings 5300 hours.

thus evaluated on 5303 hours of EEG.

In 241 of the 293 recordings (44 of 49 patients), scalp and sphenoidal electrodes were used; in the remaining 52 recordings (5 patients) intracerebral and epidural electrodes were used. Because some patients had a large number of similar seizures, averaging data from them with those of subjects having only two or three seizures would have given biased results. We therefore established a 'ceiling' for each patient and each type of seizure (Gotman 1990).

Results of the evaluation are summarized in Table 5.1. Twenty-four per cent of the 244 seizures were missed by the computer and detected only because the alarm button alone had been pressed. In 35% of seizures, both the computer and the alarm button triggered EEG sampling. In the remaining 41%, only the computer detected seizures.

It is thus clear that one cannot rely exclusively on either a patient/observer-activated alarm system or computer-based automatic detection. Using both, however, increases considerably the yield of long-term monitoring. The foregoing average detection rates do not accurately reflect the reality of individual patients. Amongst the 5 patients with intracerebral electrodes, we had 2 extreme cases: in one patient, 16 clinical seizures were recorded by the alarm button (with or without computer detection), only 3 being detected by the computer alone. In this case, the computer operated for two weeks almost continuously and yielded little additional information. In another patient, however, 21 seizures were detected by the computer alone and in one other seizure both the computer and the alarm button triggered the recording. All were clinical seizures consisting of long but quiet automatisms during which the patient stayed in bed and made no noise. Such seizures most often went unnoticed because the patient was lying in bed, but they were very disruptive in his active life. In this case the computer was extremely helpful.

The number of seizures that are missed is obviously a function of how closely the patient and the EEG are observed. If a nurse and EEG technologist observe the patient and the EEG at all times, then it is rare for any seizure to be missed. This is a very expensive procedure, however, and as the degree of observation of the patient and the EEG lessens, automatic seizure detection becomes increasingly important.

We have not given details of false-positive detections. In the majority of cases, false detections are in numbers small enough not to be disruptive and only cause EEG to be recorded unnecessarily. Such information can simply be discarded upon visual inspection. Details are given in Gotman (1990).

Limitations and future developments

Current seizure detection programs are not perfect and could be improved significantly. It would be extremely difficult, however, to detect all seizures, because some seizures have almost no EEG accompaniment and the discharge morphology is often non-specific (Ajmone Marsan 1984). The suggestion is sometimes made that performance could be improved by fine tuning the detection program to each patient's seizure, using the first seizures detected by the computer or an observer as a kind of template. Unfortunately, this introduces an unacceptable bias in detection performance toward seizures of this type recorded early in the monitoring session. In many cases, the purpose of monitoring is to document all types of seizures and particularly to see if there are also seizures *different* from those recorded early. Tailoring automated detection to a particular seizure type is only acceptable if one is interested in assessing the occurrence of that particular seizure type and is less concerned with other kinds of seizures.

In future developments, care will be given to identifying the most common causes of false detection. By reducing false detections, it will be possible to expand detection thresholds and thus improve performance. Improved detection ability with lower thresholds has been documented in an independent validation of the method (Chatrian, personal communication).

AUTOMATIC SPIKE DETECTION

Past methods

Numerous publications in the 1970s and early 1980s dealt with automatic spike detection. The usual approach consisted of: (1) selecting artefact-free EEG sections lasting 1 or 2 minutes, which included a sufficient number of spikes or sharp waves; (2) devising a method for their detection; and (3) comparing results of automatic detection with a qualified electroencephalographer's recognition of 'true' spikes. The various detection methods have been reviewed extensively (Frost 1985, Gotman 1985b). In general terms, these methods relied on one of two approaches. In the first, the EEG is broken down into elementary waves and those waves are identified that have morphological characteristics normally associated with spikes (defined by voltage, duration and sharpness). In the second, the EEG is analysed in order to find statistically improbable events of short duration. Acceptable performance was obtained with most methods, usually with 80–90% of 'true' spikes being detected and a low rate of false-positive detection. Many publications ended with statements such as: 'As computers become more powerful and less expensive, practical implementation of this method will be simple'. In fact, computers became more powerful, less expensive and faster than anybody expected but most methods did not reach practical implementation. One major reason is that the detection problem became much more complex when longer sections of EEG were analysed. In real life situations, artefacts and normal transients had to be included, and they caused numerous false detections. In addition, some methods were not readily adaptable to on-line analysis and were therefore of limited practical utility.

Difficulties of the problem

The major difficulty with spike recognition methods is their reliance on very incomplete definitions of a spike. The definition quoted by many publications is that of a 'sharp transient, easily distinguishable from the background, having a duration of less than 70 ms for a spike and 70–200 ms for a sharp wave' (Chatrian et al 1974). This definition is extremely incomplete because it lacks features that allow differentiation from transients having the same local morphology but which are not epileptiform events: eye blinks, vertex sharp waves, isolated α or spindle waves, electrode artefacts and movement artefacts to name only a few. Such transients are extremely common during prolonged EEG recordings when it would be particularly useful to have automatic spike detection.

What are the characteristics that allow a human interpreter to separate an epileptiform sharp wave from an eye blink, even though the waves themselves may have the same morphology and emerge from a similar background? These characteristics are most likely related to the overall context in which the waves appear, the concept of 'context' covering much wider space and time than that of 'background'. When interpreting a wave having the morphology of a spike, the human interpreter takes into account what happens in other channels (spatial context), and in both earlier and later parts of the recording (temporal context), and also incorporates relevant non-EEG information such as the age or clinical state of the subject. Early optimism about spike detection methods originated in the failure of investigators and engineers to appreciate how much spike identification relies on this issue of context.

It must be noted that the problems discussed above do not affect the ability to detect epileptiform discharges reliably, but they result in a large number of false-positive detections. It is thus possible to make practical use of an automatic spike detection method as long as it is conceived as a method to detect a high proportion of the spikes along with a possibly large number of non-epileptiform transients (NETs), rather than as a method to detect only spikes. Such a practical implementation was made with the spike detection algorithms developed at the Montreal Neurological Institute (Gotman et al 1979, 1985). The method has been in daily use for many years and is now also used in other institutions. It operates on-line and stores on computer disc all the sections of EEG where detections are made. These are subsequently played back on paper, and the electro-encephalographer decides which are true and which are false detections. Despite its false-positive detections, the system allows a large fraction of the spikes to be recorded and reduces data considerably. It can be combined with the automatic seizure detection described earlier in the chapter to form a system that allows automatic extraction of all epileptiform activity, ictal and interictal, during long-term epilepsy monitoring. In everyday use, such a system results in an approximate data reduction of 95%: only 5% of a 24-hour recording is retained that includes spikes, seizures and false detections.

Perspectives for improvements

Probably the only way to improve performance of spike detection methods is to make them operate more like humans, i.e. to allow them to use information 'in context'. This is a simple concept but difficult to implement, because the context encompasses a very large amount of information, and one must decide which part of that information is relevant to spike detection. It is this selection that the human electroencephalographer does so well.

Glover et al (1986, 1989) have described a context-based system aimed largely at reducing false spike detections by making use of a wide *spatial* context. Information from all EEG channels, as well as from EMG, EOG and EKG channels, is used to assess whether a transient in a particular channel is likely to be epileptiform. Figure 5.4 illustrates how genuine sharp waves are retained whereas at the same time, spindle waves, not very different in morphology, are rejected.

We have recently proposed an approach where a wide *temporal* context is used to decide on the nature of a sharp transient (Gotman & Wang 1991). We have labelled the method 'state-sensitive spike detection' because criteria for spike detection are rendered dependent on the state of the EEG. We defined five states in which we believed spike detection should be performed differently: active wakefulness, quiet wakefulness, desynchronized EEG, phasic EEG and slow wave EEG. In fact, in these different states it is not so much that spike detection has to be done differently, but rather that false detections have to be handled by different means. In active wakefulness, for example, one must be particularly aware of symmetrical frontal sharp waves which may be due to eye blinks whereas there is no such concern in the phasic EEG state. In that state, sharp waves maximal

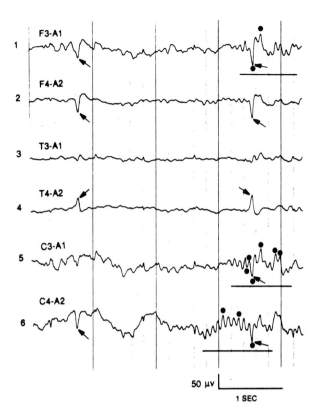

Fig. 5.4 Example of use of the spatial context in spike detection. The fact that a spindle is detected allows rejection of non-epileptiform fast transients related to the spindle, detecting nevertheless the real epileptiform activity. (From Glover et al 1989 © 1989 IEEE.)

at the vertex are a problem. The difficulty of such an approach is that, in addition to requiring methods to handle the different non-epileptiform transients, one must have a state classification procedure. An initial evaluation of such a method and of state-dependent spike detection is presented in Gotman & Wang (1991). State classification is based on spectral analysis of the EEG and recognition of eye movements in frontal–polar EEG deviations. State classification, as well as recognition of non-epileptiform transients, would be easier using non-EEG signals such as EMG, EOG or EKG, but we elected not to use them in order to avoid added discomfort to the patient during long-term recordings. In addition, all recording channels are thus available for EEG.

New methods of spike detection that are currently under investigation include neural nets. This is a very powerful pattern recognition procedure which may prove more performant than existing heuristic methods. It will nevertheless encounter the same difficulties as traditional methods, because incorporating a wide context renders its operation much more complex.

POST-DETECTION DISPLAY AND ANALYSIS

The benefits derived from computers are not only in detecting epileptiform events but also in displaying, manipulating and analysing the EEG. This is particularly true when automatic detection methods are used. Because automatic detection methods result in considerable data reduction (a 24-hour monitoring session typically being reduced to 30–60 minutes), the EEG can easily be stored on the hard disc of a personal computer. This opens many possibilities of display and analysis with inexpensive equipment. Some of these are outlined below.

Computer review of the EEG

A system that presents the EEG on the screen at about ten times the recording speed is easily implemented on a personal computer. Combining this with data reduction, it is possible to review the important information of a 24-hour recording in 3–6 minutes (30–60 minutes of EEG replayed at ten times recording speed). This does not include the time required to interpret the EEG, particularly seizures, but indicates how long it takes to have a look at the recording. Seizures may be examined on the computer screen which, unlike conventional EEG machines, are not limited to 18 or 21 channels: 32 or even 64 channels may be viewed simultaneously, greatly facilitating the interpretation of EEGs from multiple intracerebral electrodes or large subdural arrays sometimes used in pre-surgical evaluations. Modern display screens can have a resolution sufficient for meaningful and accurate EEG interpretation. Furthermore, simple manipulations such as changing gains or filters, montage reformatting or topographic mapping may be performed interactively by the electroencephalographer at the time this information is required.

Computer printers are used for writing results of computer analyses, but they may also print EEG traces. Standard laser printers have a resolution as good or better than an EEG machine (Fig. 5.5A). They can mix EEGs and other alphanumeric or graphical information. Their only drawback at present is that they are slow; only specially modified and therefore expensive printers can print EEGs as rapidly as an EEG machine.

Analysis of seizure activity

One can go beyond visual interpretation and analyse seizures in order to extract information of diagnostic or scientific interest. It is possible, for instance, to remove most of the EMG artefact that obscures many seizures recorded from the scalp (Fig. 5.5; Gotman et al 1981) or to quantify EEG changes at seizure onset (Darcey & Williamson 1985). The question that has retained the attention of most investigators, however, is seizure propagation between brain regions.

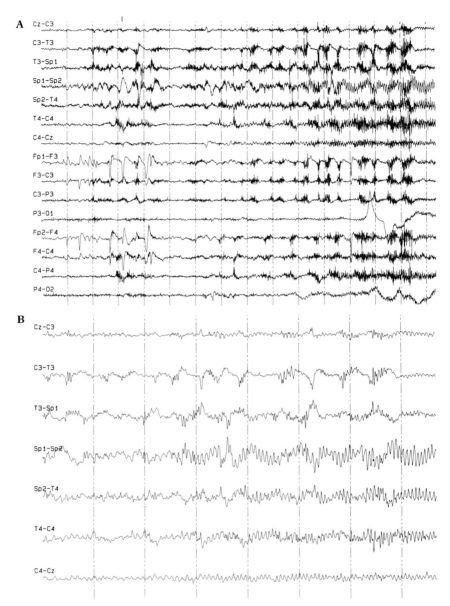

Fig. 5.5   A Onset of seizure discharge. The activity is mixed with EMG artefact. Illustration is from a laser printer. **B** Illustration of zoom and digital filter; this section is upper right quadrant of **A**, digitally filtered (low-pass, 18 Hz, FIR filter order 51) and enlarged, showing rhythmic activity in the right temporal lobe.

The study of interactions between brain regions during seizures was pioneered by Brazier (1972). She used the coherence function (derived from the cross-spectrum) to measure the strength of interaction between seizure discharges in two locations, and the phase spectrum to measure

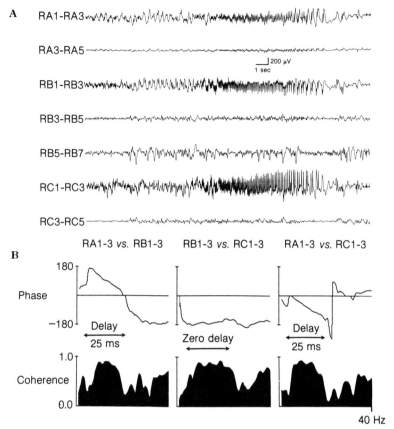

Fig. 5.6 A Short seizure localized to deep structures of the temporal lobe; electrodes are in horizontal plane with contacts 5 mm apart, contact 1 being deepest; RA aimed at amygdala, RB at anterior hippocampus, RC at middle hippocampus. **B** Phase and coherence spectra between the three pairs of deepest channels; phase is linear over frequency range where coherence is high (horizontal arrow); a time delay measurement is therefore possible, indicating a lead from RB1-3 to RA1-3 of 25 ms, from RC1-3 to RA1-3 also of 25 ms and no time difference between RB1-3 and RC1-3.

time differences between them of the order of a few milliseconds. Thus, rapid propagation of seizures could be followed. The method was made more reliable by Gotman (1981, 1983) who included in the measurement a range of frequencies rather than a single frequency. Its validity was established in experimental and human epilepsy, in cases where the location of the focus was known (Gotman 1983). This method allowed the study of interhemispheric interactions during widespread spike and wave activity (Gotman 1981) and during temporal lobe seizures (Gotman 1987, Lieb et al 1987). Figure 5.6A shows a small seizure recorded in a patient from hippocampus and amygdala. The coherence and phase spectra in Fig. 5.6B shows that the discharge in the hippocampus leads that in the amygdala by 25 ms. In other such seizures in the same patient time differences ranged from 5 to 30 ms, the hippocampus always leading the amygdala. One should be cautious in interpreting this result: it does not necessarily prove that the discharge originates in the hippocampus and propagates to the amygdala. If, however, one has to choose between amygdala and hippocampus as the most likely origin of the discharge, the coherence and phase results favour the hippocampus.

There are other methods to measure interactions during seizures. The average amount of mutual information (AAMI) has a theoretical advantage over coherence, because coherence can only detect *linear* (in the mathematical sense) relationships, whereas AAMI can also detect more complex relationships. Investigators have found, however, that coherence and AAMI most often give similar results. AAMI and other non-linear methods are described in detail in Lopes da Silva & Mars (1987). Recently, Fernandes de Lima et al (1990) compared a linear and a non-linear regression coefficient in the study of interhemispheric interactions during hippocampal seizures in the rat. They found that the non-linear measure was more robust than the linear one and could yield values of interaction when the linear one was at noise level. An important factor often not discussed when comparing these methods is that the size of the recording electrodes probably influences the type of relationship. Discharges from very small electrodes, which may record multiple unit activity, are more likely to have non-linear relationships than discharges from macroelectrodes, which record from large populations of neurones.

Analysis of interictal activity

I previously described automatic spike detection mainly in the context of data reduction, but it offers also the benefit of quantification. It is possible to edit interactively on the computer screen to eliminate false spike detections so that only valid detections remain. These can be written out on paper (Fig. 5.7) and their spatial and temporal distributions may then be presented (Fig. 5.8). Such quantification of spike activity during several days of monitoring has proved invaluable in the study of factors that might affect the rate and localization of spikes. For example, the rate of focal spiking does not change, increase or decrease, before seizures (Gotman & Marciani 1985, Katz & Spencer 1989). In contrast, there is a large increase in spiking in the days that follow most secondarily generalized seizures and many partial seizures. Surprisingly, spiking rates are unaffected by changes in antiepileptic drug levels (Gotman & Marciani 1985, Gotman & Koffler 1989). The postictal increase in spike rate and the failure of high antiepileptic drug levels to decrease spike rate have been replicated in the kindling model of epilepsy (Gotman 1984, Leung 1990, Gigli & Gotman 1991).

Spikes have also been quantified during different stages of sleep in patients undergoing evaluation for epilepsy surgery. Results from non-invasive recordings indicated that spiking is more focal during rapid eye movement

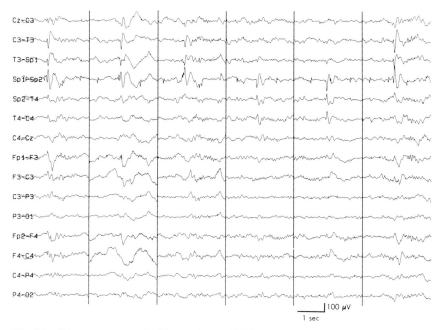

Fig. 5.7 Print-out on a standard laser printer of EEG sections recorded because of automatic spike detection. The laser printer allows printing EEG sections inexpensively and with very high resolution.

(REM) sleep than during slow-wave sleep. The localization obtained from spikes occurring in REM sleep correlates better with other tests of localization (seizure onset, radiological findings) than localization obtained during slow-wave sleep or wakefulness (Sammaritano et al 1991).

CONCLUSION

Spike and seizure detection are not simple tasks as was first thought. The electroencephalographer uses clues from a wide spatial and temporal context – clues that are difficult to encode in computer programs. Current computer methods analyse the EEG at a very local level: 10–30 seconds of EEG at a time, most often one channel at a time. It would therefore be naive to expect high reliability from automatic methods. Nevertheless, existing methods can be extremely useful if implemented in the right framework.

Seizure detection procedures are very helpful in detecting many seizures, thus greatly reducing the need for reviewing days and days of EEG paper tracings. Although the performance of seizure detection methods will improve, one important difficulty will remain: seizures are behavioural events with EEG manifestations that are sometimes poorly defined and

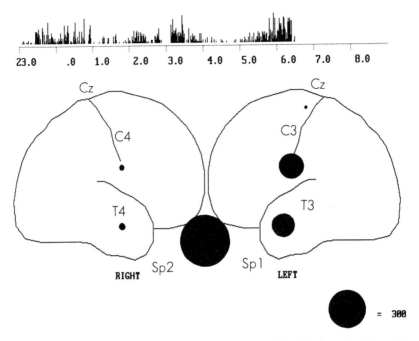

Fig. 5.8 Schematic representation of temporal and spatial distributions of spike activity detected over a period of several hours. Vertical bars represent number of spikes per minute. Circles represent number of spikes found at a particular bipolar channel (scale is at bottom right).

non-specific. It is thus mandatory always to include some form of alarm system. Conversely, patient or observer are not sufficient and automatic seizure detection helps capture numerous seizures with unobtrusive or minor clinical signs, as well as apparently subclinical seizures.

Spike detection methods are able to detect a very large fraction of spikes. The problem does not lie in the inability to detect them, but rather in the poor ability of these methods to separate epileptiform from non-epileptiform sharp transients. Non-epileptiform transients cause numerous false detections. It will only be possible to separate the two kinds of events by including a wide temporal and spatial context. It is now possible to incorporate some information from the context, and we should see significant improvement in performance in the near future.

The technological context in which automatic detection methods are implemented is rapidly changing. Existing programs can already operate on personal computers. Personal computers can be equipped with high-resolution monitors so that EEG interpretation can be done directly from the screen. Several computers may be connected via a local area network so that review of a recording can take place while the recording is in process. Given the data-reduction ability of detection programs, it is feasible to archive EEGs from a three-week monitoring session, including interictal and ictal activity, on a single optical disc.

Finally, computer analysis of seizures and spikes may provide information that is not readily available from traditional visual examination. This is primarily due to the possibility of quantifying EEG activity and of making mathematical analyses that can be related to brain function.

REFERENCES

Ajmone Marsan C 1984 Electroencephalographic studies in seizure disorders: additional considerations. J Clin Neurophysiol 1: 143–157

Babb T L, Mariani E, Crandall P H 1974 An electronic circuit for detection of EEG seizures recorded with implanted electrodes. Electroencephalogr Clin Neurophysiol 37: 305–308

Blume W T, Young G B, Lemieux J F 1984 EEG morphology of partial epileptic seizures. Electroencephalogr Clin Neurophysiol 57: 295–302

Brazier M A B 1972 Spread of seizure discharges in epilepsy: anatomical and electrophysiological considerations. Exp Neurol 36: 263–272

Chatrian G E, Bergamini L, Dondey M et al 1974 A glossary of terms most commonly used by clinical electroencephalographers. Electroencephalogr Clin Neurophysiol 37: 538–548

Darcey T M, Williamson P D 1985 Spatio-temporal EEG measures and their application to human intracranially recorded epileptic seizures. Electroencephalogr Clin Neurophysiol 61: 573–587

Fernandes de Lima V M, Pijn J P, Nunes Filipe C, Lopes da Silva F H 1990 The role of hippocampal commissures in the interhemispheric transfer of epileptiform after discharges in the rat: a study using linear and non-linear regression analysis. Electroencephalogr Clin Neurophysiol 76: 520–539

Frost J D Jr 1985 Automatic recognition and characterization of epileptiform discharges in the human EEG. J Clin Neurophysiol 2: 231–249

Gigli G, Gotman J 1991 Effects of seizures and carbamazepine on interictal spiking in amygdala kindled cats. Epilepsy Res 8: 204–212

Glover J R, Ktonas P Y, Raghavan N et al 1986 A multichannel signal processor for the detection of epileptogenic sharp transients in the EEG. IEEE Trans Biomed Eng 33: 1121–1128

Glover J R, Raghavan N, Ktonas P Y et al 1989 Context-based automated detection of epileptogenic sharp transients in the EEG: elimination of false positives. IEEE Trans Biomed Eng 36: 519–527

Gotman J 1981 Interhemispheric relations during bilateral spike and wave activity. Epilepsia 22: 453–466

Gotman J 1982 Automatic recognition of epileptic seizures in the EEG. Electroencephalogr Clin Neurophysiol 54: 530–540

Gotman J 1983 Measurement of small time differences between EEG channels: method and application to epileptic seizure propagation. Electroencephalogr Clin Neurophysiol 56: 501–514

Gotman J 1984 Relationship between triggered seizures, spontaneous seizures and interictal spiking in the kindling model of epilepsy. Exp Neurol 84: 259–273

Gotman J 1985a Seizure recognition and analysis. In: Gotman J, Ives J R, Gloor P (eds) Long-term monitoring in epilepsy. Elsevier, Amsterdam, pp 133–145

Gotman J 1985b Automatic recognition of interictal spikes. In: Gotman J, Ives J R, Gloor P (eds) Long-term monitoring in epilepsy. Elsevier, Amsterdam, pp 93–114

Gotman J 1986 Computer analysis of EEG in epilepsy. In: Lopes da Silva F H, Storm van Leeuwen W, Rémond A (eds) Handbook of electroencephalography and clinical neurophysiology, Vol 2. Elsevier, New York, pp 171–204

Gotman J 1987 Interhemispheric interactions in seizures of focal onset: data from human intracranial recordings. Electroencephalogr Clin Neurophysiol 67: 120–133

Gotman J 1990 Automatic seizure detection: improvements and evaluation.

Electroencephalogr Clin Neurophysiol 76: 317–324

Gotman J, Gloor P 1976 Automatic recognition and quantification of interictal epileptic activity in the human scalp EEG. Electroencephalogr Clin Neurophysiol 41: 513–529

Gotman J, Koffler D J 1989 Interictal spiking increases after seizures but does not after decrease in medication. Electroencephalogr Clin Neurophysiol 72: 7–15

Gotman J, Marciani M G 1985 EEG spiking activity, drug levels and seizure occurrence in epileptic patients. Ann Neurol 17: 597–603

Gotman J, Wang L-Y 1991 State-dependent spike detection: concepts and preliminary results. Electrocephalogr Clin Neurophysiol (in press)

Gotman J, Ives J R, Gloor P 1979 Automatic recognition of interictal epileptic activity in prolonged EEG recordings. Electroencephalogr Clin Neurophysiol 46: 510–520

Gotman J, Ives J R, Gloor P 1981 Frequency content of EEG and EMG at seizure onset: possibility of removal of EMG artefact by digital filtering. Electroencephalogr Clin Neurophysiol 52: 626–639

Gotman J, Ives J R, Gloor P et al 1985 Long-term monitoring at the Montreal Neurological Institute. In: Gotman J, Ives J R, Gloor P (eds) Long-term monitoring in epilepsy. Elsevier, Amsterdam, pp 327–340

Ives J R, Thompson C J, Gloor P et al 1974 The on-line computer detection and recording of spontaneous temporal lobe epileptic seizures from patients with implanted depth electrodes via a radio telemetry link. Electroencephalogr Clin Neurophysiol 37: 205

Katz A, Spencer S 1989 Spatial and temporal relations of interictal spikes and seizures. Epilepsia 5: 664

Ktonas P Y 1987 Automated spike and sharp wave (SSW) detection. In: Gevins A, Rémond A (eds) Handbook of electroencephalography and clinical neurophysiology, Vol 1: Methods of analysis of brain electrical and magnetic signals. Elsevier, Amsterdam, pp 211–241

Leung L W S 1990 Spontaneous hippocampal interictal spikes following local kindling: time-course of change and relation to behavioral seizures. Brain Res 513: 308–314

Lieb J B, Hoque K, Skomer C E, Songt X-W 1987 Inter-hemispheric propagation of human mesial temporal lobe seizures: a coherence/phase analysis. Electroencephalogr Clin Neurophysiol 67: 101–119

Lockard J S, Congdon W C, DuCharme L L et al 1980 Slow-speed EEG for chronic monitoring of clinical seizures in monkey model. Epilepsia 21: 325–334

Lopes da Silva F H, Mars N J I 1987 Parametric methods in EEG analysis. In: Gevins A, Rémond A (eds) Handbook of electroencephalography and clinical neurophysiology, Vol 1: Methods of analysis of brain electrical and magnetic signals. Elsevier, Amsterdam, pp 243–260

Prior P F, Virden R S M, Maynard D E 1973 An EEG device for monitoring seizure discharges. Epilepsia 14: 367–372

Sammaritano M, Gigli G L, Gotman J 1991 Interictal spiking during wakefulness and sleep and the localization of foci in temporal lobe epilepsy. Neurology 41: 290–297

Wieser H G 1987 Data analysis. In: Engel J Jr (ed) Surgical treatment of the epilepsies. Raven Press, New York, pp 335–360

6

Prenatal and perinatal risk factors for epilepsy

S. J. Wallace

INTRODUCTION

An understanding of the early factors which pose risks for the development of epilepsy is helped by an awareness of normal cerebral development. After conception the earliest anatomical stage is dorsal induction, which occurs maximally at three to four weeks of gestation, followed by ventral induction at five to six weeks, neuronal proliferation at two to four months, neuronal migration at three to five months, organization from six months gestation to several years postnatally, and myelination which starts in the phylogenetically oldest parts of the brain at about 12 weeks gestational age and is not complete in the forebrain until many years postnatally (Volpe 1987). If an insult to the brain occurs during development, the event undergoing maximal change is the most vulnerable. Thus the timing of an insult in relation to age can critically affect its influence. Of the events which occur during cerebral development, neuronal migration is probably the most important in the pathogenesis of epilepsy, but disorders at any stage can lead to abnormalities in which seizures are common, if not invariable.

Although it is helpful to classify prenatal and perinatal factors according to the major characteristic, multiple features are often apparent.

PRECONCEPTUAL AND PERICONCEPTIONAL FACTORS

The main preconceptual and periconceptional factors which increase the risk of epilepsy are listed in Table 6.1.

Genetically determined 'uncomplicated' epilepsy

In this context 'uncomplicated' is used to imply that epilepsy is the major symptom, and not one of a complex of other neurological conditions.

Gene identified

Benign familial neonatal convulsions have been recognized as dominantly inherited for some years. Thus the risk to children of an affected parent

Table 6.1   Preconceptional or periconceptional risk factors

Genetically determined 'uncomplicated' epilepsy
  Gene identified
  Gene not identified

Genetically determined conditions with an increased risk of epilepsy
  Neurodermatoses
  Inherited metabolic disorders

Chromosomal disorders

is one in two. In 1989, using two closely linked DNA markers, Leppert et al reported mapping of the gene for this syndrome to the long arm of chromosome 20. In addition to defining the location, they confirmed the presence of a single gene. However, they considered that further families needed to be tested for confirmation of the findings, and also for examination of the possibility that there might be mutant genes which could explain the variants in which the typical neonatal course is either followed by complete remission, or by the later occurrence of other seizures.

Juvenile myoclonic epilepsy is the other syndrome for which gene localization is at an advanced stage (Delgado-Escueta et al 1989). Tight linkage with Bf-HLA is considered to be strong evidence that the gene for juvenile myoclonic epilepsy is located on the short arm of chromosome 6 at 6p21.3. Since family members of those with juvenile myoclonic epilepsy have an increased risk of febrile seizures, absences and generalized tonic–clonic seizures (GTCS), the gene identified may be heterogeneous. The clearer definition of this gene should lead to a much better understanding of genetically determined epilepsies in general.

Gene not identified

A positive family history for seizures is recognized as an important risk factor for epilepsy (Nelson & Ellenberg 1986, Ottman et al 1985, 1988, 1989, Rocca et al 1987a, 1987b). The overall likelihood of epilepsy in children of parents with this condition is three times that in the general population (Ottman et al 1989). However, paternal epilepsy is considerably less important than a maternal history of seizures (Ottman et al 1988). The latter has been identified as one of a very small number of significant precursors of epilepsy (Nelson & Ellenberg 1986, Rocca et al 1987a, 1987b). Nevertheless, when in the National Collaborative Perinatal Project (NCPP) carried out in the USA between 1959 and 1966 the antecedents of seizure disorders in general were examined, a history of seizures in the previous five years was obtained for the mothers of only 2.3% of 386 affected children (Nelson & Ellenberg 1986).

The risk remains low when predictors for specific seizure types are assessed. In a population-based case–control study using information collected over a period of 44 years, the predictors of GTCS were examined in 53 patients (Rocca et al 1987a). The only prenatal factor found to be associated significantly with GTCS was a maternal history of febrile seizures or epilepsy, but only 3 of 53 patients had an affected mother. Similarly, when the same group of investigators assessed the predictors of complex partial seizures, although a maternal history of febrile seizures or epilepsy was present significantly more often in cases than controls, the mothers of only 4 of 82 patients had a seizure disorder (Rocca et al 1987b). In 30 patients with absence seizures who were investigated as part of the same population-based case–control study, maternal seizure disorder was not a significant predictor (Rocca et al 1987c). Conversely, parents who have had absences confer the greatest risk of seizures to their offspring (Ottman et al 1989).

The particular contribution of maternal influences on the susceptibility to seizures has been reviewed in detail by Ottman et al (1985). Neither non-paternity nor reduced fertility in men with epilepsy can fully explain the maternal–paternal differences. The formulations of the generalized single major gene locus model of inheritance attempted by Ottman et al (1985) do not elucidate the greater maternal influence on seizure susceptibility, but these authors did not exclude the possibility that other formulations might be compatible with the data found in previous studies. In addition, Ottman et al (1985) believe that maternal transmission of at least some of the epilepsies cannot be rejected.

Genetically determined conditions with an increased risk of epilepsy

Neurodermatoses

Epilepsy occurs in 90% of patients with tuberous sclerosis (TS) (Gomez 1987). In childhood, seizures, in particular infantile spasms, are the commonest presenting features of this autosomal dominant condition. There is evidence for locations of the gene for TS at both chromosome 9p34 and chromosome 11q23, and the possibility that there are two gene sites has been entertained (Editorial 1990a). In keeping with the probability that TS is a disorder of cell migration, it is of interest that both potential gene loci are near the genes for cell adhesion molecules which play an important part in migration. The risk of TS is one in two for each child of an affected parent.

In neurofibromatosis I, although disorders of neuronal migration have been reported, epilepsy occurs in only about 12% of patients (Bird 1987). Neurofibromatosis I is an autosomal dominant condition with a risk of one in two for each child of an affected parent, and a consequent risk of one in 17 for epilepsy.

Incontinentia pigmenti, an X-linked dominantly inherited abnormality of melanocyte and neuronal migration, is also associated with an increased risk of epilepsy.

Inherited metabolic disorders

Virtually any disorder which causes developmental delay or arrest in association with adverse biochemical changes can be associated with epilepsy. The majority of these conditions are inherited in an autosomal recessive manner, but a few, such as Menkes disease, are X-linked.

The metabolic causes of progressive myoclonus epilepsies have been very fully documented by Berkovic & Andermann (1986). They range through disorders of lysosomal enzymes, amino acids, copper metabolism and mitochondria to conditions where pathological rather than biochemical definition has been obtained. Pyridoxine dependency and deficiency of γ-aminobutyric acid transaminase are also associated with epilepsy (Jaeken et al 1984).

Disorders of neuronal migration are recognized in association with some of the inborn errors of metabolism (Barth 1987). In particular, microgyria is found in two of the peroxisomal disorders: Zellweger syndrome and neonatal adrenoleukodystrophy; and, verrucose dysplasia in neonatal glutaric aciduria type II. Other less specific migrational abnormalities are found in Menkes disease, GM_2 gangliosidoses and Fukuyama syndrome.

Chromosomal disorders

Chromosomal disorders can be grouped according to whether sex or autosomal chromosomes are abnormal and whether there are deletions or extra chromosomes present.

Sex chromosome abnormalities

Fragile X chromosomes are associated in the male with mental retardation, which may be profound, large ears and large testes. Connective tissue dysfunction is important in the various manifestations. Hypotonia, speech disorders, behavioural problems, hyperactivity and psychosis are common. Thirty per cent of female carriers are mentally dull. Between 28% and 42% of males with fragile X chromosomes have epilepsy (Musumeci et al 1988), but the prevalence in carrier females, whether mentally dull or not, is as yet unquantified.

Epilepsy is reported in other disturbances of sex chromosomes. In personal cases, XXY (Klinefelter's syndrome), XYY and XXX karyotypes have been found in children with epilepsy, mental retardation and behaviour disorders; and also, in a child with absence seizures and a male phenotype, an XX karyotype has been identified. The risk of epilepsy in these conditions is not well documented, but approximately 18% of XXY and 15% of XYY males who live in institutions have epilepsy (Bird 1987). Children with XXXY and XXXXY karyotypes are also reported to be prone to seizures (Kunze 1980).

Autosomal trisomies

Down's syndrome, trisomy 21, was initially thought to be associated only rarely with epilepsy, but there is increasing recognition that children with trisomy 21 have an increased risk of infantile spasms. Epilepsy as a whole occurs in up to 9% of patients with Down's syndrome (Bird 1987).

Trisomy, or partial trisomy of chromosomes 8, 13, 18 and 22, can also be associated with epilepsy. Up to 50% of patients are affected (Kunze 1980, Bird 1987). Disorders of neuronal migration are reported in both trisomy 13 and 18 (Barth 1987).

Trisomy 12p syndrome is of particular interest, since in this condition the ictal discharges are 3-Hz spike and wave (Guerrini et al 1990).

Deletions

The Miller–Dieker syndrome, in which lissencephaly and a characteristic facial appearance occur with severe epilepsy and mental retardation, is associated with partial monosomy 17p13 (Dobyns et al 1983).

Of special interest are microdeletions in chromosome 15. Prader–Willi syndrome results if the deletion is inherited from the father, and Angelman syndrome if the deletion comes from the mother (Knoll et al 1989). Epilepsy is unusual in the Prader–Willi syndrome, but common in Angelman syndrome, which is also associated with severe mental retardation. Further elucidation of the differences in phenotypic expression resulting from apparently the same deletion could be important in the understanding of the genetics of epilepsy.

Ring chromosomes

Seizures are reported to have occurred in six of seven patients with ring chromosome 14 (Schmidt et al 1981). Other features associated with this anomaly are hypo- and hyperpigmented spots and craniofacial dysmorphism.

Epilepsy has also been reported when there are ring chromosomes 4, 17, 20, 21 and 22 (Kunze 1980).

INTRAUTERINE RISK FACTORS

The main groups of conditions which can lead to an increased risk of epilepsy are listed in Table 6.2.

Table 6.2   Intrauterine risk factors

Infection
Vascular disorders
Drugs
   Therapeutic use
   Abuse
Central nervous system dysplasias
Pregnancy-related disorders

Intrauterine infection

Viral infections

Historically the infections considered most likely to cause subsequent neurological disorder and thus seizures were rubella and cytomegalovirus (CMV), but with a change in the spectrum of infections, and in most Western countries, vaccination of children against rubella, prenatal infection with human immunodeficiency virus (HIV) also now has to be considered as a potential cause of neurological illness with symptomatic seizures (Belman et al 1985).

The timing of infection with rubella is critical. If rubella is contracted in the first four months of pregnancy there is a particular risk for severe abnormalities. Seizures occur in up to 20% of affected children. They are symptomatic of cerebral pathology which may be meningoencephalitic, vascular with focal ischaemic necrosis, cytopathic with poor cellular growth or related to delayed myelination (Volpe 1987).

Prenatal infection with CMV causes recognizable neurological disorder in a minority of cases (Preece et al 1984). In those who have symptomatic infections, seizures may be prominent. Specifically, congenital CMV infection has been implicated as a potential cause of infantile spasms (Riikonen 1978). Since the pathology includes disorders of neuronal migration, expressed as polymicrogyria, in about two-thirds of cases, and lissencephaly, pachygyria and neuronal heterotopias in others, a high prevalence of epilepsy might be predicted.

The full implications of prenatal infection with HIV have probably still to be defined. Neurological illness in symptomatic acquired immunodeficiency syndrome usually takes the form of encephalopathy with or without seizures, and presents from the age of 3 months in infants with prenatal infections (Belman et al 1985).

Transplacental infection with enteroviruses can occur, but no definite evidence exists for the acquisition of Coxsackie or Echo viruses during the first or second trimesters of pregnancy. Seizures are uncommon when encephalitis is caused by Coxsackie B infection (Volpe 1987).

The destructive meningoencephalitis associated with prenatal varicella infection is complicated by early seizures and continuing epilepsy in up to 50% of cases (Volpe 1987). Early infection with herpes simplex virus is usually acquired intranatally, but transplacental acquisition, with a high incidence of neurological involvement, has been described (Volpe 1987).

Protozoan infections

Transplacental passage of *Toxoplasma gondii* in the first trimester results in significant neurological disorder in up to 60% of infected infants. Infection in the second and third trimesters is less likely to cause a symptomatic problem. Granulomatous meningoencephalitis, diffuse cerebral calcifications, periventricular inflammation and necrosis and hydrocephalus underlie the neurological symptoms and signs. Seizures are reported in up to 50% of affected children (Volpe 1987).

Spirochaetal infections

Intrauterine infection with *Treponema pallidum* is on the increase in the USA (Dorfman & Glaser 1990). Symptoms and signs are conspicuously absent in the immediate neonatal period. Presentation is usually delayed until at least two weeks, when dermatological, reticuloendothelial and skeletal findings are most obvious. Meningeal involvement is present in up to 75% of cases, and seizures are reported in about one-fifth (Volpe 1987).

Vascular disorders

Vascular disorders which might predispose to epilepsy can be considered as extracranial, particularly in relation to placental insufficiency, or intracranial and therefore closely related to the overall neurological function.

Extracranial vascular disorders

Congenital lesions of the heart and great vessels do not usually cause the fetal brain to be compromised. The competency of the placental vasculature is of more consequence. Placental insufficiency for any reason leads to intrauterine growth retardation with the subsequent births of infants who are light for gestational age. Such infants have an increased risk for neurological disorders including cerebral palsy and epilepsy (Dunn et al 1986).

Intracranial vascular disorders

When vascular insufficiency occurs in the last trimester of pregnancy, porencephalic cysts are the result. Such cysts lie within the cerebral hemispheres and may or may not communicate with the lateral ventricles. Many types of vascular disorder may be implicated. Maldevelopment of blood vessels, vasculopathies and embolic or thrombotic phenomena are itemized by Volpe (1987). The anterior cerebral circulation, especially the middle cerebral artery, is most likely to be involved. Epilepsy is a common symptom of porencephaly, and a hemiparesis often coexists. Congenital malformations of intracerebral blood vessels can be associated with epilepsy in the absence of thrombotic or haemorrhagic complications. Sturge–Weber syndrome is the most obvious example. In this condition, an angiomatous naevus involves the skin served by the frontal and possibly other divisions of the trigeminal nerve and can extend through the skull so that a comparable naevus is found on the cerebral cortex. Seizures occur in 75–90% of affected patients (Gomez & Bebin 1987). Approximately one in ten of patients with the characteristic cortical lesions have no discernible skin abnormality.

Epilepsy can also be symptomatic of non-syndromic angiomatous lesions. Prenatal intracranial haemorrhage is very unusual, but may occur in association with isoimmune thrombocytopenia, with the subsequent development of multifocal cystic lesions and presence of hydrocephalus and associated neurological deficits including epilepsy (Naidu et al 1980).

Drugs

Drugs taken during pregnancy may be for therapeutic reasons or because of dependence or addiction.

Therapeutic drug use

The drugs most likely to produce abnormalities which might later be associated with seizures are those which have effects on the central nervous system. Thus sedative, neuroleptic and antiepileptic medications are possible candidates. Nevertheless, despite sufficient abnormality of the fetal brain to cause mental retardation in those with low epoxide hydrolase activity who are exposed to phenytoin (Buehler et al 1990), continuing epilepsy does not figure prominently in reports on affected infants. Seizures secondary to withdrawal from maternal barbiturates or tricyclic antidepressants, which present in the neonatal period, rarely progress to epilepsy.

Drugs of abuse

Alcohol is the commonest drug of abuse. Of 40 children with the fetal alcohol syndrome reported from the west of Scotland, 9 had a seizure disorder (Beattie et al 1983). Although other drugs of abuse may cause fetal cerebral abnormalities, symptomatic seizures other than those which occur rarely during the neonatal withdrawal period seem to be very uncommon.

Central nervous system dysplasias

After examination of hundreds of prenatal items, Nelson & Ellenberg (1986) concluded that congenital malformations (including non-cerebral malformations) were one of the three most significant predictors of childhood epilepsy. For a large proportion of central nervous system dysplasias there is no obvious cause. Therefore, it seems most relevant to consider this group of conditions as secondary to adverse post-conception, prenatal factors.

Disorders of ventral and/or dorsal induction

The most severe degrees of holoprosencephaly are not compatible with life. Surviving infants have a high risk of epilepsy of early onset. Although the aetiology is usually obscure, cases associated with autosomal dominant or recessive inheritance or with chromosomal abnormalities have been described (Volpe 1987).

Hydrocephalus can be secondary to congenital aqueduct stenosis, associated with the Arnold–Chiari or Dandy–Walker malformations, or related to other cerebral dysplasias. When occurring as an acquired problem, it is most often preceded by periventricular haemorrhage in the premature infant. Epilepsy has been reported in 48% of 168 shunt-treated patients, and, in this group, to be unrelated to the aetiology of the hydrocephalus (Saukkonen et al 1990). This study found that 46% of those with hydrocephalus secondary to a primary malformation had epilepsy.

Disorders of proliferation

When disorders of proliferation are associated with microcephaly, mental retardation, rather than epilepsy, is the usual predominating clinical feature. However, neuronal proliferation is abnormal, and macrocephaly can be an additional finding, in some neurocutaneous syndromes in which there is an increased risk of epilepsy. In tuberous sclerosis and neurofibromatosis I, glial cells as well as neurones are involved in the proliferative disorder. Unilateral macrocephaly is characterized by abnormal neuronal proliferation in part or the whole of one hemisphere. Severe, early-onset, therapy-resistant epilepsy is the rule. Other abnormalities sometimes present in unilateral macrocephaly are abnormalities of the gyri, excessive thickness of the cortex and heterotopic collections of neurones in white matter (Volpe 1987).

Disorders of neuronal migration

A recent editorial (Editorial 1990b) has highlighted the importance of abnormalities of neuronal migration as substrates for epilepsy. When gross disorders of migration result in agyria/pachygyria, the associated epilepsy is invariably severe and resistant to conventional antiepileptic therapy. Lesser degrees of abnormality, such as those resulting in verrucose dysplasias, microgyria, heterotopias or a duplicated cortex, have variable clinical effects, but a high risk of seizures remains. Fukuyama cerebromuscular dystrophy, Bloch–Sulzberger syndrome, Zellweger syndrome, neonatal adrenoleucodystrophy and multiple acyl CoA dehydrogenase deficiency are but a few examples of genetically determined conditions in which microgyria occurs. Although some syndromes in which neuronal heterotopias are common, e.g. tuberous sclerosis, are heritable, others, for example hypomelanosis of Ito, do not seem to have genetic implications. Micro-dysgenesis has been reported in neuropathological studies of brains from patients who have suffered from infantile spasms, severe myoclonic epilepsy of infancy, the Lennox–Gastaut syndrome, partial epilepsy of temporal lobe origin and primary generalized epilepsy. Thus both minor and major migrational disorders can underlie a wide variety of epilepsies.

Disorders of neuronal organization

Defects in organization are important components of the neuropathology of Down's syndrome but, except as phenomena associated with migrational and other disorders of development, they are not related to other specific syndromes. Nevertheless, neuronal disorganization can be found as an apparently primary disturbance in children with mental retardation and seizures (Volpe 1987).

Disorders of myelination

On the whole, since myelination is at its peak after rather than before birth at term, intrauterine factors are likely to have less effect on myelination than on other aspects of brain development. However, children with aberrant myelin formation whose neurological symptoms, including seizures, were prominent in the neonatal period, and whose subsequent mental and motor development were severely impaired, have been reported (Chattha & Richardson 1977).

Pregnancy-related disorders

As part of the NCPP, Nelson and Ellenberg demonstrated that events in pregnancy, which could be identified, were only rarely predictive of epilepsy. Gestational maternal seizures were of significance, particularly when the child's epilepsy did not include 'minor motor seizures' and there was no evidence of cerebral palsy. In the same study, a relatively large head circumference in relation to birth weight was considered evidence for intrauterine growth retardation. The latter was found to be associated with a small but significant increase in the risk for a seizure disorder.

PERINATAL RISK FACTORS

Perinatal problems can be considered as occurring either during labour and delivery (intrapartum) or immediately postpartum, and, by definition, up to the age of 7 days. Possible risk factors for epilepsy are listed in Table 6.3.

Table 6.3   Perinatal risk factors

Intrapartum problems
Mode of delivery
Trauma
Asphyxia: hypoxic–ischaemic encephalopathy
Immediate postpartum problems
Asphyxia: hypoxic–ischaemic encephalopathy
Haemorrhage
Vascular occlusion
Metabolic derangement
Infection
Seizures

Intrapartum problems

In the NCPP, when low-forceps was compared with all other forms of delivery, the risk of subsequent epilepsy was decreased slightly, but significantly, to 7.2 per 1000 (Nelson & Ellenberg 1986). The rate was 9.2 per 1000 in children delivered spontaneously by the vertex and 11.3 when mid-cavity forceps had been used. In the same study, the risk of epilepsy was increased if the lowest recorded fetal heart rate was 60 or less beats per minute and if there was uterine dysfunction during labour. Both of the latter could be associated with fetal asphyxia, but this was not specifically itemized as a factor for investigation in the NCPP report. Factors found not to be predictive of later epilepsy were: induction of labour; abnormalities of the umbilical cord, including cord round the neck; polyhydramnios; placenta praevia of any degree; abruptio placentae; breech delivery; Caesarean section, whether elective or emergency; placental weight; barbiturate or phenothiazine administration during labour; generalized or local anaesthesia. Nelson and Ellenberg concluded that there seemed to be little evidence that foreseeable changes in perinatal health care would alter the frequency of childhood epilepsy.

Approximately 20% of infants who have neonatal seizures develop epilepsy later. Abnormalities of the fetal heart rate accompanied or not by meconium staining of the amniotic fluid, prolonged second stage of labour and emergency Caesarean section have been identified as intrapartum antecedents of early neonatal seizures in infants born at or after term (Minchom et al 1987). In the NCPP, not all of these factors were specifically explored. Prolongation of the second stage of labour is an event which could be amenable to intervention. The studies of Minchom et al (1987) and Nelson & Ellenberg (1986) could form the basis for prediction of which neonates who have seizures will suffer continuing epilepsy.

Hypoxic–ischaemic encephalopathy

Hypoxic–ischaemic encephalopathy can be secondary to antepartum, intrapartum, combined ante- and intrapartum and postnatal events (Volpe

1987). The contribution of the antepartum state of the infant is almost certainly underestimated. Thus it is important to emphasize that the fetus who has been subjected to pre-eclamptic toxaemia, for example, or who has suffered intrauterine growth retardation can be more vulnerable to the demands of labour and delivery. On the other hand, approximately one-third of babies who suffer hypoxic–ischaemic encephalopathy have potentially traumatic deliveries, such as difficult forceps extraction, possibly with rotation of the head; difficult breech extraction; transverse arrest leading to prolonged labour; or cord obstruction or prolapse. Seizures are an almost constant feature of the neurological picture in the neonatal period, and continuing epilepsy is usual if the long-term pathology is located in the cerebral cortex and subcortical white matter, with cavity formation in the distribution of one or more of the cerebral arteries. When the major pathological changes are in the caudate, putamen or thalamus, in the parasagittal region, predominantly posteriorly, or in the periventricular white matter, a seizure disorder is not usually one of the long-term handicaps.

Immediate postpartum problems

Asphyxia

Hypoxic–ischaemic encephalopathy is secondary to asphyxial events which occur in the very early neonatal period in about 10% of cases. Severe recurrent apnoeic spells, cardiac failure and serious pulmonary disorders are potential aetiological factors. A postnatal cause is found more often in premature rather than term infants. As for hypoxic–ischaemic encephalopathy which occurs earlier in the perinatal period, the risk of epilepsy is greatest if the residual pathology includes cavity formation secondary to the ischaemic lesions.

In a study correlating hypoxia with later epilepsy, hypoxic infants with Apgar scores of five or less after the age of 1 hour had a risk of epilepsy five times that in control infants who were born in the same geographical area during the same time period (Bergamasco et al 1984). Nevertheless, epilepsy was recorded between 4 and 12 years later in only 21 (5.6%) of 371 infants who were defined as hypoxic, suggesting that factors other than asphyxia are very important in determining the risk of subsequent seizures. Bergamasco et al addressed this point, but could attribute the epilepsy to a primary generalized cause in only 2 of 21 cases, and to a postnatal cause in 2 others. They concluded that for the remaining 17 children hypoxia was the most relevant event.

Haemorrhage

Periventricular haemorrhage (PVH) occurs almost exclusively in premature infants. When the haemorrhage from the arterial supply to the subependymal germinal matrix is entirely intraventricular, the problem is less severe. In addition to opisthotonic posturing, which is common at the onset of PVH, tonic seizures are frequent acute symptoms. In the long-term the risk of epilepsy relates to the development of ischaemic lesions associated with cavitation, in which the pathology is comparable with that following hypoxic–ischaemic encephalopathy, with the addition of changes secondary to blood products in the brain, which could themselves be epileptogenic (Willmore et al 1978).

Perinatal subarachnoid haemorrhage alone does not appear to lead to an increased risk of epilepsy. Intracerebral haemorrhage due to any cause can lead to ischaemic and subsequently infarcted lesions comparable with those seen following PVH. If cerebral contusion is found in association with subdural haemorrhage, which is most likely to be traumatic in origin, there is an increased risk of neonatal seizures and thus of later epilepsy (Volpe 1987).

Vascular occlusion

Vascular occlusion in the neonate is usually due to hypoxic–ischaemic encephalopathy or PVH with subsequent ischaemia. Thrombotic or embolic occlusion can occur in association with infection, electrolyte disorders and dehydration. There is an increased risk of later epilepsy, regardless of the aetiology of the occlusion.

Metabolic derangement

Most causes of metabolic derangement with associated long-term risks of epilepsy, which present in the neonatal period, are genetically determined, and would therefore be considered under prenatal rather than perinatal events. Of acute causes with a lasting influence on the cerebrum, the acidosis of hypoxic–ischaemic encephalopathy is undoubtedly the most important. Hypoglycaemia is usually readily correctable, but only 50% of infants who have neonatal seizures in association with hypoglycaemia do well thereafter (Bergman et al 1983). On the other hand, it is unusual for neonatal hypocalcaemia to be associated with a long-term seizure disorder. Many of the metabolic disorders which cause seizures in the immediate neonatal period are not amenable to correction, with the result that survival to an age when the term epilepsy would be applicable does not always occur.

Infection

Neonatal meningitis was one of three postnatal features identified as significantly related to later epilepsy by the NCPP (Nelson & Ellenberg 1986). When the organism involved is a group B streptococcus, approximately one-fifth of survivors have severe neurological sequelae, including persisting epilepsy (Edwards et al 1985). The risk of epilepsy following meningitis secondary to Gram-negative enteric organisms is probably comparable, but the use of recently introduced antibiotics with a more effective ability to halt the infection could alter the outlook.

Herpes simplex encephalitis is an infrequent but serious cause of acute neonatal illness and prolonged neurological disability including epilepsy. When antiviral therapy is not given, approximately three-quarters of the infants die and half of the survivors have serious sequelae, of which therapy-resistant epilepsy is one of the most distressing. The survival rate is greater following treatment with acyclovir, but persisting severe mental and motor handicap with associated epilepsy remain common residua.

Seizures in the neonatal period

Approximately 20% of newborn infants who have seizures proceed to suffer from epilepsy. In the NCPP, seizures while in the newborn nursery were associated with death in the first year of life in one-third of cases, and correlated significantly with epilepsy in those surviving to the age of 7 years (Nelson & Ellenberg 1986). Even epileptic syndromes generally considered benign, i.e. benign idiopathic neonatal convulsions (fifth-day fits) and benign familial neonatal convulsions are associated with a small but increased risk of later epilepsy (North et al 1989, Leppert et al 1989). On the other hand it is only to be expected that seizures in a neonate with an underlying structural or metabolic disorder would be followed by epilepsy in a high percentage of cases.

CONCLUSIONS

Preconceptional and intrauterine factors are very important in determining the risk of epilepsy.

Features considered adverse in the perinatal period may be present because the fetus already has a problem which is only accentuated or highlighted by events during labour and delivery.

Further investigation of the molecular biology and biochemical expression of conditions in which disorders of neuronal migration occur could lead to a better understanding of the prenatal factors which determine the development of epilepsy.

REFERENCES

Barth P G 1987 Disorders of neuronal migration. Can J Neurol Sci 14: 1–16
Beattie J O, Day R E, Cockburn F, Garg R A 1983 Alcohol and the fetus in the west of Scotland. Br Med J 287: 17–20
Belman A L, Ultman M H, Horoupin D et al 1985 Neurological complications in infants and children with acquired immune deficiency syndrome. Ann Neurol 18: 560–566
Bergamasco B, Benna P, Ferrero P, Gavinelli R 1984 Neonatal hypoxia and epileptic risk: a clinical prospective study. Epilepsia 25: 131–136

Bergman I, Painter M J, Hirsch R P et al 1983 Outcome in neonates with convulsions treated in an intensive care unit. Ann Neurol 14: 642–647

Berkovic S F, Andermann F 1986 The progressive myoclonus epilepsies. In: Pedley T A, Meldrum B S (eds) Recent advances in epilepsy 3. Churchill Livingstone, Edinburgh, pp 157–187

Bird T D 1987 Genetic considerations in childhood epilepsy. Epilepsia 29: S71–S81

Buehler B A, Delimont D, van Waes M, Finnell R H 1990 Prenatal prediction of the risk of the fetal hydantoin syndrome. N Engl J Med 322: 1567–1572

Chattha A S, Richardson E P 1977 Cerebral white matter hypoplasia. Ann Neurol 34: 137–141

Delgado-Escueta A V, Greenberg D A, Treiman L et al 1989 Mapping the gene for juvenile myoclonic epilepsy. Epilepsia 30 (Suppl 4): S8–S18

Dobyns W B, Stratton R F, Parke J T et al 1983 Miller–Dieker syndrome: lissencephaly and monosomy 17p. J Pediatr 102: 552–558

Dorfman D H, Glaser J H 1990 Congenital syphilis presenting in infants after the newborn period. N Engl J Med 323: 1299–1302

Dunn H G, Robertson A M, Crichton J V 1986 Clinical outcome: neurological sequelae and their evolution. In: Dunn H G (ed) Sequelae of low birthweight: the Vancouver study. Clinics in developmental medicine nos 95/96. MacKeith Press, London, pp 68–96

Editorial 1990a Progress in tuberous sclerosis. Lancet 336: 598–599

Editorial 1990b Epilepsy and disorders of neuronal migration. Lancet 336: 1035

Edwards E F, Rench M A, Haffer A A M 1985 Long-term sequelae of group B streptococcal meningitis in infants. J Pediatr 106: 717–722

Gomez M R 1987 Tuberous sclerosis. In: Gomez M R (ed) Neurocutaneous diseases. Butterworths, Boston, pp 30–52

Gomez M R, Bebin E M 1987 Sturge–Weber syndrome. In: Gomez M R (ed) Neurocutaneous diseases. Butterworths, Boston, pp 356–367

Guerrini R, Bureau M, Mattei M-G et al 1990 Trisomy 12p syndrome: a chromosomal disorder associated with generalised 3 Hz spike and wave discharges. Epilepsia 31: 557–566

Jaeken J, Casaer P, de Cock P et al 1984 Gamma-amino-butyric acid transaminase deficiency: a newly recognised inborn error of neurotransmitter metabolism. Neuropediatrics 15: 165–169

Knoll J H M, Nicholls R D, Magenis R E et al 1989 Angelman and Prader–Willi syndromes share a common chromosome 15 deletion but differ in the parental origin of the deletion. Am J Med Genet 32: 285–290

Kunze J 1980 Neurological disorders in patients with chromosomal anomalies. Neuropediatrics 11: 203–230

Leppert M, Anderson V E, Quattlebaum T et al 1989 Benign familial convulsions linked to chromosome 20. Nature 337: 647–648

Minchom P, Niswander K, Chalmers I et al 1987 Antecedents and outcome of very early neonatal seizures in infants born at or near term. Br J Obstet Gynaecol 94: 431–439

Musumeci S A, Colognola R M, Ferri R et al 1988 Fragile X syndrome: a particular epileptogenic EEG pattern. Epilepsia 29: 41–47

Naidu S, Messmore H, Caserta V, Fine M 1983 CNS lesions in neonatal isoimmune thrombocytopenia. Arch Neurol 40: 552–554

Nelson K B, Ellenberg J H 1986 Antecedents of seizure disorders in childhood. Am J Dis Child 140: 1053–1061

North K N, Storey G N B, Henderson-Smart D J 1989 Fifth day fits in the newborn. Aust Paediatr J 25: 284–287

Ottman R, Hauser W A, Susser M 1985 Genetic and maternal influences on susceptibility to seizures: an analytical review. Am J Epidemiol 122: 923–939

Ottman R, Annegers J F, Hauser W A, Kurland L T 1988 Higher risk of seizures in offspring of mothers than of fathers with epilepsy. Am J Hum Genet 43: 257–264

Ottman R, Annegers J F, Hauser W A, Kurland L T 1989 Seizure risk in offspring of parents with generalized versus partial epilepsy. Epilepsia 30: 157–161

Preece P M, Pearl K N, Peckham C S 1984 Congenital cytomegalovirus infection. Arch Dis Child 59: 1120–1126

Riikonen R 1978 Cytomegalovirus and infantile spasms. Dev Med Child Neurol 20: 570–579

Rocca W A, Sharbrough F W, Hauser W A et al 1987a Risk factors for generalized tonic–clonic seizures: a population-based case–control study in Rochester, Minnesota.

Neurology 37: 1315–1322

Rocca W A, Sharbrough F W, Hauser W A et al 1987b Risk factors for complex partial seizures: a population-based case–control study. Ann Neurol 21: 22–31

Rocca W A, Sharbrough F W, Hauser W A et al 1987c Risk factors for absence seizures: a population-based case–control study in Rochester, Minnesota. Neurology 37: 1309–1314

Saukkonen A-L, Serlo W, von Wendt L 1990 Epilepsy in transhydrocephalic children. Acta Paediatr Scand 79: 212–218

Schmidt R, Eviatar L, Nitowsky H M et al 1981 Ring chromosome 14: a distinct clinical entity. J Med Genet 18: 304–307

Volpe J J 1987 Neurology of the newborn, 2nd edn. Saunders, Philadelphia

Willmore L J, Sypert G W, Munson J B 1978 Recurrent seizures induced by cortical iron injection: a model of post-traumatic epilepsy. Ann Neurol 4: 329–336

7

Post-traumatic epilepsy – mechanisms and prevention

L. J. Willmore

INTRODUCTION

Epilepsy complicates head trauma in about 7% of civilians (Annegers et al 1980) and 34% of combat-injured patients (Meirowsky 1982). The risk for developing post-traumatic epilepsy is generally related to the severity of injury, or the 'brain trauma dose' (Weiss et al 1983, 1986, Caveness 1976). Patients who have sustained severe head trauma and cortical injury resulting in neurological abnormalities on physical examination, but in whom the dura mater remains intact, have an incidence of epilepsy from 7% to 39%. Dural penetration, however, increased the occurrence of epilepsy from 20% to 57% (Caveness 1976).

Several attempts have been made to refine risk factors associated with epilepsy. Feeney & Walker (1979) applied a formula using weighted trauma categories, such as the neural location, agent of injury, severity, complications, and the presence of focal neurological findings. They found that the highest numerical values of risk were associated with missile wound with dural penetration, central–parietal location, occurrence of an early seizure, and presence of an intracerebral haematoma. The Vietnam Head Injury Survey found that predictive factors associated with epilepsy risk included cortical involvement, a moderate volume of brain tissue loss, intracerebral haematoma, and retained metal fragments (Salazar et al 1985). Others have noted that prolonged post-traumatic amnesia, presence of a cortical laceration occurring with a depressed skull fracture with dural laceration, and intracerebral haematoma occur more often in patients who develop post-traumatic epilepsy (Kaplan 1961, Jennett 1975). The risk of developing seizures is also increased following haemorrhagic cerebral infarction (Richardson & Dodge 1954, DeCarolis et al 1984) and spontaneous intracerebral haematoma (Faught et al 1989), suggesting that trauma-induced haemorrhage with deposition of blood in contact with the neuropil may be an important aetiologic factor (Jasper 1970, Levitt et al 1971, Willmore et al 1978).

The latency between head injury and development of epilepsy varies, although 57% of patients have onset of seizure within one year of injury (Salazar et al 1985). Whether a seizure occurs immediately after injury, within the first week, or beyond the first week, may have prognostic significance for development of epilepsy (Jennett & Teasdale 1981).

Immediate seizures, occurring within hours after trauma or a sequence of seizures with development of post-traumatic status epilepticus, can complicate management of an injured patient by causing hypoxia, hypertension and metabolic changes. Although an immediate seizure is commonly a non-specific reaction to head trauma, an intracranial haematoma must be excluded. An *early* seizure, i.e. one that occurs during the first week after injury, increases the incidence of late epilepsy (Jennett & Teasdale 1981).

MECHANISMS OF BRAIN INJURY

Blunt impact to the head with momentary skull deformation causes transient cavitation with transmission of mechanical forces and propagation of pressure waves through neural tissue (Pudenz & Shelden 1946, Lingren 1966). Mechanical forces of head injury induce changes that depend upon acceleration of the brain, application of rotational forces, shearing injury to fibre tracts and blood vessels, and contusion (Gennarelli et al 1982). Contusional haemorrhage is an admixture of red blood cells (RBCs), coagulation necrosis and oedema caused by mechanical disruption of blood vessels or by cellular diapedesis. Histopathological studies of traumatized brain show formation of axonal retraction balls, reactive gliosis, Wallerian degeneration and microglial star formation within cystic white matter lesions (Langfitt et al 1966, Unterharnscheidt & Sellier 1966, Tornheim et al 1983).

Mechanical effects of trauma also cause bulk displacement of tissue with secondary responses that include impaired cerebral vasomotor regulation, vasospasm, altered cerebral blood flow, changes in intracranial pressure and altered vascular permeability (Willmore 1990b). Delayed effects of acute head trauma include focal or diffuse brain oedema, ischaemia, necrosis, gliosis and neuronal loss.

BIOCHEMICAL EFFECTS OF BRAIN INJURY

Contusion or cortical laceration causes extravasation of RBCs with subsequent haemolysis, and deposition of haemoglobin within the neuropil. Iron liberated from haemoglobin and transferrin, sequestered as haemosiderin, is a prominent histopathological feature of human post-traumatic epilepsy (Payan et al 1970). Iron is critical to biological functions, but iron's two stable oxidation states and its redox properties pose a biological hazard. Although oxidation of ferrous iron to ferric is a simple reaction resulting in insoluble hydroxide complexes, autoxidation reactions in aqueous solution or biological fluids, with or without chelators, causes a complicated series of one-electron transfer reactions yielding free radical intermediates (Aisen 1977). Addition of iron salts or haem compounds to solutions containing polyunsaturated fatty acids (PUFA) or to suspensions of subcellular organelles results in the formation of highly reactive free radical oxidants, including perferryl ions, superoxide radicals singlet oxygen and hydroxyl radicals (Aisen 1977, Svingen et al 1978, Fong et al 1973, 1976, Willmore et al 1983). Although free radical species probably form by iron-catalysed Haber–Weiss reactions (Czapski & Ilan 1978, Koppenol et al 1978), these oxidants are also actively generated by biologically chelated forms of iron such as in haem or with ADP (Fong et al 1976, Aust & Svingen 1982).

Free radicals react with methylene groups adjacent to double bonds of PUFA and lipids within cellular membranes, causing hydrogen abstraction and subsequent propagation of peroxidation reactions (Fong et al 1976). This non-enzymatic initiation and propagation of lipid peroxidation disrupts the membranes of subcellular organelles, degrades deoxyribose and amino acids, and yields diene conjugates and fluorescent chromophores (Baker & Wilson 1966, Niehaus & Samuelsson 1968, Triggs & Willmore 1984). Inorganic iron salts, haematin and haemoproteins stimulate peroxidation of microsomal and mitochrondrial lipids, and also change cellular thiodisulphide function (Smith & Dunkley 1962). Alkyl hydroxyl and peroxyl species of fatty acids propagate until a membrane constituent capable of electron donation without formation of a free radical is encountered and a termination reaction occurs. Such constituents include tocopherol, cholesterol, proteins or the sulphydryl group of glutathione (Aust & Svingen 1982, Willmore & Rubin 1984, Anderson & Means 1983). Pretreating animals with α-tocopherol and selenium prevents the histopathological changes that occur following injection of aqueous iron into neural tissue. This further supports the hypothesis that peroxidative reactions are important in trauma-induced brain injury responses (Willmore & Rubin 1981, 1984, Anderson & Means 1983).

CELLULAR MECHANISMS OF INJURY-RELATED EPILEPTOGENESIS

Interictal epileptiform discharges reflect stereotyped cellular events, the hallmark of which is the paroxysmal depolarization shift (PDS) (Prince & Connors 1984). Transition from interictal to ictal discharge is characterized by loss of hyperpolarization and by synchronization of neurones in the focus. Amplification of excitatory postsynaptic potentials (EPSPs) that underlie the PDS result from several mechanisms, including reduction in inhibition, frequency potentiation of EPSPs, change in the space constant of the dendrites of the postsynaptic neurone, activation of the N-methyl-D-aspartate (NMDA) receptor, and potentiation by neuromodulators (Dichter & Ayala 1987).

Biochemical injury to neurones causes a sequence of changes, ranging from frank cellular loss and gliosis to subtle alterations in neuronal plasma membranes. Membrane changes initiated by biochemical consequences of injury may critically alter the densities and distribution of ion channels on neuronal membranes so that the threshold for action potential generation is towards net excitation and cells become progressively depolarized. Cellular bursting may also develop from increases in extracellular K^+ or reduced amounts of extracellular Ca^{2+}. Development or recruitment of neurones sufficient to cause clinical manifestations requires synchronization of a critical mass of cells (Prince & Connors 1984, Dichter & Ayala 1987).

The mechanisms or critical physiological changes underlying post-traumatic epileptogenesis remain unknown. However, several processes are likely candidates for further investigation. Trauma that results in mechanical shearing of fibre tracts could lead to loss of inhibitory interneurones from anterograde trans-synaptic neuronal degeneration (Saji & Reis 1987). Trauma-induced release of aspartate or glutamate with activation of NMDA receptors (Faden et al 1989), elaboration of nerve growth factor (Gall & Isackson 1989) or enhancement of reactive gliosis may be operant as well (Nieto-Sampedro 1988). Hippocampal tissue obtained during surgical resection for temporal lobe seizures and stained for acetylcholinesterase shows enhanced staining in the outer portion of the molecular layer of the dentate gyrus (Green et al 1989). Histochemical staining of rodent kindled hippocampus shows abundant mossy fibre synaptic terminals in the supragranular region and the inner molecular layer of the dentate gyrus (Sutula et al 1989). Although speculative, synaptic reorganization may increase recurrent excitation in granule cells, which favours epileptogenesis. Experimental foci demonstrate a reduction in the number of axosomatic GABAergic terminals as represented by asymmetrical synapses. The GABAergic pericellular basket plexus, which provides tonic inhibition to pyramidal cells, was thought likely to have a high dependence on aerobic metabolism because of the large numbers of mitochondria, and may be especially vulnerable to hypoxia (Ribak et al 1979).

GENETIC FACTORS

Cellular responses to free radical oxidants that result from decompartmentalization of haemoglobin or iron-containing haem compounds include induction of protective mechanisms. For example, strains of *Escherichia coli* can be differentiated by measuring the effects caused by exposure to peroxide. Fenton-derived free radicals cause DNA damage that is repaired by enzymes critical for cell survival (Imlay & Linn 1988, Carlsson & Carpenter 1980). More speculatively, it may be that free radicals also injure membranes in ways that lead to long-term excitability changes that favour development of epileptiform activity. Thus, differences in susceptibility to develop epilepsy after a given trauma dose may be related to the effectiveness of repair response that are induced following initiation of lipid peroxidation.

Specific genetic factors that determine the brain's liability to develop post-traumatic epilepsy are presently unknown. However, one possible mechanism for genetic predisposition relates to the observation of decreased levels of serum haptoglobin in familial epilepsy (Panter et al 1985). Haptoglobins are acute-phase glycoproteins in the α_1-globulin fraction of serum that form stable complexes with haemoglobin (Gutteridge 1987). Because the extracellular fluid does not contain high concentrations of antioxidants such as superoxide dismutase and peroxidases, preventing or containing harmful oxidative reactions must depend upon effective binding of reactive metals to carrier proteins, such as transferrin, lactoferrin, ceruloplasmin and haptoglobins (Gutteridge 1987). Sequestration of free haemoglobin by haptoglobin is one mechanism to prevent induction of oxidant stress. Thus the discovery that some patients with epilepsy have a genetically impaired ability to synthesize these glycoproteins may reflect an inherent susceptibility of some individuals to developing epilepsy after head trauma.

PROPHYLAXIS AND PREVENTION

Prophylaxis is a process of reducing chances for developing a specific disease or disorder by treatment or other action that affects pathogenesis. Prevention renders a process impossible by performing an action in advance of an event (Willmore 1990a). An example of prevention is administering anticonvulsant drugs to patients with severe head trauma to prevent seizures so that complications from hypertension and hypoxia are eliminated. That is, antiepileptic drugs may be used not just to suppress seizures but to prevent complications associated with convulsive seizures. Prophylactic use of antiepileptic drugs in patients with head trauma, or for patients undergoing neurosurgical procedures on the brain, has the intent of interfering with epileptogenesis. Although using antiepileptic drugs to suppress acute seizures that occur following head injury is a practical and realistic goal (Temkin et al 1990), such treatment is unlikely to be effective prophylaxis against developing epilepsy.

Clinical reports indicating that antiepileptic drugs given prophylactically were effective in preventing the occurrence of post-traumatic epilepsy have appeared for many years (Rapport & Penry 1972). Young et al (1979) observed a 6% incidence of post-traumatic epilepsy occurrence in their treated group of head-injured patients and compared this with the incidence of post-traumatic seizures in historical controls. They concluded that early administration of antiepileptic drugs prevented the development of post-traumatic epilepsy and recommended prophylactic administration of phenytoin to patients with a 15% or greater risk of developing post-traumatic epilepsy. Rish & Caveness (1973) did not detect a difference in the occurrence of early seizures between phenytoin-treated and untreated patients. However, Wohns & Wyler (1979) reviewed patients selected because of critical trauma indicators that included depressed skull fracture,

Table 7.1   Summary of double-blind, placebo-controlled, prospective studies of the efficacy of antiepileptic drugs as prophylaxis of post-traumatic epilepsy

Authors	Drug	Percentage developing epilepsy	
		Control	Treated
Penry et al (1979)	Phenytoin Phenobarbitone	13	23
Young et al (1983)	Phenytoin	10.8	12.9
Temkin et al (1990)	Phenytoin	21.1	27.5

dural or cortical laceration, or a prolonged period of post-traumatic amnesia. Although the authors acknowledged the selection bias in their study, they concluded that antiepileptic drug administration prevented the development of post-traumatic epilepsy.

Because uncontrolled studies such as the former examples had suggested that antiepileptic drugs might be effective prophylaxis against developing epilepsy, prospective, placebo-controlled trials have been undertaken (Table 7.1). Penry et al (1979) administered phenytoin and phenobarbitone to head-injured patients in a double-blind fashion, using placebo control. Seizure probability in the treated group was 23%, and 13% in the controls – not a significant difference. They concluded that routine antiepileptic drug use did not affect the risk of developing post-traumatic epilepsy.

Young et al (1983) carried out a double-blind, prospective study of 179 head-injured patients treated with phenytoin or with placebo for 18 months. Eighty-five patients were included in the treated group, and 74 patients were enrolled as placebo controls. Seizures occurred in 12.9% of the treated patients, and in 10.8% of the control patients. The most rigorous study to date is that of Temkin et al (1990), who reported their experience with 404 patients treated prospectively. Patients with severe head trauma were assigned to receive an intravenous loading dose of either phenytoin or placebo. Serum levels were measured at regular intervals, blood levels of drug were maintained in the therapeutic range, and efforts were made to assure that evaluations were blinded. At one year there was no difference in the incidence of post-traumatic epilepsy between treated and control groups. At the same time they observed that phenytoin effectively suppressed seizures during the acute period immediately after injury. At two years, however, seizures had occurred in 27.5% of phenytoin-treated patients and in 21.1% of controls.

ALTERATION OF BRAIN INJURY RESPONSES

Because antiepileptic drugs administered prophylactically fail to inhibit epileptogenesis, are there biochemical strategies that could disrupt brain injury responses associated with development of epilepsy?

Antiperoxidants

Hydroxyl radicals, superoxide radicals and peroxides generated in biological systems by oxidative reactions or by actions of haem-containing compounds liberated within lipid systems are quenched by action of enzymes such as catalase, peroxidase and superoxide dismutase (Fridovich 1974). Glutathione peroxidase, using glutathione as a cosubstrate and selenium as a metallic cofactor, reduces intracellular formation of hydrogen peroxide and free radicals. Oxidative stress increases activity of glutathione reductase, glucose 6-phosphate dehydrogenase and glutathione peroxidase (Tappel 1973, Orlowski & Karkowsky 1976). Selenium, a metallic cofactor of glutathione peroxidase, also seems to act synergistically with α-tocopherol in preventing peroxidation of structural membrane components.

α-Tocopherol prevents peroxidative injury of sulphydryl groups of glycolipids and glycoproteins, apparently augmenting the antioxidant effects of enzyme systems such as glutathione peroxidase. Tocopherol also prevents peroxidation of unsaturated fatty acids and lipids by reaction of phenolic hydroxyl groups with propagating lipid radicals that were initiated by oxidative carbonyl hydrogen abstraction (Tappel 1972, Rehncrona et al 1980, McCay & King 1980, Witting 1980). Further, the phytyl side chain of tocopherol may intercalate within the acyl chains of polyunsaturated phospholipids, causing lipid membrane stabilization and reduction in membrane permeability (Diplock & Lucy 1973, Lucy 1972). Tocopherol may also act as a free radical scavenger and singlet oxygen quenching agent (Witting 1980). A novel non-glucocorticoid 21-aminosteroid with properties of inhibiting iron-dependent lipid peroxidation had a salutary effect on outcome following concussive injury to mice (Hall et al 1988).

Antioxidants

Superoxide radicals induce cellular and vasogenic oedema (Chan & Fishman 1980, Fishman et al 1979, Wagner & Stewart 1981). Initiation of focal oedema by cold-induced injury to the cerebral cortex of rodents causes increased levels of superoxide radicals (Chan & Fishman 1980). Administration of liposome-entrapped copper–zinc superoxide dismutase interferes with the development of cold-induced oedema, suggesting that superoxide dismutase interruption of oxygen-free radical-induced fatty acid injury may have potential for interruption of trauma-induced brain injury (Chan & Fishman 1980).

RECOMMENDATIONS

Decisions about how to manage head-injured patients to reduce the risk of post-traumatic epilepsy are confounded by the lack of specific information upon which to base recommendations. All efforts to provide prophylactic treatment should be accompanied by informed consent for patients and members of families. Misunderstanding about the intent of treatment with antiepileptic drugs may cause problems with compliance or leave the impression that discontinuation of such medication has left a patient vulnerable to development of epilepsy. Because long-term prophylaxis with conventional antiepileptic drugs has never been shown to prevent post-traumatic epilepsy, the following guidelines represent one approach to the rational use of such drugs in the management of these patients.

1. *High-risk patients*: those patients with head injury of such severity that risk of seizure occurrence is high and in whom the physiological consequences of seizures would complicate management should receive preventive phenytoin. Phenytoin effectively suppresses seizures in the acute period following injury. The patient should receive an intravenous loading dose of 18 mg/kg at a rate not to exceed 40 mg/min. A maintenance dose of 5 mg/kg per day should be given intravenously until such time that oral administration is possible. Care should be taken to avoid simultaneous feeding and drug administration via nasogastric tube. Blood levels should be maintained within the recognized therapeutic range of $10-20\,\mu g/ml$. Because an allergic rash may develop in as many as 10% of patients treated in this fashion, regular inspection of the skin should be performed. If such an allergic reaction occurs, substitution of phenobarbitone should be considered.

2. *Maintenance of prophylactic treatment*: available data suggest that treatment with phenytoin is effective only in prevention of seizures for the first month after injury. One method would be to maintain therapeutic plasma levels of phenytoin for at least three months after injury. At that time the drug should be tapered over the following six weeks. Obtaining an EEG prior to initiating drug taper may be helpful. Although the EEG has not been predictive of the potential for developing epilepsy immediately after injury, the observation of epileptiform patterns on the EEG after three months may be of value.

3. *Discontinuing treatment*: physicians choose arbitrary times after injury to discontinue medication in the absence of seizures. Patients occasionally are maintained on antiepileptic drugs for six months or up to two years. Because available data fail to support any efficacy for long-term treatment, early taper is preferred. One specific dilemma occurs when a patient has been maintained on long-term prophylaxis, occasionally for years after a head injury. In such cases, physicians often use extremely long taper times to avoid precipitating a drug withdrawal seizure. There are, however, no data to support such an approach. In addition, anxiety about drug withdrawal may confound full and informed participation by the patient in these circumstances. Special precautions regarding driving during the time of drug taper must be individualized. Realistic discussion of risk of seizure occurrence coupled with EEG assessment followed by drug

withdrawal over six weeks may be best.

4. *Natural history of post-traumatic epilepsy*: as with other forms of epilepsy, those patients with few seizures which are easily controlled tend to have the best prognosis. Walker & Erculei (1970) observed that 50% of such patients identified as having post-traumatic epilepsy would be in complete remission by 15 years after injury. Assessment and decisions about discontinuing medication after a long seizure-free interval should be governed by guidelines that apply to any patient who is a candidate for antiepileptic drug withdrawal (Callaghan et al 1988, Chadwick & Reynolds 1985).

REFERENCES

Aisen P 1977 Some physicochemical aspects of iron metabolism. Ciba Foundation Symposium. Elsevier, New York, pp 1–14

Anderson D K, Means E D 1983 Lipid peroxidation in spinal cord: $FeCl_2$ induction and protection with antioxidants. Neurochem Pathol 1: 249–264

Annegers J F, Grabow J D, Grover R V et al 1980 Seizures after head trauma: a population study. Neurology 30: 683–689

Aust S D, Svingen B A 1982 The role of iron in enzymatic lipid peroxidation. In: Pryor W A (ed) Free radicals in biology. Academic Press, New York, pp 1–28

Baker N, Wilson L 1966 Water-soluble products of UV-irradiated, autoxidized linoleic and linolenic acids. J Lipid Res 7: 341–348

Callaghan N, Garrett A, Goggin T 1988 Withdrawal of anticonvulsant drugs in patients free of seizures for two years. N Engl J Med 318: 942–946

Carlsson J, Carpenter V S 1980 The recA$^+$ gene produce is more important than catalase and superoxide dismutase in protecting *Escherichia coli* against hydrogen peroxide toxicity. J Bacteriol 142: 319–321

Caveness W F 1976 Epilepsy, a product of trauma in our time. Epilepsia 17: 207–215

Chadwick D, Reynolds E H 1985 When do epileptic patients need treatment? Starting and stopping medication. Br Med J 290: 1885–1888

Chan P H, Fishman R A 1980 Transient formation of superoxide radicals in polyunsaturated fatty acid-induced brain swelling. J Neurochem 35: 1004–1007

Czapski G, Ilan Y A 1978 On the generation of the hydroxylation agent from superoxide radical: can the Haber–Weiss reaction be the source of OH radicals? Photochem Photobiol 28: 651–653

DeCarolis P, D'Alessandro R, Ferrara R et al 1984 Late seizures in patients with internal carotid and middle cerebral artery occlusive disease following ischaemic events. J Neurol Neurosurg Psychiatry 47: 1345–1347

Dichter M A, Ayala G F 1987 Cellular mechanisms of epilepsy: a status report. Science 237: 157–164

Diplock A T, Lucy J A 1973 The biochemical modes of action of vitamin E and selenium: a hypothesis. FEBS Lett 29: 205–210

Faden A I, Demediuk P, Panter S S et al 1989 The role of excitatory amino acids and NMDA receptors in traumatic brain injury. Science 244: 798–800

Faught E, Peters D, Bartolucci A et al 1989 Seizures after primary intracerebral hemorrhage. Neurology 39: 1089–1093

Feeney D M, Walker A E 1979 The prediction of posttraumatic epilepsy: a mathematical approach. Arch Neurol 36: 8–12

Fishman R A, Chan P H, Lee J et al 1979 Effects of superoxide free radicals on the induction of brain edema. Neurology 29: 546

Fong K L, McCay B P, Poyer J L et al 1973 Evidence that peroxidation of lysosomal membranes is initiated by hydroxyl free radicals produced during flavin enzyme activity. J Biol Chem 248: 7792–7797

Fong K L, McCay P B, Poyer J L et al 1976 Evidence of superoxide-dependent reduction of Fe^{3+} and its role in enzyme-generated hydroxyl radical formation. Chem-Biol Interactions 15: 77–89

Fridovich I 1974 Superoxide dismutase. Adv Enzymol 41: 35–97

Gall C M, Isackson P J 1989 Limbic seizures increase neuronal production of messenger RNA for nerve growth factor. Science 245: 758–761

Gennarelli T A, Thibaulat L E, Adams J H et al 1982 Diffuse axonal injury and traumatic coma in the primate. Ann Neurol 12: 564–574

Green R C, Blume H W, Kupferschmid S B et al 1989 Alterations of hippocampal acetylcholinesterase in human temporal lobe epilepsy. Ann Neurol 26: 347–351

Gutteridge J M C 1987 The antioxidant activity of haptoglobin towards haemoglobin-stimulated lipid peroxidation. Biochim Biophys Acta 917: 219–223

Hall E D, Yonkers P A, McCall J M et al 1988 Effects of the 21-aminosteroid U74006F on experimental head injury in mice. J Neurosurg 68: 456–461

Imlay J A, Linn S 1988 DNA damage and oxygen radical toxicity. Science 240: 1302–1309

Jasper H H 1970 Physiopathological mechanisms of post traumatic epilepsy. Epilepsia 11: 73–80

Jennett B 1975 Epilepsy and acute traumatic intracranial haematoma. J Neurol Neurosurg Psychiatry 38: 378–381

Jennett B, Teasdale G 1981 Management of head injuries. Davis, Philadelphia

Kaplan H A 1961 Management of craniocerebral trauma and its relation to subsequent seizures. Epilepsia 2: 111–116

Koppenol W H, Butler J, van Leeuwen J W 1978 The Haber–Weiss cycle. Photochem Photobiol 28: 655–660

Langfitt T W, Weinstein J D, Kassell N F 1966 Vascular factors in head injury: contribution to brain-swelling and intracranial hypertension. In: Caveness W E, Walker A E (eds) Head injury. Lippincott, Philadelphia, pp 172–194

Levitt P, Wilson W P, Wilkins R H 1971 The effects of subarachnoid blood on the electrocorticogram of the cat. J Neurosurg 35: 185–191

Lingren S O 1966 Experimental studies of mechanical effects in head injury. Acta Chir Scand 132 (Suppl 360): 1–32

Lucy J A 1972 Functional and structural aspects of biological membranes: a suggested structural role for vitamin E in the control of membrane permeability and stability. Ann NY Acad Sci 203: 4–11

McCay P B, King M M 1980 Vitamin E: its role as a biologic free radical scavenger and its relationship to the microsomal mixed-function oxidase system. In: Machlin L J (ed) Vitamin E. Marcel Dekker, New York, pp 289–317

Meirowsky A M 1982 Notes on posttraumatic epilepsy in missile wounds of the brain. Milit Med 147: 632–634

Niehaus W G, Samuelsson B 1968 Formation of malonaldehyde from phospholipid arachidonate during microsomal lipid peroxidation. Eur J Biochem 6: 126–130

Nieto-Sampedro M 1988 Astrocyte mitogen inhibitor related to epidermal growth factor receptor. Science 240: 1784–1786

Orlowski M, Karlowsky A 1976 Glutathione metabolism and some possible functions of glutathione in the nervous system. Internat Rev Neurobiol 19: 75–121

Panter S S, Sadrzadeh S M, Hallaway P E et al 1985 Hypohaptoglobinemia associated with familial epilepsy. J Exp Med 161: 748–754

Payan H, Toga M, Berard-Badier M 1970 The pathology of post-traumatic epilepsies. Epilepsia 11: 81–94

Penry J K, White B G, Brackett C E 1979 A controlled prospective study of the pharmacologic prophylaxis of posttraumatic epilepsy. Neurology 29: 600–601

Prince D A, Connors B W 1984 Mechanisms of epileptogenesis in cortical structures. Ann Neurol 16 (Suppl): S59–S64

Pudenz R H, Shelden C H 1946 The lucite calvarium-a method for direct observation of the brain. J Neurosurg 3: 487–505

Rapport R L, Penry J K 1972 Pharmacologic prophylaxis of post-traumatic epilepsy: a review. Epilepsia 13: 295–304

Rehncrona S, Smith D S, Akesson B et al 1980 Peroxidative changes in brain cortical fatty acids and phospholipids, as characterized during Fe^{2+}- and ascorbic acid-stimulated lipid peroxidation in vitro. J Neurochem 34: 1630–1638

Ribak C E, Harris A B, Vaughn J E et al 1979 Inhibitory GABAergic nerve terminals decrease at sites of focal epilepsy. Science 205: 211–214

Richardson E P, Dodge P R 1954 Epilepsy in cerebrovascular disease. Epilepsia 3 (Series 3): 49–74

Rish B L, Caveness W F 1973 Relation of prophylactic medication to the occurrence of early seizures following craniocerebral trauma. J Neurosurg 38: 155–158

Saji M, Reis D J 1987 Delayed transneuronal death of substantia nigra neurons prevented by gamma-aminobutyric acid agonist. Science 235: 66–69

Salazar A M, Jabbari B, Vance S C et al 1985 Epilepsy after penetrating head injury. I. Clinical correlates: a report of the Vietnam Head Injury Study. Neurology 35: 1406–1414

Smith G J, Dunkley W L 1962 Initiation of lipid peroxidation by a reduced metal ion. Arch Biochem Biophys 98: 46–48

Sutula T, Cascino G, Cavazos J et al 1989 Mossy fiber synaptic reorganization in the epileptic human temporal lobe. Ann Neurol 26: 321–330

Svingen B A, O'Neal F O, Aust S D 1978 The role of superoxide and singlet oxygen in lipid peroxidation. Photochem Photobiol 28: 803–809

Tappel A L 1972 Vitamin E and free radical peroxidation of lipids. Ann NY Acad Sci 203: 12–28

Tappel A L 1973 Lipid peroxidation damage to cell components. Fed Proc 32: 1870–1874

Temkin N R, Dikmen S S, Wilensky A J et al 1990 A randomized, double-blind study of phenytoin for the prevention of post-traumatic seizures. N Engl J Med 323: 497–502

Tornheim P A, Liwnicz B H, Hirsch C S et al 1983 Acute responses to blunt head trauma. J Neurosurg 59: 431–438

Triggs W J, Willmore L J 1984 In vitro lipid peroxidation in rat brain following intracortical Fe^{++} injection. J Neurochem 42: 976–980

Unterharnscheidt F, Sellier K 1966 Mechanisms and pathomorphology of closed head injuries. In: Caveness W F, Walker A E (eds) Head injury. Lippincott, Philadelphia, pp 321–341

Wagner F C, Stewart W B 1981 Effect of trauma dose on spinal cord edema. J Neurosurg 54: 8802–8806

Walker A E, Erculei F 1970 Post-traumatic epilepsy 15 years later. Epilepsia 11: 17–26

Weiss G H, Feeney D M, Caveness W F et al 1983 Prognostic factors for the occurrence of posttraumatic epilepsy. Arch Neurol 40: 7–10

Weiss G H, Salazar A M, Vance S C et al 1986 Predicting posttraumatic epilepsy in penetrating head injury. Arch Neurol 43: 771–773

Willmore L J 1990a Prophylactic use of anticonvulsant drugs. In: Resor S R, Kutt H (eds) Medical treatment of epilepsy. Marcel Dekker, New York (in press)

Willmore L J 1990b Posttraumatic epilepsy: cellular mechanisms and implications for treatment. Epilepsia 31: S67–S73

Willmore L J, Rubin J J 1981 Antiperoxidant pretreatment and iron-induced epileptiform discharge in the rat: EEG and histopathologic study. Neurology 31: 63–69

Willmore L J, Rubin J J 1984 Effects of antiperoxidants on $FeCl_2$-induced lipid peroxidation and focal edema in rat brain. Exp Neurol 83: 62–70

Willmore L J, Sypert G W, Munson J B 1978 Recurrent seizures induced by cortical iron injection: a model of post-traumatic epilepsy. Ann Neurol 4: 329–336

Willmore L J, Hiramatsu M, Kochi H et al 1983 Formation of superoxide radicals, lipid peroxides and edema after $FeCl_3$ injection into rat isocortex. Brain Res 277: 393–396

Witting L A 1980 Vitamin E and lipid antioxidants in free-radical-initiated reactions. In: Pryor W A (ed) Free radicals in biology, Vol 4. Academic Press, New York, pp 295–319

Wohns R N W, Wyler A R 1979 Prophylactic phenytoin in severe head injuries. J Neurosurg 51: 507–509

Young B, Rapp R, Brooks W H et al 1979 Post-traumatic epilepsy prophylaxis. Epilepsia 20: 671–681

Young B, Rapp R P, Norton J A et al 1983 Failure of prophylactically administered phenytoin to prevent late post traumatic seizures. J Neurosurg 58: 236–241

8

Seizures and HIV infection

D. R. Labar

INTRODUCTION

Human immunodeficiency virus (HIV) infection and acquired immunodeficiency syndrome (AIDS) have grown to pandemic proportions in the 1980's. By 1992, it is likely that there will be 440 000 AIDS cases in the USA and 1 000 000 worldwide; 1.5 million persons are believed to be infected currently with HIV in the USA alone (i.e. HIV seropositive). Neurological manifestations are frequent (50–75% of AIDS cases, more common in children), and include disorders of the central and peripheral nervous system due to neoplasms, opportunistic infections and HIV infection itself. The neurological manifestations of HIV infection and AIDS have been reviewed recently (Elder & Sever 1988, Janssen et al 1989).

Early reports of various neurological manifestations of HIV infection and AIDS consistently noted the occurrence of seizures, but details were lacking. Among 4 children with AIDS and progressive encephalopathy, 2 had seizures (one recurrent generalized and one single focal motor). In all 4 children, electroencephalography (EEG) demonstrated diffuse background slowing, but the patient with generalized seizures had bilateral spike–wave discharges, and the patient with a focal seizure had bilateral attenuation of EEG activity in the occipital regions. Postmortem examination of the brains of these 2 children revealed diffuse atrophy and gliosis, but secondary opportunistic infections were not present (Epstein et al 1985). Among 20 children with progressive encephalopathy due to HIV infection (16 AIDS, 3 AIDS-related complex, one HIV seropositive only), 5 had seizures. These were isolated events, usually associated with a febrile illness (Epstein et al 1986). Of 46 patients with AIDS–dementia complex, 3 had seizures early in the course of their illnesses, and 6 more developed seizures late in their course. All of these underwent postmortem neuropathological examination, and none had evidence of focal brain disease or opportunistic infection (Navia et al 1986). Several other reports have noted that 12–18% of patients with neurological manifestations of HIV infection or AIDS have seizures (Belec et al 1989, Belman et al 1986, Epstein et al 1988).

These early reports raised several basic questions about seizures in patients with HIV infection and AIDS:

1. What is the occurrence rate and clinical setting of seizures in HIV infection and AIDS?
2. Do seizures, whether focal or generalized, indicate an increased risk of secondary central nervous system (CNS) disease (toxoplasmosis, lymphoma, cryptococcal meningitis), or are seizures more likely to be associated with HIV infection alone?
3. Are the seizures associated with HIV infection and AIDS more likely to be single or recurrent? Is treatment with antiepileptic drugs effective in preventing recurrence, and what medication toxicities occur?

Several recent studies have attempted to address these issues (Aronow et al 1989, Holtzman et al 1989, Rosenbaum et al 1989, Wong et al 1990), and this chapter will review these reports, especially with reference to the foregoing questions.

INCIDENCE AND CLINICAL SETTING OF SEIZURES IN HIV INFECTION

In reviewing the New York Hospital experience from 1984 to 1988, we identified 630 patients with HIV infection using hospital discharge diagnoses codes, Neurology Consult Service records, and Autopsy Service records. Diagnoses included AIDS, AIDS-related complex and seropositivity for HIV exposure. Of these 630, 70 had new-onset seizures – an incidence of 11% (Wong et al 1990). This figure is a somewhat lower occurrence rate than the 15–20% noted in smaller, earlier series. The discrepancy may reflect selection bias toward more severe cases in the earlier series, as most of those included only patients with neurological manifestations of AIDS, not the more broadly defined population we studied. Although ours was a hospital-based study, we do not believe our findings represent simply the seizure rate among the terminally ill, because a review of records for the 277 consecutive patients who died at New York Hospital in a three-month period revealed a seizure incidence of 4.7% (χ^2, 12.9; $p < 0.01$). Two other recent series (Aronow et al 1989, Holtzman et al 1989) did not address incidence questions.

Most seizures in patients with HIV infection or AIDS are generalized. In our study, 74% of patients had only generalized seizures, 20% had generalized and partial seizures, and 6% had only partial seizures (Wong et al 1990). Similarly, Holtzman et al (1989) reported that 65% of patients had generalized seizures and 35% had partial seizures, while Aronow et al (1989) indicated that 74% of seizures were generalized and 26% were partial. Partial seizures occurred in the absence of demonstrable focal brain disease, and were attributed to meningitis, systemic metabolic derangements, or HIV infection of the brain itself.

Status epilepticus has been noted frequently and may carry a poor prognosis. In one recent series, all 7 patients with status died within one

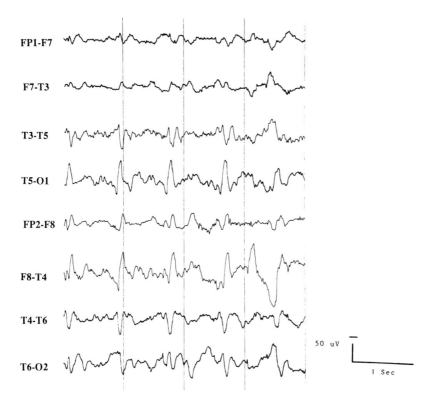

FP1-F7

F7-T3

T3-T5

T5-O1

FP2-F8

F8-T4

T4-T6

T6-O2

50 uV

I Sec

Fig. 8.1   EEG from a 29-year-old man with AIDS–dementia complex who had an acute deterioration in mental status. Findings indicate electrographic (and clinical) generalized non-convulsive status epilepticus.

month of the episode (Aronow et al 1989). We had 10 patients with status (7 convulsive, 3 non-convulsive) (Wong et al 1990), and Holtzman et al (1989) found 8 patients with status. The high frequency of generalized seizures and status epilepticus suggests that the HIV-infected brain has both a diffuse increase in cortical excitability and impaired mechanisms for terminating seizure activity.

In our series of patients with HIV infection and seizures, we had a particularly notable case of generalized non-convulsive status epilepticus. A 29-year-old man with mild dementia consistent with the AIDS–dementia complex (Navia et al 1986) suddenly developed a severe encephalopathy. He was awake but nearly mute, followed no commands, and showed no evidence of comprehension. An EEG revealed continuous, repetitive generalized sharp-wave discharges (Fig. 8.1). After treatment with intravenous diazepam, the electrographic seizure discharge disappeared, and the patient's mental status returned to baseline (Fig. 8.2). Non-convulsive status epilepticus should be considered in the differential diagnosis of acutely

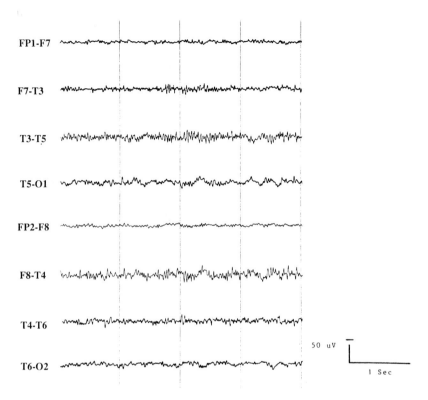

FP1-F7

F7-T3

T3-T5

T5-O1

FP2-F8

F8-T4

T4-T6

T6-O2

50 uV

1 Sec

Fig. 8.2   EEG in the same patient as Fig. 8.1 after administration of intravenous diazepam, with resolution of the electrographic seizure activity and return to baseline mental status.

altered mental status in patients with AIDS, and prompt EEG recording will lead to the correct diagnosis.

Although seizures can occur early in HIV-infected patients who have no other indication of CNS dysfunction (Rosenbaum et al 1989), most seizures are seen late in this illness. At the time of first seizure in our 70 patients, 10 were seropositive for HIV infection only, 10 had AIDS-related complex, and 50 had AIDS (Wong et al 1990). In the 100 patients reviewed by Holtzman et al (1989), 18 had seizures as the presenting symptom of HIV infection, 15 had AIDS-related complex, and 67 had AIDS. An increasing number of patients with the AIDS–dementia complex have seizures as the disease progresses. Among 46 cases, 3 had seizures early when cognitive decline was mild, but 6 other cases had seizures late, when dementia was severe (Navia et al 1986). Although overall this may reflect the increasing frequency of secondary CNS disease (infectious or neoplastic) that occurs late in the course of AIDS, that clearly was not the case in patients with AIDS–dementia complex described by Navia et al (1986), because an inclusion criterion for that study was postmortem examination of the patients' brains indicating they were free of secondary CNS diseases.

The diffuse cerebral cortical atrophy seen late in the AIDS–dementia complex (Petito 1988) suggests that HIV infection leads to progressive diffuse cortical damage producing neuronal or glial atrophy or loss, or both; this progressive cortical damage may contribute to the increased occurrence rate of seizures late in AIDS. Late widespread cortical damage also may contribute to the high incidence of generalized seizures and status epilepticus (see above). If the end result of progressive diffuse cortical damage contributes to the occurrence of status epilepticus, this may explain the observation by Aronow et al (1989) that all 7 of the patients in their series with status epilepticus died within one month after the episode of status. Thus status epilepticus may be a signature of late, severe AIDS, and the status itself may not contribute significantly to mortality.

Several clinical circumstances surrounding seizures in HIV infection appear to be of little significance. Risk factors for contracting the HIV infection in our 70 seizure patients were similar to risk factors present in the general population of AIDS patients in New York City (homosexuality 38, intravenous drug abuse 17, homosexuality and intravenous drug abuse 2, blood transfusions 4, and unknown 9) (New York City Department of Health 1987, Wong et al 1990). EEGs were performed infrequently, most likely because the responsible physicians believed that diagnosis and treatment could be reliably based on symptoms and findings on neurological examination, lumbar puncture and neuroimaging studies, without results from EEGs. In fact, those expectations were met: only 20 of our 70 patients underwent EEGs (those showed slowing in 19 and epileptiform activity in 5) (Wong et al 1990), and only 16 of the 100 patients described in the paper by Holtzman et al (1989) had EEGs (those showed slowing in 10). Using a different investigational approach, Gabuzda et al (1988) described EEG findings in 47 patients with AIDS; 28 had clinical neurological disease, 6 had seizures, and 4 of those 6 had focal slowing or sharp waves. Thus, although EEGs are usually abnormal, it appears that the findings add little new diagnostic information in patients with seizures associated with HIV infection; even patients with definite seizures may have normal studies. On the other hand, the occasional finding of epileptiform discharges in EEGs of patients with 'attacks' of unclear nature may be of diagnostic value, such as in the case of generalized non-convulsive status epilepticus described above.

CAUSES OF SEIZURES IN PATIENTS WITH HIV INFECTION AND AIDS

In the larger recent case studies describing patients with seizures and HIV infection or AIDS, neuroimaging studies were usually obtained shortly after the first seizure. In light of the well-known occurrence of opportunistic infections and neoplasms in the brains of AIDS patients, it was somewhat surprising that only 30–50% of patients had focal lesions demonstrated on computerized tomographic (CT) or magnetic resonance imaging (MRI) brain scans (Aronow et al 1989, Holtzman et al 1989, Wong et al 1990). Among the remaining patients, approximately half had diffuse atrophy, and half had normal studies.

Neuroimaging, lumbar puncture, systemic medical and postmortem neuropathological analyses were combined to determine causes of seizures. Fifty to 60% of patients had a secondary disease process which could be implicated as the seizure aetiology (systemic metabolic derangements, opportunistic brain abscess or meningitis neoplasms) (Aronow et al 1989, Holtzman et al 1989, Wong et al 1990). The other 40–50% of patients had no demonstrable cause, and cerebral HIV infection seemed to be the most likely cause of the seizures. In our series, 17 patients underwent postmortem neuropathological examination of the brain. Six of these had microglial nodules or multinucleated cells or both, supporting the diagnosis of HIV brain infection as the primary cause of seizures (Wong et al 1990). Navia et al (1986) also found that 9 patients with the AIDS–dementia complex had seizures, and their autopsies did not reveal secondary infectious or neoplastic processes. These data strongly suggest that HIV infection of the brain causes seizures, and that this is the most likely diagnosis in someone whose presenting symptom of HIV infection is a seizure (i.e. seropositive for HIV infection but no other neurological manifestations, AIDS or AIDS-related complex) (Holtzman et al 1989).

SEIZURE RECURRENCE AND TREATMENT IN PATIENTS WITH HIV INFECTION AND AIDS

Recurrent seizures are common. In one series the mean number of seizures per patient was 2.3, even though the follow-up time only averaged four months (Holtzman et al 1989). Aronow et al (1989) noted recurrent seizures in 30% of patients, and we found recurrent seizures in just over 50% of patients (Wong et al 1990). We found that single sporadic and recurrent seizures were equally distributed among patients with secondary causes (infectious, neoplastic, or metabolic) and those with only HIV infection.

The need for and effectiveness of antiepileptic drugs in patients with HIV infection and seizures is difficult to assess. Approximately 90% of our cases were treated with phenytoin (Wong et al 1990). As already noted, about 50% of patients had single seizures, while 50% had recurrent seizures. Thus, although most cases of single seizures were treated with chronic phenytoin therapy, it is unclear if lack of recurrence was the result of antiepileptic drug treatment or an isolated event that would not have recurred even if phenytoin had not been given.

The decision to treat with antiepileptic medications after a single seizure in patients with HIV infection and AIDS should not be made lightly, because there is a significant incidence of undesirable side effects from these drugs. Sixteen of 62 patients in our series (Wong et al 1990) and 12 of 87 in the Holtzman et al (1989) series treated with phenytoin had that medication discontinued due to toxicity. Untoward reactions included rashes, leucopenia, thrombocytopenia and hepatic dysfunction. Caution is warranted in ascribing these reactions solely to phenytoin, because AIDS patients can have similar complications from a large number of possible causes. Furthermore, AIDS patients often take multiple medications, and therefore phenytoin treatment may be causative, contributing, exacerbating, or unrelated. Phenobarbitone was used much less frequently, but it never had to be discontinued.

CONCLUSIONS

1. Seizures are common in patients with HIV infection and AIDS, and occur in 10–20% of cases.
2. Although seizures can occur as the presenting symptom of HIV-related disease, they are more common in the later stages of AIDS.
3. Generalized seizures are most common, but partial seizures occur even in patients without demonstrable secondary infectious or neoplastic brain disease.
4. Status epilepticus is common, including generalized non-convulsive status, and carries a poor prognosis for long-term survival.
5. In 50% of patients with seizures and HIV infection, a secondary infectious or neoplastic cause for the seizures is present. In the other 50% of patients, HIV infection itself is a sufficient cause for the seizures.
6. Recurrent seizures occur in about 50% of cases, and it is unclear whether treatment with antiepileptic drugs affects this recurrence rate.

REFERENCES

Aronow H, Feraru E, Lipton R 1989 New-onset seizures in AIDS patients: etiology, prognosis and treatment. Neurology 39: 428
Belec L, Martin P, Vohito M et al 1989 Low prevalence of neuro-psychiatric clinical manifestations in central African patients with AIDS. Trans R Soc Trop Med Hyg 83: 844–846
Belman A, Lantos G, Horoupian D et al 1986 AIDS: calcifications of the basal ganglia in infants and children. Neurology 36: 1192–1199
Elder G, Sever J 1988 AIDS and neurological disorders: an overview. Ann Neurol 23: S4–S6
Epstein L, Sharer L, Joshi V et al 1985 Progressive encephalopathy in children with AIDS. Ann Neurol 17: 488–496
Epstein L, Sharer L, Oleske J et al 1986 Neurologic manifestations of HIV infections in children. Pediatrics 78: 678–687
Epstein L, Sharer L, Goudsmit J 1988 Neurological and neuropathological features of HIV infection in children. Ann Neurol 23: S19–S23
Janssen R, Cornblath D, Epstein L et al 1989 HIV infection and the nervous system. Neurology 39: 119–122
Gabuzda D, Levy S, Chiappa K 1988 EEG in AIDS and AIDS related complex. Clin EEG 19: 1–6
Holtzman D, Kaku D, So Y 1989 New-onset seizures associated with HIV infection. Am J Med 87: 173–177

Navia B, Jordan B, Price R 1986 The AIDS–dementia complex: I. Clinical features. Ann Neurol 19: 517–524

New York City Department of Health 1987 Special AIDS issue. City Health Info 6: 1–4

Petito C 1988 Review of CNS pathology in HIV infection. Ann Neurol 23: S54–S57

Rosenbaum G, Klein N, Cunha B 1989 Early seizures in patients with AIDS without mass lesions. Heart Lung 18: 526–529

Wong M, Suite N, Labar D 1990 Seizures in HIV infection. Arch Neurol 47: 640–642

9

Medical aspects of managing seizures and epilepsy

M. L. Scheuer

INTRODUCTION

Because epilepsy is a chronic condition spanning years or an entire lifetime, virtually all patients will have a concurrent medical illness at some point. Such illness may be common, benign and self-limited, or it may be severe and life-threatening. The practitioner faced with the concurrence of two disorders must consider multiple levels of potential interaction when formulating a plan of treatment. Such potential interactions extend beyond common drug–drug interactions and also include possible direct exacerbation of epilepsy by medical illness; confounding or complicating management of the medical illness by seizures; precipitating or exacerbating the medical illness by antiepileptic drug (AED) therapy; exacerbating seizures by drugs used to treat medical disorders; and, possibly profound changes in AED disposition induced by concurrent medical illness.

While the concurrence of epilepsy and medical illness can occur at any age, it is most likely in the elderly. These individuals are subject to multiple diseases and are often treated with many medications simultaneously for their various ailments. Recent data continue to indicate that the incidence of seizures and epilepsy rises in the elderly (Loiseau et al 1990, Hauser & Kurland 1975). This, coupled with the trend towards proportionately larger aged populations in industrialized nations, suggests that the problems posed by epilepsy and concurrent illness will become increasingly prevalent.

Current knowledge of interactions between epilepsy and concurrent medical disorders derives mostly from isolated case reports or small, highly selected series. These reports usually treat epilepsy as a single entity and make no effort to distinguish between seizure types or epileptic syndromes. Further, because of the selected nature of these reports, we know little of the true incidence of reported interactions or adverse effects. A particular drug–drug interaction may occur routinely whenever certain drugs are co-administered, while another may occur only in a genetically or environmentally predisposed individual.

When treating the patient with concurrent epilepsy and medical illness, the clinician must consider all areas of potential interplay between the disorders. Therapeutic recommendations should be made only after assessment of the risk–benefit ratio of the anticipated therapy. In some cases, this ratio is unfavourable and the patient can be advised that a treatment often used for their problem should be omitted due to a low but present risk of seizure exacerbation (as in phenylpropanolamine therapy for nasal congestion). In other cases, a known and significant drug–drug interaction may be accepted given the need for specific treatment of a severe illness. Therapies which introduce interactions, even powerful ones, are not necessarily contraindicated given an appropriate indication. *Anticipation* of potential interactions, coupled with conscientious clinical observation, will minimize the likelihood of major problems arising from such interactions.

The following discussion reviews several medical disorders which often develop in the person with epilepsy, and attempts to formulate reasonable recommendations for clinical management based upon available clinical data.

GENERAL CONSIDERATIONS ON DRUG DISPOSITION

Alterations in drug disposition induced by various disease states or pharmacological therapies can substantially complicate management of concurrent epilepsy and medical illness. Unfortunately, our understanding of these interactions is based almost completely upon case reports, which results in a bias toward overestimating the magnitude or significance of such interactions. To date, there have been no prospective population-based studies designed to determine the frequency and significance of drug or disease-induced alterations in drug disposition in individuals with epilepsy. Even less is known of these problems in particular groups such as the very young or the elderly. Statements regarding potential interactions must thus be tempered by lack of firm data.

Drug disposition is the result of several processes: absorption, distribution, biotransformation and excretion (Levy & Unadkaat 1989). Drug absorption is affected by many variables, including physical properties of the drug preparation, gastric pH, motility and emptying time, duodenal pH and motility, mucosal architecture and blood flow, and the presence of drug-binding compounds within the gastrointestinal tract (Levy & Unadkat 1989, Morrelli & Melmon 1978).

Drug distribution is a complex process involving multiple body compartments which often have varying affinities for the distributing drug. Plasma albumin represents one important site of distribution for many AEDs. Phenytoin, valproate and, to a lesser extent, carbamazepine are all highly bound to plasma proteins (predominantly to albumin) (Table 9.1). Drugs which successfully compete with AEDs for protein binding sites can cause large changes in the free AED fraction. The free fraction of drug can also be increased by conditions which decrease serum albumin (severe hepatic disease or the nephrotic syndrome) or result in the accumulation of endogenous competitors for protein binding (uraemia). Because it is a free drug that is available for pharmacodynamic action, small changes in free fraction of a highly protein-bound drug can cause major clinical effects.

Table 9.1   Plasma protein binding of major AEDs

AED	% protein bound	Author
Carbamazepine	75–78	Morselli (1989)
Ethosuximide	Minimal	Chang (1989)
Phenobarbitone	45	Rust & Dodson (1989)
Phenytoin	90	Woodbury (1989)
Primidone	0–20	Cloyd & Leppik (1989)
(Phenylethylmalonamide, primidone active metabolite)	9	Cloyd & Leppick (1989)
Valproate	90	Levy & Shen (1989)

For example, a 5% increase in the free fraction of phenytoin, say from 10% to 15%, results in a 50% increase in effective concentration of the drug. To obtain a similar 50% increase in effective concentration of phenobarbitone, a moderately protein-bound drug, would require a 30% increase in free phenobarbitone fraction, from 55% to 85%.

Biotransformation of the major AEDs occurs mainly in the liver. AEDs are largely metabolized by enzymes residing in hepatocyte smooth endoplasmic reticulum (microsomal enzyme system) via the processes of oxidation, reduction, hydrolysis and conjugation. Thereafter the metabolites, some of which are pharmacologically active, are excreted in the urine or bile (Perucca & Richens 1989). In addition, variable amounts of some parent AEDs are excreted unchanged in the urine: approximately 30% of phenobarbitone; less than 20% of primidone; 10–20% of ethosuximide; and some active carbamazepine metabolites (Gambertoglio & Lauer 1981, Bennett et al 1983). Hepatic drug biotransformation is influenced by many factors, including genetic variability, net hepatocyte mass, intrinsic hepatocyte function, hepatic blood flow (and, indirectly, portal-systemic shunts), bile flow (for metabolites which undergo biliary excretion), protein binding, age, pregnancy, exposure to enzyme-inducing agents, and exposure to enzyme-inhibiting agents (Bennett 1981, Perucca & Richens 1989). While possible confounding effects of hepatic or renal disease on AED disposition are obvious, the many hepatic enzyme-inducing or inhibiting compounds are neither obvious nor easily remembered. Some drugs are highly selective in their hepatic effects, such as erythromycin's ability to cause carbamazepine accumulation by inhibiting hepatic microsomal cytochrome P-450 (Masuy 1987). This effect is not seen with other AEDs. Drugs such as isoniazid are less selective in their inhibition of hepatic AED biotransformation. Genetic factors add yet a further level of complexity to such interactions. Thus, slow acetylators of isoniazid receiving phenytoin often accumulate substantial amounts of phenytoin, while fast acetylators experience no major change in phenytoin levels (Kutt 1984). Any drug which is metabolized in the liver should be considered a potential inducer or inhibitor of hepatic microsomal enzymes. Such consideration will serve to alert the clinician to *potential* drug–drug interactions.

Alterations in drug disposition by intercurrent illness or drug–drug interactions should not pose major problems as long as the physician remains aware of such possibilities. As a corollary, patients should be informed of potential problems. Possible manifestations of drug-induced toxicities should be explained, and any reported symptoms suggesting an adverse interaction should prompt drug level determinations and, if necessary, adjustment of dosage. Free and total drug level determinations may be helpful in circumstances that alter drug protein binding. For known drug–drug interactions, routine sampling of baseline AED levels should be undertaken before the interacting drug is introduced. In the case of potent interactions, periodic sampling of drug levels is warranted until a new steady state has been achieved. The frequency of such determinations is dictated by the rate at which the interaction develops. Such determinations may lessen the likelihood of drug-induced toxicities due to drug accumulation, or of seizure exacerbation due to falling AED levels. In rare circumstances, a prophylatic change in AED dose may be warranted upon introduction of a known rapidly interacting agent. In such situations transient hospital-based observation may be indicated. Finally, one should remember that changes in drug disposition will usually return to baseline after resolution of intercurrent disease or removal of an interacting drug, necessitating cautious attention until a new steady state develops.

COMMON MINOR DISORDERS

Headaches, body aches, upper respiratory infections and seasonal viral infections ('flu') inevitably occur in the person with epilepsy as in other individuals. Limited data suggest that some medications commonly used for such problems pose possible risk to persons with epilepsy. Exposure to over-the-counter drugs designed to provide symptomatic relief of such ailments is probably common, but no good data exist regarding either the incidence of exposure to these drugs or the incidence of adverse reactions. Thus, decisions regarding use of these agents in the setting of epilepsy must be guided by estimated risk–benefit assessments (Table 9.2).

Several analgesic and antipyretic compounds interact with AEDs in certain circumstances. Aspirin successfully competes with phenytoin and valproate for serum protein binding sites. Such competition results in elevation of free AED levels, and can precipitate neurotoxicity if baseline levels of valproate or phenytoin are high (Orr et al 1982, Goulden et al 1987, Olanow et al 1981). Salicylate-induced increase in free AED is usually countered by increased hepatic clearance of the free drug, which results in a drop in total AED levels, while free (effective) levels remain little changed. Olanow et al (1981) reported on one such group of patients in whom concomitant phenytoin–aspirin therapy resulted in decreased total phenytoin levels while free levels remained unchanged; toxicity did not occur. Compensatory alterations in free and total levels might not be seen,

Table 9.2   Treatment suggestions for common respiratory infections, rhinitis and aches in the person with epilepsy (see text for references)

Symptom	Use	Use cautiously or avoid
Rhinorrhea	Pseudoephedrine Phenylephrine	Phenylpropanolamine Diphenhydramine
Myalgias, aches	Acetaminophen ± aspirin	Propoxyphene Ibuprofen Prolonged aspirin when trough PHT level high Aspirin in conjunction with VPA (primarily with high VPA levels)

Abbreviations: PHT, phenytoin; VPA, valproate.

though, in the patient treated with chronic high-dose aspirin (e.g. the patient with rheumatoid arthritis) whose baseline phenytoin levels are high. In this case, the increased free AED fraction might saturate the liver's capacity to metabolize phenytoin, resulting in accumulations of both free and total phenytoin.

Propoxyphene causes rapid and significant accumulation of carbamazepine, often resulting in significant signs and symptoms of neurotoxicity (Oles et al 1989). This is probably a relatively common consequence. Because effective alternative analgesics are readily available, the carbamazepine–propoxyphene combination should probably be avoided. Ibuprofen can also precipitate drug accumulation and neurotoxicity when co-administered with phenytoin (Sandyk 1982). Thus, ibuprofen and aspirin should be used cautiously in persons with epilepsy. Use of low initial dosages followed by gradual titration to desired clinical effect should minimize significant problems. Acetaminophen appears safer, having neither ill effects on seizure threshold nor significant interactions with AEDs. It thus represents a reasonable alternative when an analgesic or antipyretic is needed.

The non-prescription sympathomimetic drug phenylpropanolamine, commonly used as a decongestant in many proprietary cold remedies and in diet pills (Table 9.3), has precipitated seizures in several normal children (Bale et al 1984), adults (Deocampo 1979, Bernstein & Diskant 1982, Jallon et al 1986), and one probably epileptic adult (Cornelius et al 1984) at usual doses. Complex partial seizures were also exacerbated in a man with incompletely controlled epilepsy exposed to moderate therapeutic doses of phenylpropanolamine (Jallon et al 1986). Even if seizure exacerbation by this drug is infrequent, risk–benefit analysis suggests that phenyl-propanolamine use for decongestion or dieting should be avoided. Diphenhydramine is also being increasingly used in proprietary cold remedies and this drug has been reported to activate generalized spike and wave discharges, focal epileptiform discharges, and occasionally to precipitate focal or generalized convulsive seizures (Diaz-Guerrero et al 1956, Otawar et al 1963, Kitagawa & Takahashi 1980). Indications of cough, pruritus

Table 9.3   Some commonly used preparations containing phenylpropanolamine or diphenhydramine

---

Phenylpropanolamine
   Cold or allergy remedies: 4-Way Cold Tablets, Alka-Seltzer Plus Cold Medicine, Allerest, Bayer Children's Cold Tablets, Children's CoTylenol, Comtrex, Contac, Coricidin-D, Coryban-D, Deconex, Dehist, Dimetapp, Duadacin, Histabid Duracap, Naldecon Pediatric Syrup, Noraminic, Oraminic, Ornade, Sinarest, Sine-off Sinus Medicine, Sinubid, Spec-T Decongestant Lozenges, St Joseph's Cold Tablets for Children, Sucrets Cold Decongestant, Triaminic
   Diet pills: Acutrim, Control Maximum Strength, Dexatrim, Prolamine, Westrim

Diphenhydramine
   Cold, rhinitis, or pruritus preparations: Benadryl, Benylin
   Sleeping pills: Compoz, Nytol, Sleep-eze 3, Sominex

---

and nasal congestion may not merit the probably small risk of diphenhydramine-induced seizure exacerbation. Pseudoephedrine and phenylephrine have not been reported to exacerbate seizures and so represent reasonable choices when a decongestant must be prescribed.

BACTERIAL INFECTIONS

Significant antibiotic–AED interactions occur on a fairly frequent basis, and they have been the subject of many case reports. Their occurrence in clinical practice may be more common than any other type of epilepsy-related drug–drug interactions. A prime example of this class of interaction is the accumulation of carbamazepine induced by erythromycin. Erythromycin, and the related compound troleandomycin, selectively inhibit hepatic microsomal enzymes involved in carbamazepine's metabolism. This results in rapid accumulation of carbamazepine over one to several days and, usually, clinical neurotoxicity. Upon discontinuing erythromycin the interaction abates rapidly (Pippenger 1987). In general, patients treated with carbamazepine should be warned to avoid erythromycin. Such cautionary statements to the patient are necessary, because many physicians prescribing erythromycin are unaware of the interaction. When erythromycin is necessary, carbamazepine levels should be drawn daily for the first several days and dosages adjusted as appropriate; when erythromycin is discontinued, prompt titration of carbamazepine dosage to its pre-interaction baseline is necessary.

Concurrent isoniazid administration can cause accumulation of carbamazepine, phenytoin, primidone, and possibly ethosuximide through inhibition of hepatic metabolism (Kutt 1984, Pippenger 1987, van Weiringen & Vrijlandt 1983). Isoniazid's interaction with phenytoin illustrates the influence of genetic factors on the significance of a drug–drug interaction. Phenytoin accumulation is related to the patient's acetylator type; slow acetylators can accumulate substantial amounts of phenytoin, whereas metabolism is little changed in fast acetylators (Kutt 1984). In the USA, slow acetylators comprise about 50% of the population. People of certain ethnic backgrounds – North African caucasians, Jews and Scandinavians – are even more likely to be slow acetylators (Mandel & Sande 1980). Rifampicin, a drug commonly used in conjunction with INH for the treatment of tuberculosis, can substantially enhance elimination of phenytoin (Abajo 1988, Kay et al 1985). Data from one study suggest that rifampin's ability to enhance phenytoin elimination may more than offset isoniazid's ability to retard phenytoin metabolism, regardless of the patient's acetylator type (Kay et al 1985). Thus, a fall in PHT levels might be seen during combined INH–rifampicin therapy. AED levels should be obtained prior to the initiation of isoniazid, rifampicin or INH–rifampicin therapy. Thereafter, levels should be repeated several times during the first few weeks of such therapy, and dosage adjustments made as necessary.

Chloramphenicol inhibits the metabolism of phenobarbitone and phenytoin (Koup et al 1978, Rose et al 1977). The degree of inhibition varies with the dose schedule and duration of chloramphenicol treatment but can lead to clinically significant AED accumulations. The chloramphenicol–phenytoin interaction is probably often significant (Kutt 1984, Perucca & Richens 1981).

Sulphonamides inhibit phenytoin metabolism (Perucca & Richens 1981). Particular drugs implicated in this interaction include sulphadiazine, sulphamethizole and sulphamethoxazole–trimethoprim. Given sufficient dosage and duration of therapy, these agents can precipitate phenytoin intoxication. The interaction is probably most often encountered in the woman on phenytoin who is given trimethoprim–sulphamethoxazole for a urinary tract infection. Others commonly at risk are persons with localization-related epilepsy secondary to complications of acquired immunodeficiency syndrome (AIDS) who are receiving long-term sulphonamide therapy for pneumocystis pneumonia or cerebral toxoplasmosis.

Recently, treatment with the broad-spectrum β-lactam antibiotic (carbapenem class) imipenem has been reported to induce convulsive seizures (Eng et al 1989, Calandra et al 1988, Brown et al 1990). Imipenem is often used in combination with cilastatin, a drug that inhibits renal tubule brush-border enzyme. Two studies dealing with large patient populations reported that 52/1754 (3%) and 2/400 (0.5%) developed seizures while on imipenem/cilastatin (Calandra et al 1988, Brown et al 1990). As imipenem is commonly used in patients who are moderately or severely ill, often in an intensive care setting, the reported incidence of seizures is of uncertain significance. In their retrospective analysis, Calandra et al (1988) noted that 23/1702 exposed patients who did not have seizures during imipenem/cilastatin therapy had seizures when treated with other or no antibiotics. They also surveyed a group of 238 moderately or severely ill infected patients not exposed to imipenem/cilastatin and found seizure incidence to be 7%; subset analyses of their imipenem/cilastatin-treated group revealed similar seizure incidence figures. Risk factors for seizures while on imipenem therapy included renal failure, excessive imipenem/cilastatin dose, central nervous system lesions, seizure history and *Pseudomonas aeruginosa* infection. They suggested that patients with meningitis, acute seizures and poorly controlled epilepsy not be given imipenem therapy. They also suggested that head injury patients with central nervous system lesions face a potentially greater risk of seizure induction (Calandra 1988). At present the risk of imipenem-induced seizure exacerbation in the person with epilepsy is unknown. At present, imipenem therapy should be avoided if other suitable first-line antibiotics are available.

PEPTIC ULCER DISEASE

Antacid preparations containing aluminium or magnesium hydroxide, or calcium carbonate, are frequently used for the treatment of gastritis and peptic ulcer disease. They are also widely used by patients themselves in self-treatment of many non-specific gastrointestinal symptoms. Absorption of orally administered AEDs can be affected by these agents; some combinations result in impaired AED absorption while others increase absorption. Decreased phenytoin absorption has been reported during antacid therapy, but this interaction appears to be highly variable (Perucca & Richens 1981). A single report indicates that absorption of some valproate preparations can be enhanced by some antacids (May et al 1982, D'Arcy & McElnay 1987). Sucralfate, a sulphated sucrose–aluminium hydroxide complex, decreased phenytoin absorption in two studies (Smart et al 1985, Hall et al 1986); its effects on the absorption profiles of other AEDs is unknown. Such data have prompted recommendations that antacid or sucralfate administration be staggered by several hours with respect to phenytoin administration (D'Arcy & McElnay 1987), and it is probably reasonable to extend this advice to other AEDs. AEDs should probably be administered 1–2 hours before, or 2 or more hours after, antacid doses, and AED levels should be determined before and during concomitant antacid–AED therapy to screen for significant changes in drug disposition.

The H-2 receptor antagonist cimetidine inhibits certain hepatic microsomal enzymes and can cause accumulation of drugs metabolized by those enzymes (Powell & Dalton 1984). Such is the case with phenytoin and, to a lesser extent, carbamazepine. The cimetidine–phenytoin interaction often results in substantial accumulations of phenytoin, sometimes necessitating phenytoin dosage adjustments during and following concomitant therapy (Kutt 1984, Levine et al 1985). Cimetidine's effect on carbamazepine metabolism is usually less persistent and leads to a transient rise in carbamazepine levels within two days of starting cimetidine followed by return to baseline values within one week despite continued cimetidine therapy (Dalton et al 1986). The initial rise in carbamazepine levels may be accompanied by transient symptoms of neurotoxicity, but as these symptoms generally resolve rapidly there is usually no need to alter carbamazepine dosages (Levine et al 1985, Sonne et al 1983). Cimetidine has also been reported to inhibit the metabolism of valproic acid (Webster et al 1984), but the clinical significance of this interaction is unknown.

Ranitidine inhibits hepatic drug metabolism far less than cimetidine (Pippenger 1987, Dalton et al 1986, Webster et al 1984, Watts et al 1983). Only a single case report has documented possible ranitidine-induced phenytoin accumulation (Bramhall & Levine 1988). Ranitidine thus represents a reasonable first choice if an H-2 receptor antagonist must be used with an AED.

ASTHMA

Asthma and epilepsy are generally independent disorders; rarely secondary epilepsy may develop as the result of cerebral injury incurred during severe and prolonged hypoxia (Nellhaus et al 1975). Isolated seizures occasionally occur due to transient hypoxia associated with a cyanotic attack, but such seizures do not represent epilepsy. Asthmatic cough syncope is also sometimes misdiagnosed as epilepsy due to clonic movements associated with the reduction in cerebral oxygen supply and perfusion induced by paroxysmal coughing. Treatment of cough syncope consists of optimal treatment of underlying asthma; antiepileptic drugs are ineffective (Haslam & Freigang 1985). Using prevalence figures of 0.6% for active epilepsy (Hauser & Kurland 1975) and 3% for active asthma (Fanta & Ingram 1988) in the USA an estimated 40 000 persons in the USA alone suffer from both disorders.

Asthma is commonly treated with theophylline, a methylxanthine drug. Theophylline is a proconvulsant in humans over a broad range of serum concentrations. Early reports suggested that theophylline precipitated convulsive seizures in neurologically normal patients at high serum concentrations (25–70 µg/ml) (Zwillich et al 1975), but subsequent reports have suggested that theophylline also trigger seizures at therapeutic or mildly supratherapeutic levels (Covelli et al 1985, Richards et al 1985). Seizures can occur following either oral or parenteral administration (Zwillich et al 1975, Covelli et al 1985) and are often seen in the absence of typical signs and symptoms of theophylline toxicity such as apprehension, headache, abdominal pain, nausea or vomiting (Zwillich et al 1975, Covelli et al 1985, Richards et al 1985). Pre-existing neurological abnormalities may constitute an additional risk factor for induction of seizures by theophylline (Covelli et al 1985).

Studies reviewing the effect of theophylline administration on seizure frequency in patients with both asthma and epilepsy have not been published. The lack of case reports probably indicates that the risk of

Table 9.4   Tentative recommendations for treatment of the patient with concurrent asthma and epilepsy (see also Fanta & Ingram 1988, for general discussion of asthma management strategies)

1. Establish lines of communication between neurological consultant and physician managing asthma
2. Preventive measures: avoid allergens and environmental precipitants
3. Begin therapy with intermittent inhaled β-adrenergic bronchodilators for patients with occasional asthmatic attacks
4. Use regularly administered inhaled β-adrenergic bronchodilators as first-line therapy for patients with persistent asthmatic symptoms
5. If poor clinical response, add theophylline; maintain low therapeutic trough theophylline levels if such prove effective
6. If low therapeutic theophylline levels in combination with inhaled bronchodilators prove ineffective, seek pulmonary consultation (if not already obtained); consider early use of inhaled steroids or cromolyn. Maintain close collaboration between pulmonary and neurological consultants
7. Observe for drug–drug interactions and untoward effects of intercurrent illness (see text)

seizure exacerbation is small. Of interest are case reports of two depressed asthmatic patients treated with electroconvulsive therapy (ECT) who developed ECT-associated status epilepticus, a very rare occurrence, in the setting of mildly elevated theophylline levels (21.6 μg/ml and 22.6 μg/ml respectively) (Devanand et al 1988, Peters et al 1984). Despite a paucity of clinically relevant data, theophylline's proconvulsant effect warrants a cautious approach to its use in patients with epilepsy. Theophylline's elimination, like that of phenytoin, becomes non-linear as serum theophylline concentrations increase (Covelli et al 1985). Additionally, other concurrent diseases (common viral illness, upper respiratory infections, congestive heart failure or hepatic cirrhosis) or drug use (cimetidine, erythromycin) can result in high theophylline concentrations (Covelli et al 1985, Kraemer et al 1982), which may further lower seizure threshold.

Co-administration of carbamazepine, phenobarbitone or phenytoin with theophylline can result in decreased serum theophylline levels due to induction of theophylline elimination (Rosenberry et al 1983, Jonkman 1986). Simultaneous use of these drugs requires careful attention to establishing the proper dose of theophylline. Changes in AED type or dosage may change theophylline dose requirements; re-determination of theophylline levels during such changes is helpful.

Freidman et al (1982) reported a single case of possible seizure precipitation by high doses of oral terbutaline. Inhaled β-agonists have not been reported to induce seizures in humans and so are probably safe to use in the patient with asthma and epilepsy.

Given the virtual absence of sound clinical data from which to form treatment strategies for the patient with asthma and epilepsy, only tentative suggestions for treatment of concurrent asthma and epilepsy can be made (see Table 9.4).

Table 9.5 Some cardioactive drug–AED interactions

Cardioactive drug	AED	Cardiac drug level	AED level	Author
Quinidine	PHT,PB	Decreased	–	Data et al (1976), Urbano (1983)
Lidocaine	PHT,PB	Decreased	–	Heinonen et al (1970)
Digoxin	PHT	Decreased	–	Rameis (1985)
Amiodarone	PHT	?	Increased	Shackleford & Watson (1987), Gore et al (1984)
Mexiletine	PHT	Decreased	–	Begg et al (1982)
Disopyramide	PHT	Decreased	–	Aitio et al (1981)
Verapamil	CBZ	–	Increased	MacPhee et al (1986), Beattie et al (1988)
Diltiazem	CBZ	–	Increased	Eimer & Carter (1987), Brodie & MacPhee (1986)
Nifedipine	PHT	–	Increased	Ahmad (1984)

Abbreviations: CBZ, carbamazepine; PB, phenobarbitone; PHT, phenytoin.

CARDIOVASCULAR DISEASE

Congenital heart disease affects an estimated 0.8% of live births (Freidman 1984), and acquired diseases of the heart are common in persons over 60 years of age. Such disorders can cause epilepsy through secondary effects on the nervous system (cerebral embolism, ischaemic damage) (Lesser et al 1985), or they can occur as independent diseases in the patient with epilepsy. Convulsive seizures, through increased haemodynamic demand, sometimes have deleterious effects on the patient with limited cardiac reserve. Additionally, many of the drugs used to treat patients with cardiac disease interact with the AEDs, thereby complicating management of the cardiac disorder, epilepsy, or both.

Drug–drug interactions occur between various cardioactive drugs (inotropic agents, antiarrhythmic agents, antihypertensive agents, anticoagulants) and AEDs. Some reported interactions are listed in Table 9.5. Several interactions are of special note. Quinidine's half-life may be reduced by about 50% when administered concurrently with phenobarbitone or phenytoin (Data et al 1976, Urbano 1983), necessitating quinidine dosage adjustments. Amiodarone's long half-life and resulting slow accumulation can lead to rising phenytoin levels and eventual intoxication. This occurs days or weeks after the drugs are first used concurrently (Shackleford & Watson 1987, Gore et al 1984). Co-administration of verapamil frequently induces carbamazepine accumulation sufficient to cause neurotoxicity (MacPhee et al 1986, Beattie et al 1988), and reduction in carbamazepine dose may be necessary. Diltiazam's effects on carbamazepine metabolism are similar to those of verapamil (Eimer & Carter 1987, Brodie & MacPhee 1986). Increased digoxin dosages may be necessary when co-administered with phenytoin (Rameis 1985).

Generalized seizures in the critically ill patient with heart disease may tax already limited cardiac reserve sufficiently to cause further clinical deterioration. Thus, prevention of recurrent seizures is essential. Acute seizures should be terminated rapidly with intravenous diazepam unless contraindicated by individual circumstances. Long-acting AEDs should be introduced immediately or titrated to a higher blood level if already in use. Intravenous phenytoin is the drug most often used for this purpose, but its injudicious use, especially intravenously, may result in cardiotoxic side effects. Rapid intravenous administration of phenytoin can induce myocardial depression and severe hypotension even in persons with healthy hearts. This deleterious effect is much more likely in the elderly or critically ill patient. The rate of administration rather than the final total dose determines the likelihood of cardiotoxicity. Problems can even be encountered when administering a daily maintenance dose of 100–300 mg intravenously. The frequently recommended rate of 50 mg/min for intravenous phenytoin administration must often be substantially reduced in the patient with cardiovascular disease, sometimes to as little as 5–10 mg/min (Cloyd et al 1980). It is safest to begin intravenous infusion slowly (5-10 mg/min), and thereafter cautiously titrate the rate upwards as tolerated. The almost inevitable tendency to administer an entire minute's aliquot of drug over a fraction of a minute should be strictly avoided. Administering a loading dose (which may amount to 1200 mg or more) by hand at the rate of 10 mg/min is difficult. In such cases, it is often best to dilute the phenytoin to a concentration of about 5–20 mg/ml in 0.9% sodium chloride solution and administer the solution via an infusion pump. If this procedure is followed one should place a filter (0.22–0.45 μm) in the intravenous line to prevent the infusion of occasional phenytoin crystals (Cloyd et al 1980, Salem et al 1980, Cloyd et al 1978). Blood pressure and cardiac rhythm should be monitored continuously during phenytoin infusions. Some authorities have advised against using intravenous phenytoin at all in patients with severe myocardial disease, hypotension, sinoatrial block, sinus bradycardia, and second- and third-degree atrioventricular block (Browne 1983a). However, certain clinical circumstances may necessitate use of phenytoin even in the face of these recognized risks.

Warfarin's metabolism and its effect on prothrombin time are affected differently by various AEDs. Warfarin's metabolism is enhanced by carbamazepine and phenobarbitone, resulting in decreased anticoagulant effect (Udall 1975, Ross & Beeley 1980, Massey 1983). Conversely, phenytoin co-administration sometimes enhances warfarin's anticoagulant activity, apparently through inhibition of its metabolism (Perucca & Richens 1981, Nappi 1979). Adjustment of warfarin dose based on prothrombin time allows the drug to be used safely despite these interactions. If AED dose or type is changed, prothrombin times should be determined on a frequent basis to assure the desired degree of anticoagulant effect.

With the exception of calcium-channel blocker–AED interactions (discussed above), few clinically significant interactions have been observed between AEDs and antihypertensive agents. Antihypertensive therapy with the combination drug hydrochlorothiazide–amiloride has been reported to precipitate seizures occasionally due to hyponatraemia (Johnston et al 1989, Byatt 1990). An isolated case report has also suggested a hydrochlorothiazide–carbamazepine interaction as a cause of symptomatic hyponatraemia (Yassa et al 1987). Because hyponatraemia lowers seizure threshold, intermittent sampling of serum sodium concentration is prudent during diuretic treatment.

RENAL FAILURE

The concurrence of renal disease and epilepsy is usually coincidental. AED-induced nephrotoxicity is rare and most often the result of an idiosyncratic hypersensitivity reaction (Schmidt 1982, Imai et al 1989). Certain seldom-used AEDs (trimethadione, paradione, mephenytoin) occasionally induce the nephrotic syndrome (Schmidt 1982). Seizures commonly occur in the setting of severe renal disease, usually from secondary effects of renal failure of brain function. Knowledge of the effect of renal failure on AED utilization and excretion is therefore important.

Although AED metabolism occurs primarily in the liver, the kidneys contribute to the metabolism and excretion of some parent drug or their active metabolite(s). Renal insufficiency and alterations in AED protein binding induced by renal failure can therefore cause major changes in drug disposition. These changes complicate use of AEDs in the setting of acute or chronic renal failure but usually only when renal function is substantially impaired (Table 9.6).

Phenytoin binding to serum proteins progressively declines as renal function deteriorates. The compound 3-carboxy-4-methyl-5-propyl-2-furanpropanoic acid (CMPF), which accumulates in renal failure, is probably one of the endogenous substances which inhibits binding of phenytoin by albumin (Mabuchi & Nakahashi 1988). Decreased protein binding, increased drug volume of distribution and shortened drug half-life result in an overall fall in total phenytoin levels while free phenytoin levels remain fairly stable. Therefore daily phenytoin dosage requirements often do not change, even in the setting of moderately severe renal failure. In the patient with severe renal insufficiency, free serum phenytoin levels provide a more useful measure of pharmacologically active drug than do total levels. For example, at a serum creatinine of $10 \mu g/dl$, total phenytoin levels of $5–10 \mu g/ml$ correspond to 'therapeutic' free phenytoin levels of $1–2 \mu g/ml$ (Asconape & Penry 1982, Gambertoglio & Lauer 1981). Interpretation of total phenytoin levels is further complicated if there has been a substantial change in serum proteins as, for example, in the nephrotic syndrome. Equations which attempt to correct laboratory-derived total phenytoin levels in uraemic or hypoalbuminaemic patients to equivalent expected levels have proved too unreliable for clinical use (Mauro et al 1989). Thus, free phenytoin levels, signs and symptoms of dose-related neurotoxicity and drug effectiveness must guide use of phenytoin in the patient with renal disease. Free phenytoin levels of $1-2\,\mu g/ml$ are usually appropriate. A three-times-a-day dosing schedule is frequently necessary because of the drug's shortened half-life (Asconape & Penry 1982, Gambertoglio & Lauer 1981).

Assay methods used to determine phenytoin levels sometimes become unreliable in the setting of renal failure. Enzyme-multiplied immunoassay (EMIT) techniques can yield unreliably high serum phenytoin levels because the assay cross-reacts with the phenytoin metabolite 5-hydroxyphenyl-5-phenylhydantoin-glucuronide which accumulates in uraemic serum. High-performance liquid chromatography (HPLC) and fluorescence polarization immunoassay methods will give reliable phenytoin results in uraemic patients (Sirgo et al 1984).

Unlike phenytoin, alterations in protein binding of phenobarbitone associated with renal failure are usually not of clinical significance. This is most probably due to the normally large free fraction of phenobarbitone (approximately 55%). Exceptions, however, occur. Pugh (1987) reported on a burn patient with acute renal failure and severe hypoalbuminaemia who developed a 92% free fraction of phenobarbitone when his creatinine and albumin were 6.0 mg/dl and 1.9 g/dl, respectively. Careful clinical follow-up and routine determinations of total phenobarbitone levels are indicated in the uraemic patient treated with barbiturates. Phenobarbitone

Table 9.6 AED dosage adjustments in renal failure and dialysis (see Asconape & Penry 1982, Gambertoglio & Lauer 1981, Bennett et al 1983)

AED	% renal excretion	Dosage adjustment necessary? At what GFR?	Method of dosage adjustment	Removed by dialysis?
Carbamazepine	Minimal	Yes; < 10 ml/min	Decrease daily dosage by 25%	No (HD)
Ethosuximide	10–20	Yes; < 10 ml/min	Decrease daily dosage by 25%	Yes (HD)
Phenobarbitone	25–30	Yes; < 10 ml/min	Extend maintenance dosage interval by 50–100%	Yes (HD > PD)
Phenytoin	Minimal	No	Generally, use t.i.d. dosing schedule at stable baseline dosage	No (HD)
Primidone	20	Yes; < 50 ml/min	Increase dosing interval from 8 to 8–12 h for GFR 10–50, then to 12–24 h for GFR < 10	Yes (HD)
Valproate	Minimal	No	Generally no change	No (HD, PD)

Abbreviations: GFR, glomerular filtration rate; HD, haemodialysis; PD, peritoneal dialysis.

also probably poses an increased risk of cognitive and sedative side effects. Occasional monitoring of free phenobarbitone levels may be necessary in the setting of combined renal failure and hypoalbuminaemia.

Decreased plasma protein binding of valproate has been reported in uraemic patients. As with phenytoin, this can result in lower than expected total valproate levels despite unchanged free levels (Asconape & Penry 1982). Alterations in serum protein concentrations associated with the nephrotic syndrome would also be expected to result in substantial alterations in the ratio of free to total valproate. When possible, free valproate levels should be followed in the patient with significant renal impairment or hypoalbuminaemia. Free valproate levels of 8–12 μg/ml are generally appropriate.

Haemodialysis (HD) and peritoneal dialysis (PD) remove significant amounts of certain AEDs (Table 9.6) (Bennett et al 1983, Kandrotas et al 1989). Supplemental post-dialysis AED doses are sometimes required. Variables affecting the quantity of drug removed during a dialysis session include type of dialysis, initial AED concentration and duration of dialysis (Asconape & Penry 1982, Gambertoglio & Lauer 1981, Bennett et al 1983, Bennett 1981). Procedures for estimating post-dialysis supplementation needs are available but should be complemented by periodic AED level determinations to avoid gradual drug loss or accumulation. Drug level determinations should be performed just before or several hours after dialysis to avoid periods of re-equilibration (Bennett 1981, Freed 1981). Supplemental AED doses should usually be given shortly after dialysis to maintain stable AED levels.

HEPATIC DISEASE

Because the liver is the predominant site of AED metabolism, alterations in hepatic function modify AED disposition. However, because hepatic reserve capacity is very large, changes in AED metabolism usually become evident only in the setting of moderately severe to severe hepatic disease. No good measures exist by which the degree of hepatic impairment can be reliably judged in a particular patient. Assays of serum ALT (SGPT) and AST (SGOT) provide little indication of hepatic synthetic and metabolic capacities. Prothrombin time and serum albumin determinations provide some indication of the liver's synthetic capacities (Bennett 1981). Fibrinogen levels may also be indicative of synthetic capacities. These variables, though, provide little data regarding the liver's ability to metabolize drugs using normal pathways. Tanaka et al (1987) have suggested that single-dose studies of trimethadione's conversion to dimethadione might serve as an index of the liver's drug-metabolizing capabilities. However, the clinical utility of this interesting approach has not yet been validated, and correlation between this index and AED metabolism has not been studied.

Because there is no hepatic equivalent to the glomerular filtration rate to guide drug dosing in patients with hepatic disease, decisions regarding dosing must be made almost exclusively on the basis of AED levels and clinical response as assessed by signs and symptoms of neurotoxicity and seizure control. Changes in albumin concentration are common as liver disease progresses and may make determinations of free AED levels necessary, especially for highly protein bound AEDs (see Table 9.1). Every effort should be made to minimize polytherapy as this will lessen the likelihood of interactions and cumulative toxicities.

Most of the major AEDs cause serious hepatotoxicity only as a rare idiosyncratic side effect. On the other hand, minor elevations of liver enzymes (ALT and AST) are fairly common, but these are of no known clinical significance. Concern over such side effects should not interdict use of these drugs in patients with hepatic disease given an appropriate indication. There is no evidence to suggest that AED use, with the exception of valproate (see below), exacerbates existing liver disease or accelerates its course except for unpredictable idiosyncratic reactions. Discussions of AED hepatotoxicity resulting from idiosyncratic reactions are available in several recent reviews (Dreifuss & Langer 1987, Horowitz et al 1988, Gram & Bentsen 1983).

Phenytoin and phenobarbitone accumulate in the setting of severe hepatic disease (Asconape & Penry 1982, Gambertoglio & Lauer 1981). Phenytoin dose requirements are generally unchanged in the setting of mild to moderate hepatic disease; less is known regarding phenobarbitone. As patients with hepatic disease are probably at increased risk of cognitive side effects from AEDs, especially barbiturates, clinical follow-up should occur on a regular basis, and AED levels should be sampled frequently. Free phenytoin levels should be sampled as albumin levels fall, because the usual 'therapeutic range' for total serum phenytoin will no longer be applicable in this setting (Asconape & Penry 1982, Sandford et al 1987). Free phenytoin levels should generally be maintained in the $1-2\,\mu g/ml$ range (Asconape & Penry 1982, Booker & Darcey 1973).

The effects of liver disease on carbamazepine, ethosuximide and primidone disposition are largely unknown. Limited data are available regarding the phenobarbitone breakdown product of primidone, as already discussed. Given the lack of clinical data regarding use of these drugs in the setting of liver disease, careful clinical observation is mandatory. Such observation should be supplemented by frequent AED level determinations.

Only limited data are also available regarding valproate's disposition in the patient with liver disease. Klotz et al (1978) found that elimination of a single dose of valproate was slightly impaired in persons recovering from acute viral hepatitis, and was only slightly more impaired in patients with mild to moderate alcoholic cirrhosis. Gugler & von Unruh (1980) found that valproate clearance was decreased, and that valproate's half-life was increased, in patients with acute viral hepatitis. Recent recommendations are that valproate should not be administered to patients with acquired or familial hepatic disease (Dreifuss & Langer 1987, Gram & Bentsen 1983). This advice stems from concerns generated by cases of valproate-induced fatal hepatotoxicity, a rare idiosyncratic reaction (Dreifuss & Langer 1987, Gram & Bentsen 1983, Dreifuss et al 1987), possibly caused by aberrant products of valproate metabolism (Zimmerman & Kamal 1982, Rettie et al 1987, Tennison et al 1988). If valproate's use is essential dose adjustments will probably only be necessary in patients with severe hepatic impairment. Dosage requirements and total serum levels producing 'therapeutic' free valproate levels ($8-12 \mu g/ml$) will probably be substantially reduced as serum albumin levels fall. Clinical laboratory measurements (serum albumin, prothrombin time, fibrinogen, bilirubin, ALT, AST) should be checked frequently, and any complaints (of nausea, vomiting, lethargy) or change in seizure frequency should prompt rapid clinical re-evaluation to exclude the possibility of valproate-induced accelerated hepatic dysfunction.

Treatment strategies for patients with seizures and epilepsy complicating hepatic porphyrias are available in a recent review by Scheuer (in press).

SYSTEMIC LUPUS ERYTHEMATOSUS (SLE)

Seizures are fairly common in SLE, although far from ubiquitous. Published case series document highly variable seizure incidence figures which range from 2.5% to 57% (Johnson & Richardson 1968, Buchbinder et al 1988). Biased study populations undoubtedly account for much of this disparity, and the very high seizure incidence figure probably reflected terminal seizures. One longitudinal study of neuropsychiatric abnormalities associated with SLE found that 3/140 patients had recurrent seizures over a period of more than three months, while another 2/140 had recurrent seizures separated by years (Feinglass et al 1976). Epilepsy is sometimes the first neurological manifestation of SLE, and occasionally precedes even systemic manifestations by several years (Feinglass et al 1976, Johnson & Richardson 1968).

In their clinicopathological study of SLE patients with neurological manifestations, Johnson & Richardson (1968) postulated that the increased risk of seizures, epilepsy and other neuropsychiatric manifestations was related to cerebral microinfarcts and other micropathology similar to histopathological changes seen with thrombotic thrombocytopenic purpura. Seizures complicating SLE are most commonly convulsive, but simple and complex partial attacks have also been described (Feinglass et al 1976, Johnson & Richardson 1968). They are therefore most reasonably treated with carbamazepine, phenobarbitone, phenytoin or primidone.

The occurrence of a lupus-like syndrome in the person taking antiepileptic drugs always raises the possibility of a drug-induced syndrome. This must be differentiated from idiopathic SLE because treatments for these conditions are different. Carbamazepine, ethosuximide, phenytoin, pheneturide and

Table 9.7   Characteristics of drug-induced versus idiopathic lupus

	Drug-induced	Idiopathic
Onset	Weeks to 2 years post-start AED	Variable
ANAs	Common	Common
Anti-DS-DNA	Rare	Common
Anti-Sm antigen	Rare	Common
Histone-reactive ANAs	Often high titres	Variable
Hypocomplementaemia	Rare	Common
Renal involvement	Rare (but reported)	Common
CNS involvement	Rare (but reported)	Common
Course post-stop AED	sxs remit in days to weeks	No change

primidone, but not phenobarbitone, have all been reported to cause a lupus-like syndrome (Lee & Chase 1975, Weinstein 1980, Alballa et al 1987). There is only a single case of primidone-induced lupus in the literature (Ahuja & Schumacher 1966). Valproate has been implicated as an activating agent in two cases of SLE (Bleck & Smith 1990), but an alternative explanation is that those patients may have simply had coincidental flares of idiopathic SLE. Drug-induced lupus can be differentiated from idiopathic SLE by several characteristics (Table 9.7) (Lee & Chase 1975, Weinstein 1980, Harmon & Portanova 1982). When a drug-induced syndrome is strongly suspected, the offending AED should be discontinued and another drug substituted. If the diagnosis of a drug-induced lupus syndrome is correct, symptoms generally remit within weeks. A patient who experiences a lupus-like syndrome on one AED is probably not at risk of developing a similar syndrome on another of the AEDs. Laboratory abnormalities (e.g. positive ANA), though, may persist for years after resolution of clinical symptoms.

A question of some practical importance is whether AEDs exacerbate idiopathic SLE. Unfortunately there are no data that help answer this. Therefore, cautious clinical observation is warranted in the person with SLE who requires treatment with AEDs for seizures. If a flare of lupus corresponds to AED treatment, then another AED of a different chemical class should be substituted. Phenobarbitone might be a reasonable choice in such circumstances, because it is not known to induce lupus.

CHEMICAL IMMUNOSUPPRESSION

Immunosuppressive drugs are used increasingly in the treatment of many diseases. Some groups so treated are at increased risk of epilepsy (cardiac and renal transplant recipients, patients with SLE). Major interactions between AEDs and two different types of immunosuppressants – cyclosporin A and steroids – have been reported. These interactions may lead to inadequate immunosuppression and result in increased morbidity and mortality (Wassner et al 1976).

Chronic carbamazepine therapy enhances elimination of intravenous prednisolone (Olivesi 1986). Phenobarbitone can exacerbate asthma in patients whose control is steroid dependent (Brooks et al 1972). Phenobarbitone has also been implicated in decreased renal transplant survival (Wassner et al 1976), possibly because of increased prednisolone metabolism. Thus, patients receiving AEDs and requiring acute or chronic steroid treatment may need larger steroid doses to achieve the required clinical effect.

Cyclosporin A elimination is markedly enhanced by phenytoin (Keown et al 1984, Freeman 1984) and probably by carbamazepine as well (Schofield et al 1990, Hillebrand et al 1987). Hillebrand et al (1987) recommended valproate as drug of first choice therapy in patients requiring treatment of seizures. However, the effectiveness of valproate in treating partial onset seizures is unknown at present due to lack of a large well-controlled clinical trial. Thus, while valproate is appropriate for patients who have generalized seizures while receiving cyclosporin A, phenytoin and carbamazepine remain drugs of choice for patients with partial onset seizures. Use of any AED should prompt frequent cyclosporin A level measurements to allow dose adjustments as necessary to maintain therapeutic concentrations.

Seizures in transplant recipients have also been attributed to cyclosporin A (Deierhoi et al 1988, Beaman et al 1985, Shah et al 1984, Joss et al 1982, Polson et al 1985), especially when cyclosporin A levels have been high (Shah et al 1984, Beaman et al 1985, Deierhoi et al 1988). However, convulsions have also occurred in patients with cyclosporin A concentrations in the usual therapeutic range (Polson et al 1985, Appleton et al 1989). The incidence of convulsive seizures in cyclosporin A-treated kidney and bone marrow transplant recipients has been estimated at 1.5% and 5.5%, respectively (O'Sullivan 1985). Haematological malignancy, intrathecal methotrexate, whole body irradiation, hypertension, steroid treatment and impaired renal function may be predisposing conditions in some cases of cyclosporin A-associated convulsions (O'Sullivan 1985, Joss et al 1982). In contrast, a retrospective review of paediatric renal transplant recipients found no significant change in seizure prevalence (31% of transplant recipients) over the period 1965–1987, despite a change in immunosuppressive regimen from prednisone and azathioprine to cyclosporin A (McEnery et al 1989).

MAJOR PSYCHIATRIC ILLNESS

Whether major depression, mania and psychosis occur more frequently among persons with epilepsy compared with the general population remains controversial (Hauser & Hessdorfer 1990). Among persons with epilepsy followed in epilepsy clinics, however, the prevalence of depressive symptoms and use of psychotropic drugs is clearly increased (Ojemann et al 1987,

Robertson 1988). In one tertiary care epilepsy clinic, 11% of patients were treated at some time with antidepressant or antipsychotic drugs (Ojemann et al 1987). In patients with epilepsy and psychiatric illness, the effects of psychotropic agents on seizure frequency, psychoactive drug–AED interactions, and effects of epilepsy and psychiatric illness on one another are of great practical importance. Few clinical studies have specifically addressed these issues.

Psychosis

From their introduction in the 1950s, antipsychotic drugs have been reported to induce seizures in non-epileptic individuals (Logethetis 1967). There is general agreement that use of antipsychotic drugs increases the occurrence of seizures in previously seizure-free individuals. The overall risk is low, however, and seizures remain an unusual treatment complication (Logothetis 1967, Markowitz & Brown 1987, Lipka & Lathers 1987, Cold et al 1990). Haloperidol, flufenazine and thioridazine have induced seizures in previously asymptomatic individuals (Lipka & Lathers 1987, Cold et al 1990), and Logothetis (1967) reported an overall incidence of 1.2% of new onset seizures among institutionalized patients treated with phenothiazines. These seizures were most likely to occur with high drug dosages, seizure incidence approaching 10% in patients receiving the highest doses. Individuals with underlying organic brain disease were more likely to have seizures at lower drug doses (2% of 202 patients).

Few studies have systematically addressed psychosis and use of antipsychotic drugs in the setting of epilepsy. Trimble (1985) emphasized differences in treating ictal and peri-ictal psychoses compared with chronic interictal psychoses. Seizure-related psychoses require acute symptomatic treatment coupled with better seizure control; chronic interictal psychoses necessitate ongoing therapy with antipsychotic drugs. Bonafede (1955) administered chlorpromazine to 78 epileptic patients with severe behaviour problems, 60 of whom were mentally retarded. Patients were divided into three groups of 26 each. In one group, concomitant AEDs were not altered, whereas in the other two groups barbiturate dose was decreased by up to 50%. Seizure frequency increased in only 1/26 patients with unchanged AEDs, but increased seizures occurred in 17/52 patients whose barbiturate dose had been decreased. Tarjan et al (1957) reported on the effects of chlorpromazine in 278 mentally deficient patients (IQ less than 50 in 80%), 82 of whom had pre-existing epilepsy. They found that 12/278 experienced increased seizure frequency while on chlorpromazine, but noted that in 10 patients phenobarbitone had been tapered or discontinued when chlorpromazine was started. Pauig et al (1961) treated 100 children and adults with epilepsy using both AEDs and thioridazine. They found that 64% had fewer seizures, and 36% had no change in seizure frequency compared to pre-thioridazine baseline rates. Baldwin & Kenny (1966) used thioridazine to treat 23 epileptic children with behaviour disorders and found no change or improved seizure control in 22/23. James (1986) retrospectively reviewed the records of 26 chronically hospitalized patients with severe mental handicaps who were treated with neuroleptics. Despite incomplete and ambiguous data, his study indicated a low probability of seizure exacerbation in patients with pre-existing epilepsy who had 'adequate' serum antiepileptic drug levels at the time of neuroleptic treatment. Ojemann et al (1987) retrospectively analysed major tranquillizer use (chlorpromazine, thioridazine, thiothixene and haloperidol) in 13 patients treated at their epilepsy centre. In 12 patients, seizure control was improved or unchanged. The single patient whose seizures worsened had had similar seizure frequencies at times before thiothixene was prescribed.

Based upon these data, neuroleptic drug treatment of psychosis in persons with epilepsy can be undertaken with low probability of seizure exacerbation if therapeutic serum AED levels are maintained. Because available data suggest that seizures are more likely to occur with very high antipsychotic drug doses or with rapid increases in dose (Logothetis 1967), careful titration is indicated. Should seizures increase in frequency or severity during neuroleptic treatment, AED levels should be checked and the dosages adjusted as tolerated. If such adjustments fail to control seizures adequately, or if unacceptable symptoms of neurotoxicity develop, then another antipsychotic agent of a different class should be used. There are virtually no data regarding the effects of combination treatment with two or more antipsychotic drugs on seizure frequency.

Depression

Antidepressant drugs occasionally induce seizures in individuals without a history of epilepsy (Robertson 1988). Estimates of the incidence of seizures induced by tricyclic antidepressant (TCA) drugs vary considerably and range from 0.1% to 4% (Jick et al 1983, Leyberg & Denmark 1959, Lowry & Dunner 1980). Seizures have been attributed to virtually all TCAs (Robertson 1988). Many of the newer non-tricyclic antidepressants have also been reported to induce seizures, including trazadone (Lefkowitz et al 1985, Bowdan 1983, Robertson 1988), fluoxetine (Ware & Stewart 1989, Cooper 1988), maprotiline (Kim 1982, Bernad & Levine 1986, Dessain et al 1986, Robertson 1988) and amoxapine (Koval et al 1982). These newer agents may be more likely than tricyclics to induce seizures in normal individuals, especially maprotiline when used in doses greater than 200 mg per day (Dessain et al 1986, Robertson 1988). Most monoamine oxidase inhibitors have little epileptogenic potential, and iproniazide, isocarboxazide and tranylcypromine have not been reported to cause seizures (Robertson 1988).

While the relative risk of major depression in persons with epilepsy compared to the general population is unknown, the risk in patients seen at specialty epilepsy clinics is increased (Hauser & Hesdorffer 1990). Despite the apparently high prevalence of major depression among certain patient groups with active epilepsy, little data exist regarding optimal treatment of depression and concurrent epilepsy. In a retrospective review of patients with carefully documented clinic records, Ojemann et al (1983) noted improved seizure control in 15/19 and no change in 2/19 patients treated with doxepin for depression diagnosed by DSM III criteria. In a subsequent retrospective review, Ojemann et al (1987) reported that 29/32 patients with epilepsy treated with doxepin had improved or stable seizure control. Those with worse control while on doxepin had had similar or higher seizure frequencies at some time prior to treatment with the antidepressant. Robertson & Trimble (1985) conducted a prospective double-blind trial in which amitriptyline, nomifensine and placebo were compared in patients with coexisting depression and epilepsy. One of 42 patients entered in the trial withdrew because of an unacceptable increase in seizure frequency over the first month of amitriptyline treatment. In the 39 patients who completed the trial, there was no statistical difference in seizure frequency among equal groups receiving placebo, amitriptyline and nomifensine. In a study of amitriptyline for agitation following severe head injury, none of 20 treated patients developed seizures (Mysiw et al 1988). In an uncontrolled study of tricyclic antidepressant therapy in 68 severely head-injured patients, 7 had incident seizures without a previous seizure history, and 5 with prior seizures had slight increases in seizure frequency (Wroblewski et al 1990). Absence of an untreated control population in this group of patients at high risk for epilepsy makes interpretation of these results difficult.

Fromm et al (1978) carried out a small double-blind, placebo-controlled crossover study and discovered that imipramine was effective in reducing occurrence of intractable absence and myoclonic–astatic seizures. This finding raises the interesting possibility that some psychotropic drugs may affect different epilepsies and seizure types in substantially different ways.

As with the antipsychotic agents, the known but relatively infrequent pro-convulsant effects of many antidepressant drugs warrant a cautious approach to their use in persons with epilepsy. The need for antidepressant drug treatment should be unambiguous. Available clinical data indicate that the majority of patients treated with antidepressant drugs will not experience deterioration in seizure control; some may even benefit. Antidepressant agents should be started at a low dose, gradually titrating the dose to achieve the desired clinical effect. Doxepin may be a reasonable agent of first choice, but its sedative effects must be weighed in light of possible similar side effects from co-administered AEDs. Because maprotiline seems more likely to induce seizures in normal individuals, its use should probably be minimized in persons with epilepsy. If seizure control deteriorates under treatment, a change to an antidepressant drug of a different chemical class would be reasonable. Because monoamine oxidase inhibitors do not seem to be epileptogenic, they represent alternatives to the more commonly used agents. Finally, electroconvulsive therapy is an option for severe cases of depression, but little is known about its effects in the person with epilepsy (Robertson 1988).

Bipolar disorder occasionally occurs in persons with epilepsy (Shukla et al 1988) and lithium is generally the treatment of choice. Conflicting data have attributed both proconvulsant and antiepileptic properties to lithium. Convulsive and non-convulsive seizures have occurred in patients treated with therapeutic concentrations of lithium (Demers et al 1970, Baldessarini & Stephens 1970, Moore 1981). Jus et al (1973) reported that 3 of 8 women with temporal lobe epilepsy had major clinical deterioration in seizure control after less than two weeks of lithium despite levels of 0.58 mEq/l or lower. The authors did not comment whether these women were also being treated with antipsychotic drugs. Typical absence seizures were markedly exacerbated in a 14-year-old treated with lithium for one week (Moore 1981). In contrast, other reports suggest that lithium has either antiepileptic properties or no significant effect on seizure frequency. Gershon (1968) found that 21 patients with epilepsy experienced improved seizure control while being treated with lithium but few clinical details were provided. Erwin et al (1973) reported that 10 of 15 patients with active epilepsy treated with lithium had fewer seizures than before lithium was started. Four other patients had unchanged seizure frequency and one worsened. Shukla et al (1988) noted that none of eight bipolar patients with epilepsy had worse seizure control while taking lithium.

In the appropriate patient with partial or secondarily generalized seizures, treatment of concurrent bipolar disorder might first utilize carbamazepine as therapy for both epilepsy and the psychiatric disorder. Clinical studies indicate that carbamazepine is an effective alternative or adjunct to lithium therapy for the acute and prophylactic therapy of bipolar disorder (Ballenger & Post 1980, Post 1988). Valproate, usually as an adjunct to lithium, may also be useful in the treatment of mania (Post 1988). Thus, treating the patient with both generalized seizures and mania might be effectively accomplished using a combination of lithium and valproate.

Psychotropic drug–AED interactions

Various interactions between AEDs and psychotropic drugs have been reported (Table 9.8). Many of these reports are only of a few cases, and their relevance to the general population of interest is uncertain. Combined therapy with AEDs and antidepressant or antipsychotic drugs usually proceeds without clinically significant interactions. Baseline AED levels should be obtained before instituting psychotropic therapy, and any unexpected patterns of clinical response (e.g. failure of psychotropic effect, seizure exacerbation or other neurotoxic symptoms) should prompt determination of AED and psychotropic drug levels.

Table 9.8   Some reported interactions between AEDs and psychotropic drugs

Psychotropic drug	No. of patients studied	AED	Interaction	Author
Chlorpromazine		PHT	PHT accumulation	Kutt (1975)
	6	VPA	Inhibition of VPA metabolism	Ishizaki et al (1984)
Thioridazine	2	PHT	PHT accumulation	Vincent (1980)
	27	PHT	No significant PHT change	Sands et al (1987)
	9	PHT, PB, PHT + PB	Thioridazine level unchanged, mesoridazine active metabolite decreased	Linnoila et al (1980)
	6	PHT	Generally no significant PHT level changes	Gay & Madsen (1983)
	5	PB	Relatively decreased PB levels	Gay & Madsen (1983)
Haloperidol	9	PHT, PB, PHT + PB	Decreased haloperidol levels	Linnoila et al (1980)
	7	CBZ	Decreased haloperidol levels	Arana et al (1986)
	1	CBZ	Decreased haloperidol levels	Fast et al (1986)
	6	VPA	No significant effect	Ishizaki et al (1984)
Desipramine	2	PHT	Decreased desipramine levels	Fogel & Haltzman (1987)
Imipramine	2	PHT	PHT accumulation	Perucca & Richens (1977)
Trazadone	1	PHT	PHT accumulation	Dorn (1986)
Lithium	5	CBZ	Encephalopathy, tremor at acceptable drug levels	Shukla et al (1984)

Abbreviations: CBZ, carbamazepine; PB, phenobarbitone; PHT, phenytoin; VPA, valproate.

REFERENCES

Abajo F J 1988 Phenytoin interaction with rifampicin. Br Med J 297: 1048
Ahmad S 1984 Nifedipine–phenytoin interaction. J Am Coll Cardiol 3: 1582
Ahuja G K, Schumacher G A 1966 Drug-induced systemic lupus erythematosus. J Am Med Assoc 198: 669–671
Aitio M L, Mansury L, Tala E et al 1981 The effect of enzyme induction on the metabolism of disopyramide in man. Br J Clin Pharmacol 11: 279–285
Alballa S, Fritzler M, Davis P 1987 A case of drug induced lupus due to carbamazepine. J Rheumatol 14: 599–600
Appleton R E, Farrell K, Teal P et al 1989 Complex partial status epilepticus associated with cyclosporin A therapy. J Neurol Neurosurg Psychiatry 52: 1068–1071
Arana G W, Goff D C, Friedman H et al 1986 Does carbamazepine-induced reduction of plasma haloperidol levels worsen psychotic symptoms? Am J Psychiatry 143: 5–6
Asconape J J, Penry J K 1982 Use of antiepileptic drugs in the presence of liver and kidney diseases: a review. Epilepsia 23 (Suppl 1): S65–S79
Ayus J C, Krothapalli R K, Arieff A I 1985 Changing concepts in the treatment of severe symptomatic hyponatremia: rapid correction and possible relation to central pontine myelinolysis. Am J Med 78: 897–902
Baldessarini R J, Stephens J H 1970 Lithium carbonate for affective disorders. Arch

Gen Psychiatry 22: 72–77

Baldwin R W, Kenny T J 1966 Thioridazine in the management of organic behavior disturbances in children. Curr Ther Res 8: 373–377

Bale J F, Fountain T, Shaddy R 1984 Phenylpropanolamine-associated CNS complications in children and adolescents. Am J Dis Child 138: 683–685

Ballenger J C, Post R M 1980 Carbamazepine in manic-depressive illness: a new treatment. Am J Psychiatry 137: 782–790

Basciewicz A M 1986 Carbamazepine drug interactions. Ther Drug Monit 8: 305–317

Beaman M, Parvin S, Veitch P S, Walls J 1985 Convulsions associated with cyclosporin A in renal transplant recipients. Br Med J 290: 139–140

Beattie B, Biller J, Mehlhaus B, Murray M 1988 Verapamil-induced carbamazepine neurotoxicity: a report of two cases. Eur Neurol 28: 104–105

Begg E J, Chinwah P M, Webb C et al 1982 Enhanced metabolism of mexiletine after phenytoin administration. Br J Clin Pharmacol 14: 219–223

Bennett W M 1981 Altering drug dose in patients with diseases of the kidney and liver. In: Anderson R J, Schrier R W (eds) Clinical use of drugs in patients with kidney and liver disease. Saunders, Philadelphia, pp 16–29

Bennett W M, Aronoff G R, Morrison G et al 1983 Drug prescribing in renal failure: dosing guidelines for adults. Am J Kidney Dis 3: 155–193

Bernad P G, Levine M S 1986 Maprotiline-induced seizures. South Med J 79: 1179–1180

Bernstein E, Diskant B M 1982 Phenylpropanolamine: a potentially hazardous drug. Ann Emerg Med 11: 311–315

Bivins B A, Rapp R P, Griffen W O et al 1978 Dopamine–phenytoin interaction: a cause of hypotension in the critically ill. Arch Surg 113: 245–249

Bleck T P, Smith M C 1990 Possible induction of systemic lupus erythematosus by valproate. Epilepsia 31: 343–345

Boenigk H E, Lorenz J H, Jurgens U 1986 Experience to date using bromide in the treatment of generalized epilepsies. Epilepsia 27: 586

Bonafede V I 1955 Chlorpromazine (thorazine) treatment of disturbed epileptic patients. Arch Neurol Psychiatry 74: 158–162

Booker H E, Darcey B 1973 Serum concentrations of free diphenylhydantoin and their relationship to clinical intoxication. Epilepsia 14: 177–184

Bowdan N D 1983 Seizure possibly caused by trazodone HCl. Am J Psychiatry 140: 642

Bramhall D, Levine M 1988 Possible interaction of ranitidine with phenytoin. Drug Intell Clin Pharm 22: 979–980

Brodie M J, MacPhee G J 1986 Carbamazepine neurotoxicity precipitated by diltiazem. Br Med J 292: 1170–1171

Brooks S M, Werk E E, Ackerman S J et al 1972 Adverse effects of phenobarbital on corticosteroid metabolism in patients with bronchial asthma. N Engl J Med 286: 1125

Brown R B, Sands M, Morris A B 1990 Seizure propensity with imipenem. Arch Intern Med 150: 1551

Browne T R 1983a Status epilepticus. In: Browne T R, Feldman R G (eds) Epilepsy: diagnosis and management. Little, Brown, Boston, pp 341–354

Browne T R 1983b Paraldehye, acetazolamide, trimethadione, paramethadione, and phenacemide. In: Browne T R, Feldman R G (eds) Epilepsy: diagnosis and management. Little, Brown, Boston, pp 247–258

Buchbinder R, Hall S, Littlejohn G O, Ryan P F 1988 Neuropsychiatric manifestations of systemic lupus erythematosus. Aust NZ J Med 18: 679–684

Byatt C M 1990 Hyponatraemia and moduretic-grand mal seizures. J R Soc Med 83: 200

Calandra G, Lydick E, Carrigan J et al 1988 Factors predisposing to seizures in seriously ill infected patients receiving antibiotics: experience with imipenem/cilastatin. Am J Med 84: 911–918

Chalk J B, Ridgeway K, Brophy Tro R, Yelland J D N, Eadie M J 1984 Phenytoin impairs the bioavailability of dexamethasone in neurological and neurosurgical patients. J Neurol Neurosurg Psychiatry 47: 1087–1090

Chang T 1989 Ethosuximide: absorption, distribution, and excretion. In: Levy R H, Mattson R, Meldrum B et al (eds) Antiepileptic drugs. Raven Press, New York, pp 671–678

Cloyd J C, Leppik I E 1989 Primidone: absorption, distribution, and excretion. In: Levy R H, Mattson R, Meldrum B et al (eds) Antiepileptic drugs. Raven Press, New York, pp 391–400

Cloyd J C, Bosch D E, Sawchuk R J 1978 Concentration–time profile of phenytoin after admixture with small volumes of intravenous fluids. Am J Hosp Pharm 35: 45–48

Cloyd J C, Gumnit R J, McLain L W 1980 Status epilepticus: the role of intravenous phenytoin. JAMA 244: 1479–1481

Cold J A, Wells B G, Froemming J H 1990 Seizure activity associated with antipsychotic therapy. Drug Intell Clin Pharm 24: 601–606

Cooper G L 1988 The safety of fluoxetine: an update. Br J Psychiatry 153: 77–86

Cornelius J R, Soloff P H, Reynolds C F 1984 Paranoia, homicidal behavior, and seizures associated with phenylpropanolamine. Am J Psychiatry 141: 120–121

Covelli H D, Knodel A R, Heppner B T 1985 Predisposing factors to apparent theophylline-induced seizures. Ann Allergy 54: 411–415

Dalton M J, Powell J R, Messenheimer J A, Clark J 1986 Cimetidine and carbamazepine: a complex drug interaction. Epilepsia 27: 553–558

D'Arcy P F, McElnay J C 1987 Drug–antacid interactions: assessment of clinical importance. Drug Intell Clin Pharm 21: 607–617

Data J L, Wilkinson G R, Nies A S 1976 Interaction of quinidine with anticonvulsant drugs. N Engl J Med 294: 699–702

Deierhoi M H, Kalayoglu M, Sollinger H W, Belzer F O 1988 Cyclosporine neurotoxicity in liver transplant recipients: report of three cases. Transplant Proc 20: 116–118

Demers R, Lukesh R, Prichard J 1970 Convulsion during lithium therapy. Lancet ii: 315–316

Deocampo P D 1979 Convulsive seizures due to phenylpropanolamine. J Med Soc NJ 76: 591–592

Dessain E C, Schatzberg A F, Woods B T, Cole J O 1986 Maprotiline treatment in depression. Arch Gen Psychiatry 43: 86–90

Devanand D P, Decina P, Sackeim H A, Prudic J 1988 Status epilepticus following ECT in a patient receiving theophylline. J Clin Psychopharmacol 8: 153

Diaz-Guerrero R, Feinstein R, Gottlieb J S 1956 EEG findings following intravenous injection of diphenhydramine hydrochloride (benadryl). EEG Clin Neurophysiol 8: 299–306

Donaldson J O 1986 Does magnesium sulfate treat eclamptic convulsions? Clin Neuropharmacol 9: 37–45

Dorn J M 1986 A case of phenytoin toxicity possibly precipitated by trazodone. J Clin Psychiatry 47: 89–90

Dreifuss F E 1989 Bromides. In: Levy R H, Dreifuss F E, Mattson R H et al (eds) Antiepileptic drugs. Raven Press, New York, pp 877–879

Dreifuss F E, Bertram E H 1986 Bromide therapy for intractable seizures. Epilepsia 27: 593

Dreifuss F E, Langer D H 1987 Hepatic considerations in the use of antiepileptic drugs. Epilepsia 28 (Suppl 2): S23–S29

Dreifuss F E, Santilli N, Langer D H et al 1987 Valproic acid hepatic fatalities: a retrospective review. Neurology 37: 379–385

Eimer M, Carter B L 1987 Elevated serum carbamazepine concentrations following diltiazem initiation. Drug Intell Clin Pharm 21: 340–342

Eng R H K, Munsif A N, Yangeo B G et al 1989 Seizure propensity with imipenem. Arch Intern Med 149: 1881–1883

Erwin C W, Gerber C J, Morrison S D, James J F 1973 Lithium carbonate and convulsive disorders. Arch Gen Psychiatry 28: 646–648

Fanta C H, Ingram R H 1988 Asthma. In: Rubenstein E, Federman D D (eds) Scientific American medicine. Scientific American, New York, 14(II), pp 1–18

Fast D K, Jones B D, Kusalic M, Erickson M 1986 Effect of carbamazepine on neuroleptic plasma levels and efficacy. Am J Psychiatry 143: 117–118

Feinglass E J, Arnett F C, Dorsch C A et al 1976 Neuropsychiatric manifestations of systemic lupus erythematosus: diagnosis, clinical spectrum, and relationship to other features of the disease. Medicine 55: 323–339

Fogel B S, Haltzman S 1987 Desipramine and phenytoin: a potential drug interaction of therapeutic relevance. J Clin Psychiatry 48: 387–388

Freed C R 1981 Clinical pharmacology for the clinician. In: Anderson R J, Schrier R W (eds) Clinical use of drugs in patients with kidney and liver disease. Saunders, Philadelphia, pp 1–15

Freeman D J, Laupacis A, Keown P A et al 1984 Evaluation of cyclosporin–phenytoin interaction with observations on cyclosporin metabolites. Br J Clin Pharmacol 18: 887–893

Friedman R, Zitelli B, Jardine D, Fireman P 1982 Seizures in a patient receiving terbutaline. Am J Dis Child 136: 1091–1092

Freidman W F 1984 Congenital heart disease in infancy and childhood. In: Braunwald E B (ed) Heart disease. Saunders, Philadelphia, pp 941–1023

Fromm G H, Wessel H B, Glass J D et al 1978 Imipramine in absence and myoclonic–astatic seizures. Neurology 28: 953–957

Gambertoglio J G, Lauer R M 1981 Use of neuropsychiatric drugs. In: Anderson R J, Schrier R W (eds) Clinical use of drugs in patients with kidney and liver disease. Saunders, Philadelphia, pp 276–295

Gay P E, Madsen J A 1983 Interaction between phenobarbital and thioridazine. Neurology 33: 1631–1632

Gershon S 1968 Use of lithium salts in psychiatric disorders. Dis Nervous System 29: 51–55

Gore J M, Haffajee C I, Alpert J S 1984 Interaction of amiodorone and diphenylhydantoin. Am J Cardiol 54: 1145

Goulden K J, Dooley J M, Camfield P R 1987 Clinical valproate toxicity induced by acetylsalicylic acid. Neurology 37: 1392–1394

Gram L, Bentsen K D 1983 Hepatic toxicity of antiepileptic drugs: a review. Acta Neurol Scand S97: 81–90

Gugler R, von Unruh G E 1980 Clinical pharmacokinetics of valproic acid. Clin Pharmacokinet 5: 67–83

Hall T G, Cuddy P G, Glass C J, Melethil S 1986 Effect of sucralfate on phenytoin bioavailability. Drug Intell Clin Pharm 20: 607–611

Hantman D, Rossier B, Zohlmann R et al 1973 Rapid correction of hyponatremia in the syndrome of inappropriate secretion of antidiuretic hormone: an alternative treatment to hypertonic saline. Ann Intern Med 78: 870–875

Harmon C E, Portanova J P 1982 Drug-induced lupus: clinical and serological studies. Clin Rheumatic Dis 8: 121–135

Haslam R H A, Freigang B 1985 Cough syncope mimicking epilepsy in asthmatic children. Can J Neurol Sci 12: 45–47

Hauser W A, Hesdorffer D C 1990 Intellectual and psychological factors. In: Hauser W A, Hesdorffer D C (eds) Epilepsy: frequency, causes, and consequences. Demos, New York, pp 245–271

Hauser W A, Kurland L T 1975 The epidemiology of epilepsy in Rochester, Minnesota, 1935 through 1967. Epilepsia 16: 1–66

Heinonen J, Takki S, Jarho L 1970 Plasma lidocaine levels in patients treated with potential inducers of microsomal enzymes. Acta Anaesth Scand 14: 89–95

Hillebrand G, Castro L A, Van Scheidt W et al 1987 Valproate for epilepsy in renal transplant recipients receiving cyclosporine. Transplantation 43: 915–916

Horowitz S, Patwardhan R, Marcus E 1988 Hepatotoxic reactions associated with carbamazepine therapy. Epilepsia 29: 149–154

Hughs G R 1982 The treatment of SLE: the case for conservative management. Clin Rheum Dis 8: 299–313

Imai H, Nakamoto Y, Hirokawa M et al 1989 Carbamazepine-induced granulomatous necrotizing angiitis with acute renal failure. Nephron 51: 405–408

Ishizaki T, Chiba K, Saito M et al 1984 The effects of neuroleptics (haloperidol and chlorpromazine) on the pharmacokinetics of valproic acid in schizophoric patients. J Clin Psychopharmacol 4: 254–261

Jallon P, Louiset P, Loiseau P 1986 Epileptiques, gare aux rhumes: danger des medicaments contenant de la phenylpropanolamine. Presse Med 15: 1877–1878

James D H 1986 Neuroleptics and epilepsy in mentally handicapped patients. J Ment Defic Res 30: 185–189

Jick H, Dinan B J, Hunter J R et al 1983 Tricyclic antidepressants and convulsions. J Clin Psychopharmacol 3: 182–185

Johnson R T, Richardson E P 1968 The neurological manifestations of systemic lupus erythematosus. Medicine 47: 337–369

Johnston C, Webb L, Daley J, Spathis G S 1989 Hyponatraemia and moduretic-grand mal seizures: a review. J R Soc Med 82: 479–483

Jonkman J H 1986 Therapeutic consequences of drug interactions with theophylline pharmacokinetics. J Allergy Clin Immunol 78: 736–742

Joss D V, Barrett A J, Kendra J R, Lucas C F, Desai S 1982 Hypertension and convulsions in children receiving cyclosporin A. Lancet i: 906

Jus A, Villeneuve A, Gautier J et al 1973 Some remarks on the influence of lithium carbonate on patients with temporal epilepsy. Int J Clin Pharmacol 7: 67–74

Kandrotas R J, Oles K S, Gal P, Love J M 1989 Carbamazepine clearance in hemodialysis and hemoperfusion. Drug Intell Clin Pharm 23: 137–140

Kaplan P W, Lesser R P, Fisher R S et al 1988 No, magnesium sulfate should not be used in treating eclamptic seizures. Arch Neurol 45: 1361–1364

Kay L, Kampmann J P, Svendsen T L et al 1985 Influence of rifampicin and isoniazid on the kinetics of phenytoin. Br J Clin Pharmacol 20: 323–326

Keown P A, Laupacis A, Carruthers G et al 1984 Interaction between phenytoin and cyclosporine following organ transplantation. Transplantation 38: 304–305

Kim W Y 1982 Seizures associated with maprotiline. Am J Psychiatry 139: 845

Kitagawa T, Takahashi K 1980 EEG activation of 3 Hz spike and wave complexes, especially activation with diphenhydramine (benadryl). Folia Psychiatr Neurol Jpn 34: 327–328

Klotz U, Rapp T, Muller W A 1978 Disposition of valproic acid in patients with liver disease. Eur J Clin Pharmacol 13: 55–60

Koup J R, Gibaldi M, McNamara P et al 1978 Interaction of chloramphenicol with phenytoin and phenobarbital. Clin Pharmacol Ther 24: 571–575

Koval G, VanNuis C, Davis T D 1982 Seizures associated with amoxapine. Am J Psychiatry 139: 845

Kraemer M J, Furukawa C T, Koup J R et al 1982 Altered theophylline clearance during an influenza B outbreak. Pediatrics 69: 476–480

Kutt H 1975 Interactions of antiepileptic drugs. Epilepsia 16: 393–402

Kutt H 1984 Interactions between anticonvulsants and other commonly prescribed drugs. Epilepsia 25 (Suppl 2): S118–S131

Lamon J M, Bennett M, Frykholm B C et al 1978 Prevention of acute porphyric attacks by intravenous haematin. Lancet ii: 492–494

Lee S L, Chase P H 1975 Drug-induced systemic lupus erythematosus: a critical review. Semin Arthritis Rheum 5: 83–103

Lefkowitz D, Kilgo G, Lee S 1985 Seizures and trazodone therapy. Arch Gen Psychiatry 42: 523

Lesser R P, Luders H, Dinner D S, Morris H H 1985 Epileptic seizures due to thrombotic and embolic cerebrovascular disease in the elderly. Epilepsia 26: 622–630

Levine M, Jones M W, Sheppard I 1985 Differential effect of cimetidine on serum concentrations of carbamazepine and phenytoin. Neurology 35: 562–565

Levy R H, Shen D D 1989 Valproate: absorption, distribution, and excretion. In: Levy R H, Mattson R, Meldrum B et al (eds) Antiepileptic drugs. Raven Press, New York, pp 583–600

Levy R H, Unadkat J D 1989 Drug absorption, distribution, and elimination. In: Levy R H, Mattson R, Meldrum B et al (eds) Antiepileptic drugs. Raven Press, New York, pp 1–22

Leyberg J T, Denmark J C 1959 The treatment of depressive states with imipramine hydrochloride (Tofranil). J Ment Sci 105: 1123–1126

Linnoila M, Viukari M, Vaisanen K, Auvinen J 1980 Effect of anticonvulsants on plasma haloperidol and thioridazine levels. Am J Psychiatry 137: 819–821

Lipka L J, Lathers C M 1987 Psychoactive agents, seizure production, and sudden death in epilepsy. J Clin Pharmacol 27: 169–183

Livingston S, Pearson P H 1953 Bromides in the treatment of epilepsy in children. Am J Dis Child 86: 717–720

Logothetis J 1967 Spontaneous epileptic seizures and electroencephalographic changes in the course of phenothiazine therapy. Neurology 17: 869–877

Loiseau J, Loiseau P, Duche B et al 1990 A survey of epileptic disorders in southwest France: seizures in elderly patients. Ann Neurol 27: 232–237

Lowry M R, Dunner F J 1980 Seizures during tricyclic therapy. Am J Psychiatry 137: 1461–1462

Mabuchi H, Nakahashi H 1988 A major inhibitor of phenytoin binding to serum protein in uremia. Nephron 48: 310–314

MacPhee G J, Thompson G G, McInnes G T, Brodie M J 1986 Verapamil potentiates carbamazepine neurotoxicity: a clinically important inhibitory interaction. Lancet i: 700–703

Mandell G L, Sande M A 1980 Drugs used in the chemotherapy of tuberculosis and leprosy. In: Gilman A G, Goodman L S, Gilman A (eds) The pharmacologic basis of therapeutics. Macmillan, New York, pp 1200–1221

Markowitz J C, Brown R P 1987 Seizures with neuroleptics and antidepressants. Gen Hosp Psychiatry 9: 135–141

Mason J W 1987 Amiodarone. N Engl J Med 316: 455–466

Massey E W 1983 Effect of carbamazepine on coumadin metabolism. Ann Neurol 13: 691–692

Mauro L S, Mauro V F, Bachmann K A, Higgins J T 1989 Accuracy of two equations in determining normalized phenytoin concentrations. Drug Intell Clin Pharm 23: 64–68

May C A, Grnett W R, Small R E, Pellock J M 1982 Effects of three antacids on the bioavailability of valproic acid. Clin Pharm 1: 244–247

McEnery P T, Nathan J, Bates S R, Daniels S R 1989 Convulsions in children undergoing renal transplantation. J Pediatr 115: 532–536

McGuire G M, Macphee G J, Thompson G G et al 1988 Effects of sodium valproate on haem biosynthesis in man: implications for seizure management in the porphyric patient. Eur J Clin Invest 18: 29–32

Messing R O, Simon R P 1986 Seizures as a manifestation of systemic disease. Neurol Clin 4: 563–584

Moore D P 1981 A case of petit mal epilepsy aggravated by lithium. Am J Psychiatry 138: 690–691

Moore M R, McColl K E L, Rimington C, Goldberg A 1987 Disorders of porphyrin metabolism. Plenum, New York, pp 81–117

Morrelli H F, Melmom K L 1978 Drug interactions. In: Melmon K L, Morrelli H F (eds) Clinical pharmacology. Macmillan, New York, pp 982–1107

Morselli P L 1989 Carbamazepine: absorption, distribution, and excretion. In: Levy R H, Mattson R, Meldrum B et al (eds) Antiepileptic drugs. Raven Press, New York, pp 473–490

Mysiw W J, Jackson R D, Corrigan J D 1988 Amitriptyline for post-traumatic agitation. Am J Phys Med Rehabil 67: 29–33

Nappi J M 1979 Warfarin and phenytoin interaction. Ann Int Med 90: 852

Nellhaus G, Neuman I, Ellis E, Pirnat M 1975 Asthma and seizures in children. Pediatr Clin North Am 22: 89–100

Ojemann L M, Baugh-Bookman C, Dudley D L 1987 Effect of psychotropic medications on seizure control in patients with epilepsy. Neurology 37: 1525–1527

Ojemann L M, Friel P N, Trejo W J, Dudley D L 1983 Effect of doxepin on seizure frequency in depressed epileptic patients. Neurology 33: 646–648

Olanow C W, Finn A L, Prussak C 1981 The effects of salicylate on the pharmacokinetics of phenytoin. Neurology 31: 341–342

Oles K S, Mirza W, Penry J K 1989 Catastrophic neurologic signs due to drug interaction: tegretol and darvon. Surg Neurol 32: 144–151

Olivesi A 1986 Modified elimination of prednisolone in epileptic patients on carbamazepine monotherapy, and in women using low-dose oral contraceptives. Biomed Pharmacol 40: 301–308

Orr J M, Abbott F S, Farrell K et al 1982 Interaction between valproic acid and aspirin in epileptic children: serum protein binding and metabolic effects. Clin Pharmacol Ther 31: 642–649

O'Sullivan D P 1985 Convulsions associated with cyclosporin A. Br Med J 290: 858

Otawar S, Kajiya T, Shimo M et al 1963 Study on the activation of the electroencephalogram by diphenhydramine in children. Acta Paediatr Jpn 67: 583–592

Pauig P M, DeLuca M A, Osterheld R G 1961 Thioridazine hydrochloride in the treatment of behavior disorders in epileptics. Am J Psychiatry 117: 832–833

Perucca E, Richens A 1977 Interaction between phenytoin and imipramine. Br J Clin Pharmacol 4: 485–486

Perucca E, Richens A 1981 Drug interactions with phenytoin. Drugs 21: 120–137

Perucca E, Richens A 1989 Biotransformation. In: Levy R H, Mattson R, Meldrum B et al (eds) Antiepileptic drugs. Raven Press, New York, pp 23–48

Peters S G, Wochos D N, Peterson G C 1984 Status epilepticus as a complication of concurrent electroconvulsive and theophylline therapy. Mayo Clin Proc 59: 568–570

Pippenger C E 1987 Clinically significant carbamazepine drug interactions: an overview.

Epilepsia 28 (Suppl 3): S71–S76

Plum F, Posner J B 1980 The diagnosis of stupor and coma, 3rd edn. Davis, Philadelphia, p 228

Polson R J, Powell-Jackson P R, Williams R 1985 Convulsions associated with cyclosporin A in transplant recipients. Br Med J 290: 1003

Post R M 1988 Approaches to treatment-resistant bipolar affectively ill patients. Clin Neuropharmacol 11: 93–104

Powell J R, Dalton K H 1984 Histamine H2 antagonist drug interactions in perspective: mechanistic concepts and clinical implications. Am J Med 77 (S5B): 57–84

Pugh C B 1987 Phenytoin and phenobarbitol protein binding alterations in a uremic burn patient. Drug Intell Clin Pharm 21: 264–267

Rameis H 1985 On the interaction between phenytoin and digoxin. Eur J Clin Pharmacol 29: 49–53

Rettie A E, Rettenmeier A W, Howald W N, Baillie T A 1987 Cytochrome P-450-catalyzed formation of delta-4-VPA, a toxic metabolite of valproic acid. Science 235: 890–892

Reza M J, Dornfeld L, Goldberg L S 1975 Hydralazine therapy in hypertensive patients with idiopathic systemic lupus erythematosus. Arthritis Rheum 18: 335–338

Richards W, Church J A, Brent D K 1985 Theophylline-associated seizures in children. Ann Allergy 54: 276–279

Robertson M M 1988 Depression in patients with epilepsy reconsidered. In: Pedley T A, Meldrum B S (eds) Recent advances in epilepsy. Churchill Livingstone, Edinburgh, pp 205–240

Robertson M M, Trimble M R 1985 The treatment of depression in patients with epilepsy: a double-blind trial. J Affective Disord 9: 127–136

Rose J Q, Choi H K, Schentag J J et al 1977 Intoxication caused by interaction of chloramphenicol and phenytoin. JAMA 237: 2630–2631

Rosenberry K R, Defusco C J, Mansmann H C, McGeady S J 1983 Reduced theophylline half-life induced by carbamazepine therapy. J Pediatr 102: 472–474

Ross J R, Beeley L 1980 Interaction between carbamazepine and warfarin. Br Med J 280: 1415–1416

Rust R S, Dodson W E 1989 Phenobarbital: absorption, distribution, and excretion. In: Levy R H, Mattson R, Meldrum B et al (eds) Antiepileptic drugs. Raven Press, New York, pp 293–304

Salem R B, Yost R L, Torosian G et al 1980 Investigation of the crystallization of phenytoin in normal saline. Drug Intell Clin Pharm 14: 605–608

Sandford N L, Murray N, Keyser A J, Reynolds T B 1987 Phenytoin toxicity and hepatic encephalopathy: simulation or stimulation? J Clin Gastroenterol 9: 337–341

Sands C D, Robinson J D, Salem R B et al 1987 Effect of thioridazine on phenytoin serum concentration: a retrospective study. Drug Intell Clin Pharm 21: 267–272

Sandyk R 1982 Phenytoin toxicity induced by interaction with ibuprofen. SA Med J 62: 592

Scheuer M L (in press) The medical patient with epilepsy. In: Resor S R, Kutt H (eds) Medical treatment of epilepsy. Dekker, New York

Scheuer M L, Pedley T A 1990 The evaluation and treatment of seizures. N Engl J Med 323: 1468–1474

Schmidt D 1982 Disorders of the kidneys. In: Schmidt D (ed) Adverse effects of antiepileptic drugs. Raven Press, New York, p 111

Schofield O M V, Camp R D R, Levene G M 1990 Cyclosporin A in psoriasis: interaction with carbamazepine. Br J Dermatol 122: 425–426

Shackleford E J, Watson F T 1987 Amiodorone–phenytoin interaction. Drug Intell Clin Pharm 21: 921

Shah D, Rylance P B, Rogerson M E et al 1984 Generalised epileptic fits in renal transplant recipients given cyclosporin A. Br Med J 289: 1347–1348

Shukla S, Godwin C D, Long L E B, Miller M G 1984 Lithium–carbamazepine neurotoxicity and risk factors. Am J Psychiatry 141: 1604–1606

Shukla S, Mukherjee S, Decina P 1988 Lithium in the treatment of bipolar disorders associated with epilepsy: an open study. J Clin Psychopharmacol 8: 201–204

Sirgo M A, Green P J, Rocci M L Jr, Vlasses P H 1984 Interpretation of serum phenytoin concentrations in uremia is assay-dependent. Neurology 34: 1250–1251

Smart H L, Somerville K W, Williams J et al 1985 The effects of sucralfate upon phenytoin absorption in man. Br J Clin Pharmacol 20: 238–240

Sonne J, Luhdorf K, Larsen N E, Andreasen P B 1983 Lack of interaction between cimetidine and carbamazepine. Acta Neurol Scand 68: 253–256

Tanaka E, Ishikawa A, Ono A et al 1987 Trimethadione metabolism in patients with normal liver and in patients with chronic liver disease. J Pharmacobiodyn 10: 499–502

Tarjan G, Lowery V E, Wright S W 1957 Use of chlorpromazine in two hundred and seventy-eight mentally deficient patients. Am J Dis Child 94: 294–300

Taylor R L 1981 Magnesium sulfate for AIP seizures. Neurology 31: 1371–1372

Tennison M B, Miles M V, Pollack G M et al 1988 Valproate metabolites and hepatotoxicity in an epileptic population. Epilepsia 29: 543–547

Trimble M R 1985 The psychoses of epilepsy and their treatment. Clin Neuropharmacol 8: 211–220

Udall J A 1975 Clinical implications of warfarin interactions with five sedatives. Am J Cardiol 35: 67–71

Urbano A M 1983 Phenytoin–quinidine interaction in a patient with recurrent ventricular tachyarrhythmias. N Engl J Med 308: 225

van Weiringen A, Vrijlandt C M 1983 Ethosuximide intoxication caused by interaction with isoniazid. Neurology 33: 1227–1228

Vincent F M 1980 Phenothiazine-induced phenytoin intoxication. Ann Intern Med 93: 56–57

Ware M R, Stewart R B 1989 Seizures associated with fluoxetine therapy. Drug Intell Clin Pharm 23: 428

Wassner S J, Pennisi A J, Malekzadeh M H, Fine R N 1976 The adverse effect of anticonvulsant therapy on renal allograft survival. J Pediatr 88: 134–137

Watts R W, Hetzel D J, Bochner F et al 1983 Lack of interaction between ranitidine and phenytoin. Br J Clin Pharmacol 15: 499–500

Webster L K, Mihaly G W, Jones D B et al 1984 Effect of cimetidine and ranitidine on carbamazepine and sodium valproate pharmacokinetics. Eur J Clin Pharmacol 27: 341–343

Weinstein A 1980 Drug-induced systemic lupus erythematosus. Prog Clin Immunol 4: 1–21

Werman H A, Davis E A, Rund D A 1987 Abdominal pain and seizures in a young man. Ann Emerg Med 16: 425–433

Woodbury D M 1989 Phenytoin: absorption, distribution, and excretion. In: Levy R H, Mattson R, Meldrum B et al (eds) Antiepileptic drugs. Raven Press, New York, pp 177–196

Wroblewski B A, McColgan K, Smith K et al 1990 The incidence of seizures during tricyclic antidepressant drug treatment in a brain-injured population. J Clin Psychopharmacol 10: 124–128

Yassa R, Nastase C, Camille Y et al 1987 Carbamazepine, diuretics, and hyponatremia: a possible interaction. J Clin Psychiatry 48: 281–283

Zimmerman H J, Kamal I G 1982 Valproate-induced hepatic injury: analysis of 23 fatal cases. Hepatology 2: 591–597

Zwillich C W, Sutton F D, Neff T A et al 1975 Theophylline-induced seizures in adults: correlation with serum concentrations. Ann Intern Med 82: 784–787

10

Management of epilepsy in developing countries

N. A. Kshirsagar   P. U. Shah

INTRODUCTION

The management of epilepsy in developing countries differs markedly from that in developed countries. This arises not only because of population variation and differences in disease pattern but more significantly through the economic and cultural differences in the respective populations.

Several excellent reviews on epilepsy in developing countries have been published (Shorvon & Farmer 1988, Bittencourt 1988, Chandra 1988, Meinardi 1988).

This review, which analyses the relative importance of the above-mentioned determinants, may help practitioners in developing countries in planning effective health care delivery systems for epilepsy and to improve control of seizures and the overall quality of life.

POPULATION VARIATION

Of the total estimated world population of 5246 million, 4036 million are in developing countries. In developed countries 25% live in rural areas, while in developing countries 60–75% are in rural areas (Tabibzadeh et al 1989). Literacy rates differ in rural and urban areas. In India 29% of those in villages are literate whilst 57% of those in cities can read and write (Rural Health Statistics 1988). The large population, its unequal distribution between urban and rural areas and its heterogeneity, particularly with respect to economic standards, literacy rate and orthodoxy, is partly responsible for the observed differences in disease prevalence and aetiology.

Prevalence of epilepsy

Shorvon & Farmer (1988) have critically analysed studies from various countries and brought out the importance of survey methodology, patient cooperation and current practices in obtaining a correct estimate of disease patterns. Prevalence rates as low as 1.5 per 1000 in Nigata city (Sato 1964) and as high as 31 per 1000 in Melipilla in Chile (Chiofalo et al 1979) have been reported. It is claimed that the prevalence of epilepsy in developing countries is twice that in the developed nations.

Prevalence of epilepsy has been reported to differ in rural and urban populations in Nigeria, being 5.3/1000 in a town compared to 37/1000 in a village (Osuntokun et al 1987). Non-availability of effective primary health care, greater incidence of childhood infections and poor antenatal care may be responsible for the higher incidence in villages. Such a marked difference has, however, not been found in other studies. Gourie-Devi et al (1987) in India found a prevalence of 5.6 per 1000 in rural and 2.5 per 1000 in semi-urban communities. In a rural population in Kashmir the rate was found to be 2.47 per 1000 (Kaul et al 1988). In the Parsi community in Bombay, in a door-to-door survey using a questionnaire that had a sensitivity of 100% in a pilot study, 3.6 per 1000 were found to have active epilepsy (Bharucha et al 1988).

In the USA, epidemiological studies show racial variation in the incidence and prevalence of epilepsy, these being higher in blacks than in whites (Shamansky & Glaser 1979, Haerer et al 1986).

Aetiology

The proportion of cases with identifiable aetiology depends largely on the rational use and availability of investigations. In studies from developed countries, the aetiology of epilepsy can be established in about one-third of all cases (Sander & Shorvon 1987). The aetiological profile of epilepsy in different parts of the world shows true variation (Shorvon & Farmer 1988). In developing countries many of the causes of epilepsy (e.g. infections, infestations and birth injuries) are preventable (Bittencourt 1988, Ogunniyi et al 1987). In recent years with the advent of computed tomography (CT) and magnetic resonance imaging (MRI) more cases of secondary epilepsy due to tuberculoma and cysticercosis are being detected. However, there is also a large number of cases in which there is a diagnostic dilemma about aetiology, as in 'disappearing CT lesions'.

Some of these important causes and details of the 'disappearing CT lesions' are described.

Tuberculosis

The risk of tuberculous infection is a hundred times higher in the developing countries (World Health Statistics 1989, Vengsarkar et al 1986). There has been a downward trend in the incidence of tuberculosis, but the position is far from satisfactory. Lalitha et al (1980) found that in the children's wards of a teaching hospital in Bombay admissions due to neurotuberculosis fell from 4.4% per year during 1951–1960 to 1.9% per year by 1971. Post-mortem study shows that there was a decline in the number of tuberculomas of the brain from 30.5% of all intracranial space-occupying lesions in 1963 to 21.5% in 1968, 17.6% in 1972 and 12.3% in 1974 (Lalitha & Dastur 1980).

Diagnosis. Tuberculosis of the central nervous system manifests as basal meningitis, vasculitis, encephalopathy, tuberculoma, spinal meningitis and rarely intraspinal tuberculoma. The diagnosis of neurotuberculosis depends on clinical features, cerebrospinal fluid (CSF) findings and CT scan. In tuberculous meningitis, the demonstration of acid-fast bacilli has been possible in less than 30% of cases (Wadia 1989). Many attempts have been made to detect specific antibody, antigen or antigen–antibody complex (Ranadive & Banerjee 1989). Brooks et al (1990) reported a frequency-pulsed electron capture gas–liquid chromatographic (GLC) method for profiling carboxylic acid C2–C22 along with identification of tuberculostearic acid. The test had a sensitivity of 95% and specificity of 91%. Elisa test for detection of IgG antibody against *Mycobacterium tuberculosis* in CSF of tuberculous meningitis patients was found to have a specificity of 93–100% and sensitivity of 92–95% (Dole et al 1989). These tests are, however, not yet available routinely. For the diagnosis of tuberculoma, CT scan has become the investigation of choice (Vengsarkar et al 1986). In cases of tuberculous meningitis, asymptomatic microtuberculoma have been demonstrated with CT scan (Bhargava and Tandon 1980).

Treatment. Protocols for therapy have varied. The selection of drugs and duration of therapy are often left to the clinician's fancy and the demands of each case (severity of the disease, affordability, drug availability). Most favour a four-drug regimen comprising streptomycin, isoniazid, rifampicin and pyrazinamide for three months, followed by a variable combination of two to three drugs for 12–18 months. There is also considerable variation in the extent and duration of steroid treatment. Ramachandran et al (1986, 1989) studied three regimens. The first consisted of streptomycin, isoniazid and rifampicin for two months followed by ethambutol and isoniazid for ten months. In the second regimen pyrazinamide was added in the first two months and in the third regimen rifampicin was reduced to twice a week. The response was comparable in the three regimens (27% died of tuberculous meningitis, 39% had neurological sequelae and 34% recovered completely). Prognosis was noted to be dependent on the stage of the disease rather than the regimen, thus emphasizing the need for early diagnosis and treatment. A cautionary note has been sounded about the use of a short-term regimen in tuberculous meningitis as a disastrous flare-up of the disease may follow on stopping treatment in some patients (Pandya 1987).

As regards the treatment for tuberculomas, in the pre-streptomycin and isoniazid era total surgical excision was carried out wherever possible. Incomplete removal was followed by the development of tuberculous meningitis with high morbidity and mortality. With the advent of bactericidal drugs total excision of tuberculomas became unnecessary. Small tuberculomas regress with medical treatment. When the granuloma is large and in vital areas, decompressive surgery can now be safely attempted under the cover of drugs without the complication of meningitis (Bhagwati 1986).

Regularity in treatment, especially in the first three months, is crucial to good prognosis. Hepatotoxicity due to antitubercular drugs may, at times, hinder the continuity of full-dose treatment (Ramachandran et al 1989).

Parasitosis

Parasitosis is common in developing countries. Seizures may complicate parasitosis acutely or later as sequelae to infection and brain scarring, the severity and characteristics of seizure disorder varying with the disease stage and the individual's seizure threshold. Epilepsy is a well-recognized consequence of cysticercosis, toxoplasmosis and hydatid cyst but it is unclear how frequently it occurs as a chronic sequela to malaria, schistosomiasis or trypanosomiasis. (The reader is referred to the exhaustive review by Bittencourt et al (1988) on cysticercosis and other parasitic diseases causing epilepsy.)

Cysticercosis. Cysticercosis is common in Latin America, southern Africa and eastern Asia. Ahuja and Mohanta in New Delhi (1982) found cysticercosis in 5.1% of 233 patients evaluated for epilepsy of recent onset. Diagnosis of cysticercosis is based on CT and MRI findings. Attempts are being made to develop immunological tests for rapid diagnosis (Correa et al 1989). Praziquantel (PZQ) is effective in decreasing cyst size and number in the cerebral parenchyma. The usual regimen is 50 mg/kg per day for 15–21 days (Sotelo et al 1984). Episodes of meningeal reaction and increased intracranial pressure have led to occasional deaths during therapy (Sotelo et al 1984). Judicious use of steroids, diuretics and ventriculoperitoneal shunt can minimize complications during treatment (Bittencourt et al 1988). Wadia et al (1988) noted severe reaction to PZQ in patients with disseminated cysticercosis and recommend 'priming' of patients with dexamethasone and a small initial dose of PZQ. The experience of Chinese neurologists with similar patients has been different. They have used doses up to 120–180 mg/kg per day without running into any problem (Zhu and Xu 1983), thus raising the question of ethnic susceptibility among Indians to the drug. Albendazol (ALB), a new broad-spectrum antihelminthic, is currently the drug of choice. The efficacy of different regimens of therapy for parenchymal brain cysticercosis either with PZQ or with ALB was compared in 114 patients. Three months after therapy both ALB and PZQ were effective, as shown by disappearance of cystic lesions on CT. ALB was more effective for both full-term (15 mg/kg per day × 30) and short-term (15 mg/kg per day × 8) therapy compared to PZQ full-term (50 mg/kg per day × 15) and short-term (50 mg/kg per day × 8) therapy (85% versus 60% and 85% versus 48% disappearance of lesions), respectively. These authors recommended an eight-day course of ALB as treatment for parenchymal brain cysticercosis. A 15-day course of PZQ can be used in those patients who show a partial response to ALB (Sotelo et al 1990). In another study ALB 15 mg/kg per day was given for three days or one month. The authors concluded that both regimens were equally effective (Escalante & Duena 1989).

Dilemma of 'disappearing CT lesions'

With the availability of CT scans, there have been reports from India of hypodense lesions in the plain scan, and ring or disc-like enhancement surrounding the hypodensity on contrast scan in patients with epilepsy. Tandon & Bhargava (1980) first reported these lesions and suggested tuberculomas on the basis of histology in some cases and association with tuberculous meningitis in several others. Sethi et al (1985) reported that in some patients such lesions disappeared after three months without any antituberculous therapy, the patient being treated only with antiepileptic drugs (AED). These lesions are not likely to be due to seizures per se as reports from Western countries have not described CT changes persisting over a long duration after seizures (Sethi et al 1985). Wadia et al (1987) investigated 150 patients with simple partial seizures and found such disappearing lesions in 40% of children below 15 years of age and in 19% of adults.

The dilemma of aetiology can be solved by biopsy. However, biopsy at first diagnosis seems unnecessary and unwarranted as many of these lesions may clear with anticonvulsant therapy. Some of the excision biopsy studies carried out have shown the aetiology to be variable. Chandy & Rajshekhar (1988) reported biopsy findings in 6 patients, all of whom showed non-specific chronic inflammatory lesions. Nagarajaswamy (1989) biopsied the lesions seen on CT scans in 13 selected patients and found cysticercosis in 6, pyogenic abscess in 2, tuberculoma in 1, lymphocytic infiltration in 2, astrocytoma in 1 and gliosis in 1. Bansal et al (1989) postulate that these disappearing lesions may be small infarcts or follow transient disruption of the blood–brain barrier. Thomas et al (1989) reported on 10 stereotaxic biopsies where chronic inflammatory tissue was found. In 18 subsequent cases 17 showed cysticercosis and 1 a tuberculoma. Katrak (unpublished) found larval granuloma of *spirometra mansoni* – a tapeworm of cats and dogs (sparganosis) – on biopsy of such a lesion in one patient. Bhatia & Tandon (1988) have come across identical lesions caused by histoplasmosis, blastomycosis, sarcoidosis and infectious vasculitis. MRI scan differentiates between tuberculomas and cysticercosis in some patients (Desai 1990, personal communication).

There is no standard treatment protocol for such lesions. A practical approach may be to observe the patient on anticonvulsant therapy for three months and repeat the CT scan. Thereafter specific treatment, based on presumptive diagnosis, may be started if the lesion persists. (As shown by Diwate & Apte (1988), the presence of tuberculosis elsewhere in the body does not necessarily indicate that the lesion is tuberculous.) Biopsy is indicated only in non-responders to therapy.

Reflex epilepsies

Certain peculiar forms of seizures such as 'hot-water epilepsy' and 'eating epilepsy' may be more prevalent in India and Sri Lanka (Mani et al 1968). Hot-water epilepsy was observed in 4.4% of complex partial and generalized tonic–clonic seizures (Satishchandra et al 1988). Studies comparing the incidence of photosensitive epilepsy have shown that it is relatively rare in Africans. In the UK there is evidence of seasonal variation of photosensitive epilepsy – less in summer than in winter. Danesi (1988) showed that photoparoxysmal discharges (PPD) are less in summer than in winter.

Febrile seizures

The general guidelines to manage febrile seizures as practised in developed countries are also followed in developing countries. However, lack of easy access to emergency medical care and poor educational status of the parents, at times, force the treating physicians to start phenobarbitone on a continuous basis, even in the absence of risk factors.

Drug pharmacokinetics

Exposure to diseases peculiar to developing countries, malnutrition, dietary habits and ethnic differences in genetic polymorphisms have been shown to affect the pharmacokinetics of several drugs (Krishnaswamy & Teoh 1980, Kshirsagar et al 1987). Interpopulation differences and effects of nutritional deficiencies on AED pharmacokinetics have been investigated.

   The frequency of slow hydroxylation of phenytoin in Western populations is 1 in 500 (Inaba 1990). Dam et al (1977) have indicated that ethnic differences may have a significant influence on plasma clearance of AED. Anecdotal evidence from India suggests that effective AED dosage may be lower in Indians (Mani 1987). However, Peiris et al (1988) found no significant differences in the relative serum concentration of AED in Sri Lankan and matched European populations. Joshi et al (1990) found that phenytoin V_{max} and K_m values in the Indian population were comparable to reports from Western populations. There was no big difference between the actual phenytoin plasma values and the values predicted using nomograms derived from pharmacokinetic data from Western populations (Perucca & Richens 1981).

   In developing countries 45–75% of the population is malnourished and/or anaemic. This can affect the pharmacokinetics of, and the extent of adverse reactions to, AEDs. Singh et al (1987) reported that the steady-state phenobarbitone levels were significantly higher in children with grade II protein energy malnutrition, and clinical toxicity (viz. sedation, behavioural problems) was seen in two-thirds of the patients. Iron deficiency anaemia, although initially reported to affect pharmacokinetics (Desai et al 1982), has not been found to affect drug metabolism substantially (Kshirsagar et al 1988). Absorption and other pharmocokinetic parameters of phenytoin are not significantly altered in patients with iron deficiency anaemia (Joshi et al 1991). Thus no substantial AED pharmacokinetic differences have been found between developing and developed countries. This similarity is of practical importance as it justifies application of established dosage rules in developing countries (Joshi et al 1990, Osuntokun et al 1987). However, there is a paucity of data in children and neonates. At present, dosage adjustment based on pharmacokinetic principles is not yet practised in all developing countries. Clinicians and clinical pharmacologists often do not work together.

Adverse drug reactions

The AEDs have a narrow margin of safety and even in therapeutic doses produce adverse reactions. Considering the subnormal nutritional status in developing countries, one would expect a higher incidence of AED-induced folic acid and calcium deficiency particularly during pregnancy. However, the literature does not unequivocally substantiate this.

The effect of phenytoin on folic acid has been reviewed by Eadie & Tyrer (1989). Phenytoin intake at times causes reduced folate levels and, rarely, megaloblastic anaemia. Contrary to earlier studies it has been shown that administration of folic acid does not alter behaviour, personality or seizure control (Eadie & Tyrer 1989). Dastur & Dave (1987) found that serum folic acid levels were significantly lower in epileptic patients in Bombay receiving prolonged phenytoin/phenobarbitone treatment. None of the patients suffered from megaloblastic anaemia. Dansky et al (1987) found that blood folate levels were significantly lower in pregnancies with abnormal outcome than in those with normal outcome. However, Ramamurthi (1989a) did not find evidence of increased teratogenicity in 5325 children born to 3500 Indian women taking AEDs. The incidence of gingival hyperplasia is linked to folate status (Backman et al 1989). There are no reports of the incidence being different in developing countries.

Low serum calcium levels and raised serum alkaline phosphatase have been reported in patients taking phenytoin (Eadie & Tyrer 1989). Livingstone et al (1973) found no osteomalacia or metabolic disorder in 5500 epileptic patients from an affluent society in the USA. Mosenkilde & Melsen (1976) identified low dietary vitamin D intake, exposure to sunlight and anticonvulsant combination as risk factors for developing AED-induced osteomalacia. Out of 27 patients from a low socio-economic background in Bombay, 4 females were found to have clinical and radiological evidence of osteomalacia (Dastur & Dave 1987). Ganapathy et al (1973) found evidence of osteomalacia in 71% of iliac crest biopsy samples of patients on long-term AED. In northern India serum calcium was decreased in 11.4% of patients (Ganapathy et al 1973), and in southern India Snehlata & Ramamurthi (1972) found reduced serum calcium in 1.92% of patients. Malnutrition has been shown to predispose to hepatotoxicity induced by antitubercular drugs (Ramachandran et al 1989).

Several drug–drug interactions have been reported with AEDs. Interaction between antitubercular drugs and phenytoin is especially important. Isoniazid inhibits drug metabolism, while rifampicin stimulates it. Abajo (1988) reported an increase in phenytoin levels after withdrawal of rifampicin and ethambutol. Kay et al (1985) have reported that phenytoin clearance doubled after two weeks of treatment with rifampicin in volunteers.

ECONOMIC AND CULTURAL ASPECTS

Prevailing attitudes and beliefs, the use of traditional remedies and the economics of health care delivery play a major role in early and proper diagnosis, compliance with treatment and social acceptance, which are the mainstays of successful management.

Attitudes and beliefs

There is a reluctance on the part of the patient and family members to divulge information about seizures, and more so when the patient is a young girl. Generalized tonic–clonic seizures are not missed by people but there is considerable ignorance about recognition of absence or partial seizures and misbelief about the aetiology. Shorvon & Farmer (1988) have reviewed the beliefs prevailing in different cultures. In Sri Lanka, 30% of the preschool teachers who were being trained for the epilepsy programme believed epilepsy to be an affliction due to supernatural forces (Chandra 1988). Nigerians, including medical students, believe that epilepsy is contagious. The traditional healers seem to be the current repository and the propagators of this belief (Awaritefe 1989).

In some cultures 80% of the subjects first consult the traditional medical practitioner and may never be seen in modern hospitals (Osuntokun 1985). All cases in one study were treated by herbal remedies (Osuntokun et al 1987). Large cities in some countries have a different scenario, possibly due to increasing awareness. In one large, Indian, urban survey, 92% of patients had taken modern AEDs initially. However, as the importance of continued drug therapy was not emphasized, many were not actually receiving AED at the time of the survey or had turned to alternative systems or were combining drugs from multiple systems (Shah & Krishnaswamy, unpublished). (The medicinal properties of many plants and their interactions with modern drugs have been investigated and are reviewed below.)

Patients commonly receive proper treatment only after a valuable time period is lost and the disease achieves chronicity, which then leads to various economic and social problems for the patient. The existence of such chronically ill patients perpetuates the feeling of 'non-curability' or 'non-controllability' among others. This then increases the overall non-acceptance of the disease in society.

The social disadvantage for the person with epilepsy depends on how he sees himself and how he is seen by his peers. In Ethiopia, patients are treated as lepers and banished from the community. In Africa patients are forced to work due to economic reasons, often in areas not safe for epileptics, resulting in burns in many patients (Shorvon & Farmer 1988). In Kenya and Equador, people stated that they would not let their children play with known epileptics or marry them. In India, a woman known to have epilepsy has virtually no chance of an arranged marriage. Many hide their illness after the marriage, get recurrence of seizures due to non-compliance and then are sent back to their parents (Shorvon & Farmer 1988). On the other hand, in Iran 53% of the female patients were married (Afkhami et al 1989). The non-acceptance of patients, particularly the females, arises out of a strong belief in the role of heredity in the genesis of epilepsy and the teratogenic effects of AEDs during pregnancy.

The protection, sometimes even overprotection, given by the family is dependent on culture. In a house-to-house survey in Bombay by one of us (Shah), it was observed that 92% of the epileptic patients were reasonably well protected by the family; 5% were, in fact, overprotected. This is done in many families at a considerable economic burden for the family. Overprotection often results in negligence of other sibs economically and emotionally. Close family ties, cohesive cultural backgrounds and faith in advice tendered by the physician often prompt poor relatives to take excellent care of epileptic individuals. Under such circumstances it is very important for the physician to use available resources judiciously so as to avoid imposing unbearable burdens on the patient or family.

Economics of health care delivery

Caretaker team

There is a shortage of different members of the caretaker team. Epilepsy is treated by family physicians, paediatricians, physicians, psychiatrists and neurologists. In India there are 4 medical officers per 80 000 population at community health centres and 1 per 30 000 at primary health centres (Rural Health Statistics 1988) and 1 neurologist per 3 million population. The available doctors and specialists are concentrated in cities. Paramedical persons such as social workers are also in short supply. There is also a lack of expertise and training to diagnose and treat epilepsy satisfactorily.

Investigations

There is difficulty in following the 1985 ILAE classification in developing countries on account of the sophistication needed for the diagnosis of subtypes of 'symptomatic localization related epilepsies' – presently a privilege of investigators using depth electrodes (Bittencourt 1988a).

Electroencephalogram (EEG). The routine eight-channel EEG is the most widely used investigation. Its role in diagnosis is over-emphasized in developing countries. We are witness to a proliferation of laboratories without a similar proliferation of trained neurophysiologists (Bittencourt 1988). Video monitoring, telemetry and ambulatory EEG are either not available or are found in just a few places (Maheshwari 1982). Treatment of epilepsy is based by many solely on abnormal EEG findings without clinical correlation. Normal EEG may dissuade some patients from long-term compliance.

Neuroimaging. CT scanners are to be found only in cities with more than 300 000 inhabitants (Bittencourt 1988). There are no positron emission tomography (PET) scanners in the Third World. SPECT and magnetic resonance scanners are scarce. As the cost of a CT scan is high, its use is restricted to patients who can afford it and where the history suggests seizures with a focal onset.

Therapeutic drug monitoring. EEG and CT scan facilities are available in large cities, and in some countries at district headquarters, but a therapeutic drug-monitoring facility is available only at very few centres. In India the number of technicians available for clinical chemistry constitutes only 10% of the calculated requirement (Rural Health Statistics 1988). Even at those centres where such facilities are available, their reliability is questionable because of the absence of internationally acceptable quality control (Bittencourt 1988).

Nearly 50% of patients receiving phenytoin have plasma levels outside the therapeutic range (Ionnides Demos et al 1988, Kshirsagar & Shah 1990). It is possible to adjust dosage by increasing the dose slowly until response or toxicity occurs (Bittencourt 1988). In practice the low physician–patient ratio, ignorance amongst patients and poor follow-up do not allow optimum dosage adjustment. There is a great need for reliable and cheap monitoring kits (Ramamurthi 1989b). It is estimated that 20% of patients receiving phenytoin will benefit from drug monitoring but for developing countries the cost is the important deterrent.

Drug treatment

The treatment gap in developing countries is 80–94% (Shorvon & Farmer 1988). Even the low cost of phenobarbitone and phenytoin (the cost in India is equivalent to US $20–30 for a year's supply) is not affordable by many with low socio-economic status (the per capita income in India is equivalent to US $110 per year (Rural Health Statistics 1988).

A recent community-based programme in a rural and semi-urban region of Kenya showed that primary health workers administering carbamazepine or phenobarbitone to previously untreated patients with chronic epilepsy achieved good compliance and seizure control, with more than 50% of patients becoming seizure free (Feksi et al 1991).

Choice of antiepileptic drug. Ideally, choice of the drug should depend on the type of seizure and age of the patient, but in the present situation the cost of the drug and its easy availability are the major determinants. Ease of unmonitored use, level of expertise available, acceptability of side effects, the patient's status in society and prevailing practices also govern the selection of the drug.

The cost of phenytoin and phenobarbitone are comparable ($1\frac{1}{2}$-fold difference) while that of carbamazepine is 20-fold higher. For generalized tonic–clonic seizures it may be preferable to use phenobarbitone in a rural setting, especially in a patient who is a casual labourer, where control of seizures is important and some effect on cognition is acceptable. As the level of expertise provided by medical practitioners improves through education and when phenytoin tablets containing 25 mg of the drug become available, its use can be advocated more freely. Use of carbamazepine and sodium valproate is restricted to the well-to-do at present.

Availability. Ensuring a regular supply of drugs is vital. Regulations which are intended to ensure supply and avoid misuse actually result in short supply. In India the use of phenobarbitone is strictly regulated because it has been misused by addicts and by those intending to commit suicide. The pharmacist is required to keep detailed records of stocks and sales. Since the margin of profit on this drug is small, most pharmacists do not stock it. Thus a cheap drug is often unavailable.

In many countries appropriate formulations of AEDs are not available. Drug-monitoring studies have shown that 30% of patients on phenytoin need additional fractional doses of 50 mg or 25 mg. The use of 100-mg tablets results in subtherapeutic or toxic levels (Kshirsagar et al 1990). As the profit margin on this drug is low, no pharmaceutical company is prepared to market 25-mg tablets of phenytoin. Liquid preparations of phenytoin are marketed in the concentration of 25 mg/ml, making its correct use difficult as patients are required to measure 1 ml accurately using a syringe (instead of using a teaspoon). Preparations with 5 mg/ml would prove easier to use.

Contrary to usual belief, major differences in bioavailability have not been demonstrated. The comparative bioavailability of two products was investigated in normal volunteers by Naik & Marton (1989). One of the products had a small but significantly higher bioavailability. Multiple-dose studies showed that changes from one product to another did not produce any significant differences in steady-state phenytoin levels.

Traditional medicines. As mentioned above, patients in developing countries turn to alternative systems for a variety of reasons. Sack (1990) reviewed traditional therapeutic practices in Ethiopia. Patients with psychosis, headache and fits had frequently used traditional treatment before turning to modern medicine. A community-based survey in a rural area of Ethiopia found that most patients received treatment with local herbs, holy water and amulets and only 1.6% had received recognized antiepileptic drugs (Tekle-Haimanot et al 1990).

Controlled trials of herbal medicines are not available. Many, however, have been investigated in animal studies using maximal electroshock seizures (MES), pentylene tetrazole (PTZ) or strychnine-induced convulsions. In a recent review as many as 25 plants were reported to have anticonvulsant activity (Chauhan et al 1988). Anticonvulsant activity was found in the roots of *Cichorium intybus*. An alcoholic extract of *Convolvulus pleuricaulis* was found to shorten the duration of extensor seizures in MES rat model (Sharma et al 1965). *Nardostachys jatamansi* is a plant commonly used in India for mental disorders, insanity and epilepsy by Ayurvedic physicians. Jatamansone, an essential oil of jatamansi, abolishes hindlimb extension in MES (Arora et al 1958). A methanol extract of root of *Boerhavia diffusa* produces 100% protection in the PTZ seizure model (Adesina 1979). An acetone-soluble fraction of *Withania somnifera* leaves exacerbates PTZ convulsion, but protects against MES (Prasad & Malhotra 1968). *Nymphaea lotus alba* rhizomes counteract strychnine-induced convulsions (Delphaut & Balansard 1943). *Convolvulus arvensis* (with chemical constituents umbelliferone, scopoletin and isoferulic acid), *Marsilea rajasthanensis* (containing marsiline) and *Canscora decussata* have been shown to possess anticonvulsant activity (Chauhan et al 1988). In Ghana, *Annona arenaria* is used in epilepsy (Oliver Bever 1983). *Acorus calamus* contains neutral and aromatic essential oils which are reported to be effective against PTZ-induced seizures (Madan et al 1960). Angelecin isolated from *Selinum vaginatum* shows marked tranquillizing, anticonvulsant and muscle relaxant activity (Chandoke & Ray Ghatak 1975).

Many marketed preparations of indigenous drugs contain mixtures of several plants. Thus Shankhapushpi, a marketed preparation, contains eight different plants. Interestingly, two of these, viz. convolvulus and alkaloidal fraction of jatamansi, have shown anticonvulsant activity in animal studies, while *Bacopa monniera* has been shown to possess convulsant effect in mice (Das et al 1961).

There are no clinical studies reported on these plants except one report from China: Chinese workers have reported antiepilepsirine obtained from plants to be useful clinically (Wang et al 1989).

In one study 30% of the patients have been found to opt for combining modern medical treatment in India with the traditional system (Pruthi et al 1979). Out of 3000 plants screened for biological activity in the Indo-US PL480 project, CNS activity was observed in 17.6% (CDRI 1988). It is therefore likely that interactions occur between modern drugs and traditional herbal remedies. In one study coadministration of one herbal preparation

(Shankhapushpi) was reported to lead to breakthrough seizures in patients (Kshirsagar et al 1990). Administration of Shankhapushpi resulted in more than 50% reduction in efficacy of phenytoin in MES seizure model in rats; the antagonism occurred with a single dose as well as multiple doses (Dandekar et al 1991).

SUGGESTED STRATEGIES FOR TREATMENT OF EPILEPSY IN DEVELOPING COUNTRIES

The goal of management is to:

1. Improve quality of service and provide reliable health care to those 5–15% who come for medical management
2. Educate and inform the population using modern means of mass education and enlarge the segment covered by medical treatment
3. Stress preventable causes
4. Improve social attitudes towards epilepsy, with special reference to schooling, employment and marriage.

These goals can be achieved by:

1. Ensuring easy availability of correctly formulated AEDs at low prices at all times
2. Integration of management of epilepsy into the existing systems of health care delivery
3. Emphasis on management of epilepsy at undergraduate level
4. Active, intensive and sustained training of health personnel at primary health centre level
5. Education of public, tribal and local leaders
6. Research for developing long-acting, cheap and safe anticonvulsants (Osuntokun 1979).

In developed countries the establishment of multidisciplinary epilepsy centres has been advocated to provide medical care to epileptic patients (Silfvenius & Olivecrona 1988). However, in developing countries the burden of treatment will be largely on the family physician or primary health doctor (Chandra 1988). Educating or re-educating them in the right approach to management is crucial to successful treatment. A few advanced centres in large city hospitals should help to develop the basic details of primary health care centres, train the personnel, provide sophisticated facilities and carry out research in traditional systems.

Reddy (1986) has reported on the utility of satellite clinics as extensions of large city-based hospitals with community involvement.

CONCLUSION

Eighty per cent of the epileptic population is in the age range 0–35 years – an economically productive population in the formative years of life.

Appropriate treatment is important as it will lessen the socio-economic burden on society and the nation. The main variants and determinants of management of epilepsy in developing countries are the population differences, economic backwardness and sociocultural heterogeneity.

The major population differences relate to the aetiology of secondary epilepsy. Major advances have been in methods of diagnosis (e.g. for tuberculosis, cysticercosis and 'disappearing CT scan lesions'), and treatment (e.g. clinical trials of different regimens for tuberculosis and cysticercosis).

Several studies have now shown that there are no major pharmacokinetic differences for AEDs in populations of developed and developing nations and data from developed countries can be extrapolated to those in developing countries. There is a general paucity of data from children and neonates.

The most important problems are: (1) the lack of patient awareness of the need for early diagnosis and for continued prolonged treatment; (2) the lack of expertise for clinical, investigational and pharmacotherapeutic aspects; (3) the irregular drug supply and high cost of the drugs; (4) the use of traditional systems without documented efficacy; and (5) sociocultural barriers.

The strategies for management involve linking the management of patients with epilepsy to the total health care structure: a three-tier referral system of primary health centre doctor, district level services and city hospital. The education of patients and proper training of doctors is very important. Successful management requires active patient participation and has to be by means acceptable to the people.

ACKNOWLEDGEMENTS

The authors are greatly indebted to Dr S. K. Pandya, Professor, Head of the Department of Neurosurgery, K.E.M. Hospital, Bombay, and Dr D. Bakhle, Glaxo Laboratories, Bombay; to Mrs S. L. Chinnappa, National Informatics Centre, New Delhi and Dr S. C. Karande for their help in preparing this manuscript; to Mr U. M. Godhwani and Mrs Shirke for secretarial assistance; and to Dr P M Pai, Dean, K.E.M. Hospital, for permitting us to carry out studies referred to in this paper at the K.E.M. Hospital.

REFERENCES

Abajo F J 1988 Phenytoin interaction with rifampicin. Br Med J 297: 1048
Adesina S K 1979 Anticonvulsant properties of rootbark of *Boerhavia diffusa* L. Q J Crude Drug Res 17: 84–86
Afkhami A, Barahmand U, Sarandi P 1989 A study of demographic, socioeconomic features and prognosis in epileptic patients in the state of Azarbaijan in Iran. 18th International Epilepsy Congress, New Delhi, Abstract No. 404
Ahuja G K, Mohanta A 1982 Late onset epilepsy: a prospective study. Acta Neurol Scand 66: 216–226

Arora R B, Sharma P L, Kapila K 1958 Antiarrhythmic and anticonvulsant activity of Jatamansone. Indian J Med Res 46: 782–789

Awaritefe A 1989 Epilepsy: the myth of contagious disease. Cult Med Psychiatry 13: 449–456

Backman N, Holm A K, Hanstrom L et al 1989 Folate treatment of diphenylhydantoin induced gingival hyperplasia. Scand J Dent Res 97: 222–232

Bansal B C, Dua A, Gupta R, Gupta M S 1989 Spontaneously disappearing CT shadows in focal generalised epilepsy. 18th International Epilepsy Congress, New Delhi. Abstract No. 379

Bhagwati S N 1986 Intracranial tuberculoma. Editorial. Neurology (India) 34: 161–163

Bhargava S, Tandon P N 1980 CNS tuberculosis: lessons learnt from CT studies. Neurology (India) 28: 207–212

Bharucha N E, Bharucha E P, Bhise A V, Schoenberg B S 1988 Prevalence of epilepsy in Parsi community in Bombay. Epilepsia 29: 111–115

Bhatia R, Tandon P N 1988 Solitary microlesions in a clinical study and followup. Neurology (India) 36: 139–150

Bittencourt P R M 1988 Epilepsy in Latin America. In: Laidlaw J, Richens A, Oxley J (eds) A textbook of epilepsy, 3rd edn. Churchill Livingstone, Edinburgh, pp 518–527

Bittencourt P R M, Gracia C M, Lorenzana P 1988 Epilepsy and parasitosis of the central nervous system. In: Pedley T A, Meldrum B S (eds) Recent advances in epilepsy 4. Churchill Livingstone, Edinburgh, pp 123–160

Brooks J B, Daneshwar M I, Haberberger R L, Mikhail I A 1990 Rapid diagnosis of tuberculous meningitis by frequency pulse electron capture gas liquid chromatographic detection of carboxylic acid in CSF. J Clin Microbiol 28: 989–997

CDRI Publications 1988 Screening of Indian plants for biological activity. Central Drug Research Institute, Lucknow

Chandoke N, Ray Ghatak B J 1975 Pharmacological investigation of Angelecin: a tranquillosedative and anticonvulsant agent. Indian J Med Res 63: 833–841

Chandra B 1988 Epilepsy in Indonesia. In: Laidlaw J, Richens A, Oxley J (eds) A textbook of epilepsy, 3rd edn. Churchill Livingstone, Edinburgh, pp 511–517

Chandy M J, Rajshekhar V 1988 Focal epilepsy in India. J Neurol Neurosurg Psychiatry 51: 1242

Chauhan A K, Dophal M P, Joshi B C 1988 A review of medicinal plants showing anticonvulsant activity. J Ethnopharmacol 22: 11–23

Chiofalo N, Kirschbaum A, Fuentes A et al 1979 Prevalence of epilepsy in Melipilla Chile. Epilepsia 10: 261–266

Correa D, Sandoval M A, Harrison E J 1989 Human neurocysticercosis, comparison of enzyme immunoassay capture technique based on monoclonal and polyclonal antibodies for the detection of parasite products in CSF. Trans R Soc Trop Med Hyg 83: 811–816

Dam M, Larsen L, Christiansen J 1977 Phenytoin: ethnic differences in plasma levels and clearance. In: Gardener T, Janz D, Meinardi H, Pippenger C E (eds) Antiepileptic drug monitoring. Pitman, Tunbridge Wells, pp 73–79

Dandekar U P, Chandra R S, Kshirsagar N A et al 1991 Analysis of a novel clinically important interaction between phenytoin and an ayurvedic preparation. Indian J Med Res (in press)

Danesi M A 1988 Seasonal variation in the incidence of photoparoxysmal response to stimulation among photosensitive epileptic patients: evidence from repeated recordings. J Neurol Neurosurg Psychiatry 51: 875–877

Dansky L V, Andermann E, Rosenblatt D et al 1987 Anticonvulsants, folate levels and pregnancy outcome: a prospective study. Ann Neurol 21: 176–182

Das P K, Malhotra C C, Dhalla N S 1961 Studies on alkaloid of Herpestic Monniera linn. Indian J Physiol Pharmacol 5: 136–139

Dastur D K, Dave U P 1987 Effect of prolonged anticonvulsant medication in epileptic patients on serum lipids, vitamin B6, B12 and folic acid: proteins and fine structure of liver. Epilepsia 28: 147–159

Delphaut J, Balansard J 1943 Recherches pharmacologiques sur le nenuphar blanc (N. alba L.). Rev Phytotherapie 7: 83–85

Desai N K, Karbhari K, Paul T et al 1982 Prolongation of antipyrine half life after correction of severe anaemia due to hookworm infestation. Br J Clin Pharmacol 13: 745–747

Diwate P G, Apte C A 1988 Focal epilepsy in India (letter). J Neurol Neurosurg Psychiatry 51: 1365–1366

Dole M, Maniar P, Lahiri K, Shah M D 1989 Elisa for detection of *M. tuberculosis* specific IgG antibody in the CSF in cases of tuberculous meningitis. J Trop Pediatr 35: 218–220

Eadie M J, Tyrer J H 1989 Anticonvulsant therapy: pharmacological basis and practice, 3rd edn. Churchill Livingstone, Edinburgh, pp 51–137

Escalante A F, Duena L 1989 Neurocysticercosis: short course of treatment with albendazole. Arch Neurol 46: 1231–1236

Ganapathy G R, Krishna Rao G V G, Gourie-Devi M 1973 Bone changes after long term anticonvulsant therapy. Neurology (India) 21: 159–164

Feksi A T, Kaamugisha J, Sander J W A S, Gatiti S, Shorvon S D 1991 Comprehensive primary health care antiepileptic drug treatment programme in rural and semi-urban Kenya. Lancet 337: 407–409

Gourie-Devi M, Rao V N, Prakash R 1987 Neuroepidemiological studies in semi-urban and rural areas in south India: pattern of neurological disorders including MND. In: Gourie-Devi M (ed) Motor neurone disease. Oxford and IBM Publishing Co, Pvt Ltd, New Delhi, pp 11–23

Haerer A F, Anderson D W, Schoenberg B S 1986 Prevalence and clinical features of epilepsy in a biracial US population. Epilepsia 27: 66–75

Inaba T 1990 Phenytoin pharamacogenetic polymorphism of 4-hydroxylation. Pharmacol Ther 46: 341–347

Ionnides Demos L L, Horne M K, Tong N et al 1988 Impact of a pharmacokinetic service on clinical outcomes in an ambulatory care epilepsy clinic. Am J Hosp Pharm 45: 1549–1551

Joshi M V, Pohujani S M, Kshirsagar N A, Jain S K et al 1990 Phenytoin dosage adjustment in Indian population. Neurology (India) (in press)

Joshi M V, Pohujani S M, Mehta B C, Kshirsagar N A 1991 Effect of iron deficiency and its treatment on single dose phenytoin pharmacokinetics. Eur J Clin Pharmacol (in press)

Kaul R, Razdan S, Motta A 1988 Prevalence and pattern of epilepsy in rural Kashmir, India. Epilepsia 29: 116–122

Kay L, Kampman J P, Svendsen T L et al 1985 Influence of rifampicin and isoniazid on the kinetics of phenytoin. Br J Clin Pharmacol 20: 323–326

Krishnaswamy K, Teoh D C 1980 Diseases of a tropical environment. In: Avery G S (ed) Drug treatment, 2nd edn. Churchill Livingstone, Edinburgh, pp 1174–1180

Kshirsagar N A, Shah P U 1990 Therapeutic drug monitoring: antiepileptic drugs. J Gen Med 2: 41–46

Kshirsagar N A, Pohujani S M, Takle M R et al 1987 Sulphadimidine acetylation status in Gujarati and Marathi population. J Postgrad Med 33: 128–133

Kshirsagar N A, Saraf Y S, Joshi M V et al 1988 Effect of iron deficiency anaemia and its treatment on the absorption and elimination of phenformin. Xenobiotica 18: 1185–1189

Kshirsagar N A, Dalvi S S, Joshi M V et al 1990 Phenytoin and Ayurvedic preparation: clinically important interaction in epileptic patients. J Assoc Physicians India (in press)

Lalitha V S, Dastur D K 1980 Tuberculosis of the central nervous system. II: Brain tuberculomas vis-à-vis intracranial space occupying lesions 1953–1978. Neurology (India) 28: 202–206

Lalitha V S, Marker F E, Dastur D K 1980 Tuberculosis of the central nervous system. Neurology (India) 28: 197–206

Livingstone S, Berman W, Pauli L L 1973 Anticonvulsant drugs and vitamin D metabolism. JAMA 226: 787

Madan B R, Arora R B, Kapila K 1960 Anticonvulsant, antiveratrisic and antiarrhythmic activity of *Acorus calamus*, an Indian indigenous plant. Arch Int Pharmacodyn Ther 124: 201–211

Maheshwari M C 1982 Electroencephalography in the management of epilepsies. Indian Pediatr 19: 361–374

Mani K S 1987 Collaborative epidemiological study on epilepsy in India: final report of the Bangalore centre, Bangalore. Department of Neurology, NIMHANS

Mani K S, Gopalkrishnan P N, Vyas J N, Pillai M S 1968 Hot water epilepsy: a peculiar type of reflex epilepsy. A preliminary report. Neurology (India) 16: 107–110

Meinardi H 1988 Epilepsy in developing countries. In: Laidlaw J, Richens A, Oxley J (eds) A textbook of epilepsy, 3rd edn. Churchill Livingstone, Edinburgh, pp 528–532

Mosenkilde L, Melsen F 1976 Anticonvulsant osteomalacia determined by quantitative analysis of bone changes: population study and possible risk factors. Acta Medica Scand

199: 349–355

Nagarajaswamy A S 1989 18th International Epilepsy Congress, New Delhi. Abstract No. 136

Naik D, Marton D J 1989 A comparative bioavailability of 2 oral solid phenytoin dosage forms. Cent Afr J Med 35: 384–388

Ogunniyi A, Osuntokun B O, Bademosi O et al 1987 Risk factors for epilepsy: case control study in Nigerians. Epilepsia 28: 280–285

Oliver Bever B 1983 Medicinal plants in tropical West Africa. II. Plants acting on the nervous system. J Ethnopharmacol 7: 1–93

Osuntokun B O 1979 Treatment of epilepsy with special reference to developing countries. Prog Neuropsychopharmacol Biol Psychiatry 31: 81–84

Osuntokun B O 1985 Community based research in neurology: Nigerian experience. West Afr J Med 4: 111–124

Osuntokun B O, Adeuju A O G, Nottidge V A et al 1987 Prevalence of epilepsy in Nigerian Africans: a community based study. Epilepsia 28: 272–279

Pandya S K 1987 Is short term therapy justified in tuberculous meningitis? Editorial. Neurology (India) 35: 185–186

Peiris J B, Karunanayake E H, Joice D D T M et al 1988 Relationship between dose and serum concentrations of carbamazepine, phenytoin, phenobarbital and primidone in a Sri Lankan population compared with European population. Epilepsia 29: 564–570

Perucca E, Richens A 1981 Antiepileptic drugs: clinical aspects. In: Richens A, Marks V (eds) Therapeutic drug monitoring. Churchill Livingstone, Edinburgh, pp 320–348

Prasad S, Malhotra C L 1968 *Withania ashwagandha*: effect of alkaloidal fractions (acetone, alcohol, water soluble) on the central nervous system. Indian J Physiol Pharmacol 12: 175–181

Pruthi N, Dhir A, Srinivas Murthy R 1979 Rural community attitude to epilepsy. Neurology (India) 27: 170–173

Ramachandran P, Duraipandian M, Nagarajan M et al 1986 Three chemotherapy studies in tuberculous meningitis in children. Tubercle 67: 17–29

Ramachandran P, Duraipandian M, Reetha A M 1989 Long term status of children treated for tuberculous meningitis in south India. Tubercle 70: 235–239

Ramamurthi B 1989a Anticonvulsants, teratogenesis and pregnancy. 18th International Epilepsy Congress, New Delhi. Abstract No. 129

Ramamurthi B 1989b The future of neurosciences in India. In: Pandya S K (ed) Neurosciences in India: retrospect and prospect. Neurological Society of India, Trivandrum; Council of Scientific and Industrial Research, New Delhi, pp 5–22

Ranadive S N, Banerjee K 1989 Recent advances in serodiagnosis of tuberculosis. ICMR Bull 19: 11–13

Reddy G N N 1986 Extension of mental health service by satellite clinics as a model. NIMHANS J 4: 71–75

Rural Health Statistics in India Dec 1988 Ministry of Health and Family Welfare, Nirman Bhavan, New Delhi

Sack G 1990 Traditional treatment procedures in neurologic and psychiatric diseases in Ethiopia. Psychiatr Neurol Med Psychol Beih 42: 96–101

Sander J W A S, Shorvon S D 1987 Incidence and prevalence studies in epilepsy and their methodological problems: a review. J Neurol Neurosurg Psychiatry 50: 829–839

Satishchandra P, Shivaramakrishna, Kaliaperumal V G, Schoenberg B S 1988 Hot water epilepsy: a variant of reflex epilepsy in southern India. Epilepsia 29: 52–56

Sato S 1964 The epidemiological and clinicostatistical study of epilepsy in Nigata city. Rinsho Shinkeigaku 4: 413–424

Satyavati G V 1986 Pharmacology of medicinal plants and other natural products in India. Part I. ICMR Bull 16: 115–123

Sethi P K, Kumar B R, Madan V S, Mohan V 1985 Appearing and disappearing CT scan abnormalities and seizures. J Neurol Neurosurg Psychiatry 48: 866–869

Shamansky S L, Glaser G H 1979 Socioeconomic characteristics of childhood disorders in New Haven area: an epidemiological study. Epilepsia 20: 457–474

Sharma V N, Barar F K S, Khanna N K, Mahawar M M 1965 Some pharmacological actions of *Convolvulus pleuricaulis*, an Indian indigenous herb. Indian J Med Res 53: 871–876

Shorvon S D, Farmer P J 1988 Epilepsy in developing countries: a review of epidemiological, sociocultural and treatment aspects. Epilepsia 29 (Suppl 1): 538–554

Silfvenius H, Olivecrona M 1988 Epilepsy in Sweden as revealed by mortality, disability pensions and drug consumption, 1971–1984. Acta Medica Scand (Suppl) 117: 15–23

Singh L M, Mehta S, Vohra R M, Nair C K 1987 Monitoring of phenobarbitone in epileptic children. Int J Clin Pharmacol Ther Toxicol 25: 15–22

Snehlata C, Ramamurthi B 1972 Calcium metabolism during anticonvulsant therapy. Neurology (India) 20: 94–98

Sotelo J, Escibedo F, Rodriguez-Carbajal J et al 1984 Therapy of parenchymal brain cysticercosis with praziquantel. N Engl J Med 310: 1001–1007

Sotelo J, Del Brutto O H, Penogos P 1990 Comparison of therapeutic regimes of anticysticercal drugs for parenchymal brain cysticercosis. J Neurol 237: 69–72

Tabibzadeh I, Espagnet Rossi A, Maxwell R 1989 Spotlight on the cities improving urban health in developing countries. WHO, Geneva

Tandon P N, Bhargava S 1980 CNS tuberculosis lessons learnt from CT Studies. Neurol India 28: 207–212

Tekle-Haimanot R, Forsgren L, Abebe M, Gebre-Mariam A, Heijbel J, Holmgren G, Ekstedt J 1990 Clinical and electroencephalographic characteristics of epilepsy in rural Ethiopia: a community based study. Epilepsy Res 7: 230–239

Thomas J, Shanker P, Singh J P et al 1989 CT guided stereotaxic localization and excision of solitary lesions in the treatment of focal epilepsy in India. 18th International Epilepsy Congress, New Delhi. Abstract No. 35

Vengsarkar U S, Pispaty R P, Parekh B et al 1986 Intracranial tuberculoma and the CT scan. J Neurosurg 64: 568–574

Vohora S B, Shah S A, Dandiya P C 1990 Central nervous system studies on an ethanol extract of *Acorus calamus* rhizome. J Ethnopharmacol 28: 53–62

Wadia N H 1989 Clinical neurology. In: Pandya S K (ed) Neurosciences in India: retrospect and prospect. Neurological Society of India, Trivandrum; Council of Scientific and Industrial Research, New Delhi, pp 437–508

Wadia N H, Desai S, Bhatt M 1988 Disseminated cysticercosis. Brain 111: 597–614

Wadia R S, Bakhale C N, Kelkar A V, Grant K B 1987 Focal epilepsy in India with special reference to lesions showing ring or disc enhancement on contrast computed tomography. J Neurol Neurosurg Psychiatry 50: 1298–1301

Wang L, Zhao D Y, Zhang Z H et al 1989 Double blind cross over study on antiepilepsirine. Chung Hua I Hsueh Tsa Chih 102: 79–85

World Health Statistics 1989 Annual. WHO, Geneva

Zhu D, Xu W 1983 Effect of biltricide on cysticercosis cellulosae with muscular pseudohypertrophy, a report of three cases. Chung Kuo Chi Sheng Chung Hsueh Yu Chi Sheng Chung Ping Tsa Chih (Chinese J Parasitol Parasitic Dis) 1: 185–186

11

Vigabatrin

H. A. Ring   E. H. Reynolds

INTRODUCTION

Vigabatrin (γ-vinyl GABA) is a synthetic analogue of GABA designed to enhance inhibitory neurotransmission. As a specific irreversible inhibitor of GABA transaminase, the enzyme responsible for the catabolism of GABA, it increases concentrations of GABA in the brain and this effect is presumed to be responsible for its antiepileptic action. In the last 18 months the drug was licensed in the UK, Denmark, Ireland and Sweden for clinical use in the treatment of epileptic patients who are refractory to standard antiepileptic drugs. In this chapter we will review the rapidly accumulating data on the clinical pharmacology, efficacy and toxicity of vigabatrin and its present use in clinical practice. Earlier experience has been summarized by Schechter (1986), Richens (1989), Reynolds (1990) and the *Lancet* (Editorial 1989).

BACKGROUND

γ-Aminobutyric acid (GABA) is an inhibitory neurotransmitter widely distributed in the brain (McGeer & McGeer 1989). As pointed out by Gale (1989), this does not necessarily mean that increasing GABA transmission always results in net inhibition of brain excitability. In some regions GABA neurones impinge on one another in series, resulting in net disinhibition of a target area. Nevertheless, it is the inhibitory effects of GABA activity on the presumed neuronal hyperexcitability of an epileptic discharge that led to consideration of the manipulation of this system as a therapeutic approach to the treatment of epilepsy. The role of GABA in human epilepsy is uncertain (Chadwick & Crawford 1986). It has been demonstrated experimentally that impairment of GABAergic inhibition leads to focal or generalized seizures, whilst enhancement of this inhibition has antiepileptic effects (Meldrum 1984).

A number of mechanisms have been considered for the pharmacological enhancement of GABA-mediated neuronal inhibition. GABA itself is not an effective anticonvulsant because following systemic administration it does not readily cross the blood–brain barrier, except in neonates (McGeer

177

& McGeer 1989). Studies of the use of pro-drugs, direct agonists or inhibitors of GABA reuptake have not yet produced clinically useful results. On the other hand benzodiazepines, which act by allosteric enhancement of affinity of GABA recognition sites (McGeer & McGeer 1989) have proven efficacy as anticonvulsants. Likewise phenobarbitone, which acts on the receptor–chloride ionophore complex to augment the inhibitory action of GABA, is a long-established anticonvulsant in clinical practice (Olsen 1982). Concentrations of GABA at the synapse may also be increased by inhibiting the enzyme GABA transaminase (GABA-T) that is responsible for GABA catabolism. It was the search for a specific GABA-T inhibitor that led to the synthesis of vigabatrin. This rational approach to the search for a new antiepileptic treatment contrasts with earlier empirical methods involving the screening of diverse compounds in animal models of epilepsy.

MODE OF ACTION

Vigabatrin is a γ-amino acid with a structure similar to GABA. It is an irreversible inhibitor of GABA-T, the activated drug binding covalently to the active site of the enzyme (Lippert et al 1977). In vitro when vigabatrin is withdrawn from culture, GABA-T activity slowly returns to pre-treatment levels over four to six days (Larsson et al 1986). This time course correlates with synthesis of new enzyme. In vivo vigabatrin has been shown to increase cerebral GABA concentrations in rodents (Jung et al 1977) and cerebrospinal fluid (CSF) GABA in patients with epilepsy (Schechter et al 1984). The effect on brain GABA is dose dependent and cumulative (Jung et al 1977, Schechter et al 1984). Gram et al (1989) investigated the effects of clinically active S and inactive R enantiomers of vigabatrin on selectively cultured neurones and astrocytes. It was found that only the form of the drug with anticonvulsant activity in animal models of epilepsy inhibited GABA-T and that there was preferential inhibition of the neuronal rather than the glial form of the enzyme. The authors conclude that their findings substantiate a direct GABAergic mechanism of action of vigabatrin. The marketed drug is a racemic form and the presence of the inactive enantiomer does not interfere with the therapeutic effect.

If the elevation of GABA concentrations by vigabatrin underlies its anticonvulsant activity, then it may be predicted that those patients in whom vigabatrin does not have this effect are less likely to derive therapeutic benefit. This hypothesis was examined in 75 patients with complex partial seizures (Riekkinen et al 1989a). Fifty-five per cent of patients showed a greater than 50% reduction in seizure frequency after three months of treatment. The CSF of both 'responders' and 'non-responders' was examined for vigabatrin levels and for concentrations of markers of GABA neurotransmission: total GABA, free GABA and homocarnosine. There was no difference in vigabatrin levels between the two groups, implying that it was not variable penetration of the drug across the blood–brain barrier that determined response. However, the 'responders' had significantly higher levels of total GABA and homocarnosine. Riekkinen et al (1989b) therefore suggest that non-responders may already have greater destruction of GABA-synthesizing neurones, thus resulting in lower GABA levels even in the presence of vigabatrin-induced GABA-T inhibition. The situation is more complex since it is GABA concentrations in particular regions such as the substantia nigra that seem to determine seizure threshold, rather than activity across the brain as a whole as reflected in CSF GABA concentrations (Gale 1989).

NEUROCHEMICAL SPECIFICITY

Unlike other experimental GABA-T inhibitors, vigabatrin has only a small inhibitory effect on the activity of glutamate decarboxylase, the enzyme responsible for GABA synthesis (Jung et al 1977). Thus far there has been no clear experimental evidence for a direct effect of vigabatrin on other neurochemical systems. However, the observation of enhanced GABA-mediated tonic inhibition of the hippocampal cholinergic system in mice receiving vigabatrin (Miller & Richter 1986) suggests that there are effects secondary to changes in GABAergic systems. With regard to the dopamine system, however, Beart et al (1985) found that 7–14 days of vigabatrin administration in rats did not alter striatal dopamine, dihydroxyphenylacetic acid or homovanillic acid levels, despite producing a 44% increase in striatal GABA concentrations.

A number of clinical studies have investigated the degree of neurochemical specificity of vigabatrin for the GABAergic system (Schechter et al 1984, Pitkanen et al 1988, Beart et al 1985, Halonen et al 1988). The effects of single and repeated doses of vigabatrin on CSF concentrations of neurotransmitters and their metabolites have been examined. Riekkinen et al (1989a) reported a dose-dependent two- to threefold increase in CSF free and total GABA and homocarnosine over six months of regular treatment with 1.5 g and 3 g per day of vigabatrin. They also noted a small increase in the concentration of glycine but did not find any consistent change in markers of other neurotransmitter systems including the cholinergic, dopaminergic, serotonergic and peptidergic systems, or in concentrations of excitatory amino acids. A similar lack of effect on CSF excitatory amino acid concentrations was noted by Halonen et al (1988). In a dose-interval study of 11 patients Ben-Menachem (1989) observed a brief but significant increase in CSF homovanillic acid after a single dose of 50 mg/kg and a significant decrease in CSF 5-hydroxyindoleacetic acid, a marker of serotonergic neurotransmission, after one month of treatment with vigabatrin in a daily dose of 50 mg/kg. There were no other sustained changes except increases in total GABA and homocarnosine.

ELECTROPHYSIOLOGICAL EFFECTS OF VIGABATRIN

Electroencephalographic (EEG) studies

The effects of vigabatrin on brain electrical activity have been studied in experimental seizure models and in patients. Four hours after the administration of vigabatrin to amygdala-kindled rats the drug appeared to be pro-convulsant, prolonging behavioural seizures and electrographic afterdischarges (Loscher et al 1989). However, one to three days after administration the drug produced a dose-dependent reduction in seizure severity and duration and in afterdischarge duration. It was suggested that these different effects could be related to differences in the time-course of nerve terminal GABA increases in selective brain regions such as amygdala and corpus striatum.

In patients with epilepsy, EEG studies have sought to correlate seizure control with alterations of electrical epileptiform activity during treatment. Ben-Menachem & Treiman (1989) examined EEG changes in patients with intractable complex partial seizures who were participating in a single-blind add-on trial of vigabatrin. In 8 of the subjects who continued treatment for at least a year there was no significant overall correlation of alteration in seizure frequency with EEG changes. Similarly, a study of serial EEGs recorded in 15 patients undergoing a controlled clinical trial of vigabatrin failed to detect any drug-related changes in intrinsic brain rhythms (Hammond & Wilder 1985b). It was, however, noted by these authors that 3 patients did show a consistent reduction in the amount of epileptiform activity compared to pre-treatment recordings. The conclusion that vigabatrin has no consistent effect on the surface EEG of patients with epilepsy is supported by a study comparing vigabatrin and carbamazepine monotherapy. Whilst carbamazepine was associated with occipital slowing vigabatrin was not associated with any systematic EEG changes (Mervaala et al 1989). It should be noted, however, that a recent review of EEG findings in trials of standard antiepileptic drugs concluded that the EEG is of doubtful value as an outcome variable in clinical anticonvulsant trials (Van Wieringen et al 1987).

Evoked potential studies

Evoked potential measurements are of special interest because they have been claimed to provide an index of the species-specific pathological changes of reversible myelin microvacuolation associated with some chronic high-dose vigabatrin studies (Liegeois-Chauvel et al 1989). In dogs vigabatrin-induced neurotoxicity following 12 weeks of treatment with a daily dose of 300 mg/kg is associated with prolongation of the central conduction time of somatosensory evoked potentials (SEPs) (Arezzo et al 1989). These SEP changes returned to normal over 17 weeks following the cessation of vigabatrin.

Evoked potential studies of patients with epilepsy have not demonstrated any abnormalities. A seven-week study of patients receiving between 1 and 3 g of vigabatrin did not reveal any changes in SEPs, visual or brainstem auditory evoked potentials (Cosi et al 1988). Longer-term studies for up to 3.5 years of vigabatrin daily at doses of 1–4 g per day have also failed to demonstrate any significant change in evoked potential parameters (Cosi et al 1989, Liegeois-Chauvel et al 1989). In these studies the patients were treated with vigabatrin in addition to their regular anticonvulsant medication, making it difficult to assess electrophysiological effects of vigabatrin alone. However, in a double-blind cross-over study that compared evoked potentials in 17 patients taking carbamazepine with repeated measurements in 7 of these who were blindly switched to vigabatrin monotherapy, it was also found that there was no significant increase in latencies on vigabatrin, although such a finding in SEPs was noted during treatment with carbamazepine (Mervaala et al 1989). Unfortunately since all patients started on carbamazepine an order effect cannot be excluded.

THE CLINICAL USE OF VIGABATRIN

Pharmacokinetics

Vigabatrin is rapidly absorbed following oral administration in normal volunteers and epileptic patients (Schechter 1989), but the rate of absorption is reduced in the elderly (Haegele et al 1988). Vigabatrin is not bound to plasma proteins and no metabolites have been found in man (Rimmer & Richens 1989). The plasma elimination half-life in normal volunteers is between 5 and 7 hours. Vigabatrin is excreted primarily via the kidneys with about 65% of an administered dose detected unchanged in the urine within 24 hours. In the elderly the rate of renal clearance of vigabatrin was less than one-fifth of that in young healthy volunteers, perhaps accounting for the poor tolerance to a single oral dose of 1.5 g in the older group (Haegele et al 1988).

Drug interactions

Because it is neither plasma protein bound nor metabolized by the liver, vigabatrin demonstrates limited potential to interact with other drugs. Such a property is important because patients with resistant epilepsy, who will comprise the group treated with vigabatrin, are generally already taking other anticonvulsants. However, a fall in plasma phenytoin levels of between 20% and 30% has been noted in several studies (Rimmer & Richens 1984, Browne et al 1987, Luna et al 1989, Tartara et al 1989, Tassinari et al 1987). A study designed to investigate this phenomenon found that after more than four weeks of treatment with a dose of 3 g daily mean plasma phenytoin concentrations fell significantly by 23% (Rimmer & Richens

1989). As expected, there was no evidence to suggest that this was a result of hepatic enzyme induction or displacement of phenytoin from plasma protein binding sites, and the mechanism remains to be elucidated. In the study by Browne et al (1987) smaller but significant falls in serum phenobarbitone (7% decrease) and primidone (11% decrease) were also reported.

Efficacy of vigabatrin

Short-term studies

The efficacy of vigabatrin has been evaluated in four single-blind studies (Table 11.1) and seven double-blind, placebo-controlled studies (Table 11.2). Six of the double-blind trials were cross-over in design and one was a parallel group study. The evidence for efficacy was remarkably similar in all these studies. The drug was administered in doses ranging from 2 g to 4 g for between 7 and 12 weeks in between 15 and 30 patients, or 89 patients in the multicentre study by Browne et al (1987, 1989). All the patients were adults with intractable epilepsy resistant to one, two or more standard antiepileptic drugs. As is usually the case in such populations the great majority had complex partial seizures with or without secondary generalization. Overall approximately half the patients studied experienced a greater than 50% fall in seizure frequency. Some of these 50% of patients achieved much greater benefit and between 0 and 7% of the patients entering these studies showed complete seizure control. Those experiencing greatest benefit usually have partial seizures with or without secondary generalization. Because most patients with intractable epilepsy have partial seizures vigabatrin has been evaluated in far fewer patients with primary generalized epilepsy. Michelucci & Tassinari (1989) reviewed the published

Table 11.1   Short-term single-blind efficacy studies

Study	No. of patients	Design	Dose (g/day)	Treatment duration (weeks)	Efficacy (%)
Gram et al (1983)	15	Single-blind placebo lead-in	1–3	12	50[a]
Schechter et al (1984)	10	Single-blind placebo follow-up	1–2	4	60[b]
Browne et al (1987)	89	Single-blind placebo lead-in	up to 4	12	51[c]
Cocito et al (1989)	19	Single-blind placebo lead-in	2	8	53[d]

[a] Percentage change in median seizure frequency from placebo to active treatment.
[b] Percentage of patients achieving complete seizure control.
[c] Percentage of patients completing the study who achieved at least a 50% reduction in seizure frequency during vigabatrin treatment compared to baseline.
[d] Overall mean percentage change in median seizure frequency from baseline.

Table 11.2 Short-term double-blind placebo-controlled efficacy studies

Study	No. of patients entered	Seizure type PS[a]	Design	Dose (g/day)	Treatment duration (weeks)	Efficacy[b] (%)
Rimmer & Richens (1984)	24	24?	Cross-over	3	9	67
Gram et al (1985)	21	21?	Cross-over	3	12	44
Loiseau et al (1986)	23	19	Cross-over	3	10	58
Tartara et al (1986)	23	17	Cross-over	2–3	7	60
Remy et al (1986)	19	11	Cross-over	3	12	37[c]
Tassinari et al (1987)	31	30	Cross-over	2–3	12	33
Ring et al (1990)	31	30	Parallel Amery design	3	8	48[d]

[a] Number of patients with partial seizures ± secondary generalization.
[b] Efficacy = percentage of patients completing each study who achieved at least a 50% reduction in seizure frequency during active treatment.
[c] Overall decrease in seizure frequency compared to placebo.
[d] Mean reduction during the last six weeks of the dose optimization phase.

literature relating to 18 cases of primary generalized epilepsy and 435 patients with partial seizures. Overall it was found that vigabatrin was more effective in partial than in primary generalized epilepsy. In the group with partial epilepsy 49% achieved at least a 50% reduction in seizure frequency. Response was best in patients with only one seizure type, lower seizure frequency, unifocal EEG abnormalities and absence of mental impairment. Of the 18 patients with primary generalized epilepsy 39% experienced at least a halving in their seizure frequencies.

In the studies reported in Tables 11.1 and 11.2 all patients were given vigabatrin as add-on therapy to an existing antiepileptic treatment regimen. It is conceivable that differences in this concomitant medication may have affected response to vigabatrin. However, there was no evidence for any difference in efficacy between patients taking one and those taking two additional anticonvulsants (Ring et al 1990).

Long-term studies

The development of tolerance to anticonvulsant treatment, for example with benzodiazepines, can pose a problem in the management of epilepsy. Although vigabatrin acts through the GABAergic system in a quite separate manner to that of the benzodiazepines it is important to establish whether or not its use is also associated with the development of tolerance. From the long-term studies detailed in Table 11.3, it can be seen that in the majority of trials, after a period of dose optimization and the subsequent exclusion of non-responders, fewer than 30% of patients went on to

Table 11.3   Open long-term efficacy studies

Study	No. of patients	Duration of treatment (months)	Dose (g/day)	Entry design	Seizure breakthrough No. (%) of patients	Clinical benefit[a] number (%)
Pedersen et al (1985)	36	Mean 9.3	Mean 2.6	Unselected	2 (6%)	20 (56%)
Brown et al (1987)	66	Median 16.7	Median at entry 3.2	Responders	10 (15%)	26 (40%)
Matilainen et al (1988)	29	7	Mean 2.64	Responders[c]	?	15 (52%)
Cocito et al (1989)	16	13–15	Mean 3	Responders	2 (12.5%)	12 (63%)
Dam (1989)	62	Maximum of 36	?	Unselected	21[b] (34%)	At 36 months, median % of baseline seizures in remaining patients was <20%
Remy & Beaumont (1989)	254	Mean 22.7	Mean 3.1	Responders	26 (10.2%)	Median seizure frequency on vigabatrin maintained at 35% of baseline
Tartara et al (1989)	25	Median 22	Median 47 mg/kg	Responders	3 (12%)	18 (72%)
Sander et al (1990)	128	Mean 7.5	Mean 3.2	Unselected (28 with severe side effects withdrawn)	5 (4%)	41 (32%)
Reynolds et al (1991)	17	14–16	3	Responders	0	Mean % reduction in total seizure frequency compared to baseline = −53%

[a] Number of patients demonstrating at least a 50% reduction in seizure frequency at the end of the study compared to their baseline frequency.
[b] Total of patients withdrawn for all reasons including loss of efficacy and adverse effects.
[c] Includes patients who showed a 'global improvement' in the absence of a 50% reduction in seizure frequency.

experience a deterioration in seizure control sufficient to warrant a change of anticonvulsant therapy. However, there are a number of pit-falls in the interpretation of these longer-term follow-up studies. For example, Dam (1989) reported the outcome in an initial cohort of 62 patients after one, two and three years of treatment with vigabatrin as add-on therapy to existing anticonvulsant medication. By the end of the first year of treatment 21 patients had left the study for various reasons but it is not clear exactly how many were withdrawn due to loss of seizure control. For the majority of patients who continued treatment beyond this first year, there was no overall loss of efficacy. In a long-term treatment phase follow-up of 16 patients for 13–15 months, 63% maintained a greater than 50% reduction in seizure frequency and only 2 patients were withdrawn because of increasing seizure frequency (Cocito et al 1989). The latter authors point out that these figures are similar to the response rates seen in the published short-term efficacy studies. But as in this study, only proven responders entered the long-term phase, a sustained response rate in 63% in fact represents some deterioration from the initial two-month single-blind study period.

Reynolds et al (1991) analysed long-term seizure frequency in 17 patients who successfully completed a double-blind study (i.e. responded with at least a 50% reduction in seizure frequency) and were then followed up for a further year. This period was divided into two equal epochs of six months each. In the first of these periods the mean percentage reduction in total seizure frequency compared to baseline was -49% and in the second -53%. There was thus no evidence of any loss of efficacy up to one year. The persistent efficacy of vigabatrin was also suggested by Tartara et al (1989), who found a mean percentage reduction in seizure frequency of 56% after initial exposure to vigabatrin, compared to a mean reduction of 60% during the last two months of long-term therapy in the same patients. As the authors point out, the results of long-term follow-up studies tend to be biased because those who show the best response to treatment will remain on it for longer. Hence analysing seizure frequencies of patients on long-term treatment will overestimate efficacy unless an end-point analysis is performed including patients withdrawn because of loss of efficacy. Overall it appears that although a small minority of patients do experience a loss of efficacy on continued treatment, the majority maintain worthwhile benefit from vigabatrin.

Dosage: initiation and withdrawal

The anticonvulsant response to vigabatrin is dose dependent. In a dose-reduction study 1.5 g per day has been shown to significantly reduce seizure frequencies from baseline rates, although 3 g per day was clearly more effective (Sivenius et al 1987). Our practice in adults is to start treatment at 0.5 g twice daily, subsequently increasing by 0.5-g increments according to clinical progress. Although 3 g per day is the most commonly advised dose ceiling, some patients have derived greater benefit by increasing the dose to 4 g per day (Cocito et al 1989). The evidence suggests that there is an optimally effective dose for each patient.

Ben-Menachem et al (1989) investigated the efficacy of daily, alternate day and third day dosing regimens. Seizure frequency progressively decreased with decreasing dosing interval.

In the early clinical trials of vigabatrin it was assumed that because experimental evidence indicated GABA-T regenerates only slowly after stopping vigabatrin, the whole dose could be withdrawn at once. However, sudden cessation of vigabatrin has been clearly associated with exacerbation of seizures (Rimmer & Richens 1984, Ring et al 1990). In the study by Ring et al (1990), in the group of patients blindly randomized to switch abruptly to placebo after eight weeks of vigabatrin, seizure frequency was observed to increase to 18% above baseline in the month after this change and one patient went into status epilepticus.

Adverse effects in short-term use

The reported side effects of vigabatrin are in many respects similar to those of the standard anticonvulsant drugs. In double-blind placebo-controlled trials somnolence and fatigue were the most common adverse events both on vigabatrin and to a lesser extent when placebo was added to conventional anticonvulsant therapy. The range of side effects and their incidence in these studies are summarized in Table 11.4. Similar side effects were reported during single-blind and open studies of the drug (Browne et al 1987, Gram et al 1983, Ring et al 1990). The only adverse event that has been reported to increase with prolonged treatment is weight gain, which Tartara et al (1989) reported to increase by 5–16% of initial body weight in 40% of their 25 patients over the first three to six months of vigabatrin treatment before tending to reach a plateau. Effects outside the central nervous system are unusual. Systematic changes in metabolic or haematological parameters have rarely been reported. In five mentally handicapped adults a greater than 50% decrease in granulocyte count was observed but not thought to be significant (Matilainen et al 1988). Adverse effects of vigabatrin have not been observed to be any more common in patients already taking two than in those taking just one additional antiepileptic drug (Ring et al 1990).

Psychiatric effects

The use of vigabatrin has been associated with the occasional development of psychiatric symptoms independent of any overall confusional state.

Psychosis. Sander et al (1991) report a series of 14 patients developing a schizophrenia-like psychosis out of approximately 210 patients that they

Table 11.4   The incidence of the ten most commonly reported adverse effects in six double-blind placebo-controlled trials[a]

Adverse event	Incidence (%)	
	Vigabatrin add-on	Placebo add-on
Somnolence	27.2	12.9
Fatigue	7.5	6.1
Irritability	5.4	4.8
Dizziness	5.4	1.4
Headache	4.1	4.1
Depression	4.1	2.7
Confusion	3.4	0.7

[a] Total number of patients in these studies = 147. Studies included Gram et al (1985), Loiseau et al (1986), Remy et al (1986), Rimmer & Richens (1984), Tartara et al (1986), Tassinari et al (1987).

had treated with vigabatrin. Ten of the affected patients suffered from complex partial seizures with or without secondary generalization. The duration of vigabatrin treatment prior to the development of psychosis varied between five days and 32 weeks and the mean dose at the onset of the disturbance was 2580 mg. Four patients became psychotic after a cluster of seizures following a period of almost total seizure control and a further 4 became seizure free and then developed a psychosis between ten days and six weeks following the onset of this seizure remission. In 5 patients there was no relationship with seizure pattern. In all cases the psychosis resolved after withdrawal of vigabatrin. The different patterns of emergence of psychosis preclude any single explanation of this effect. The doses of vigabatrin given to these patients were not unduly high and the majority had normal neurological examinations and computerized tomography brain scans. It was observed, however, that 8 of the affected patients had a significant past psychiatric history. It should be noted, however, that in other series the incidence of psychosis is lower than that reported by Sander et al (1991). Dam (1990) reported 2 cases of frank psychosis in 117 patients, many of whom had been on vigabatrin for up to eight years. Betts & Thomas (1990) described the development of a mild paranoid psychosis in just one patient out of 75 treated. The latter two reports suggest that the difference in incidence is due to differences in the nature of the patients treated. Psychosis has also been reported to occur following sudden withdrawal of treatment (Brodie & McKee 1990, Ring & Reynolds 1990). In the latter report the patient described was the only one to become psychotic out of 60 patients treated with vigabatrin by the authors.

Depression. From Table 11.4 it may be seen that in 6 double-blind trials the incidence of depression was 4%. However, in the study by Ring et al (1990) 8 of the 33 patients entering the study were observed to become depressed during the initial six-week open dose optimization phase. In 4

Table 11.5   Side effects leading to withdrawal of vigabatrin in 16 patients[a] (from the 305 patients receiving treatment in the single and double-blind short-term efficacy studies)

Effect	Number of reports
Confusion	4
Depression	4
Drowsiness	4
Headache	3
Ataxia	2
Dizziness	2
Nausea	1
Abdominal pain	1
Psychosis	1
Vertigo	1

[a] Some patients were described to have several effects leading to the decision to withdraw treatment, hence number of reports > than 16.

patients with the most severe mood disturbance these changes were progressive as treatment continued and only remitted after vigabatrin was withdrawn. Furthermore, of 16 patients withdrawn from vigabatrin because of side effects (Table 11.5), depression was a factor in 25%, confirming that when this effect does occur it may be important. It is well known that phenobarbitone may induce depression (Robertson et al 1987). Like vigabatrin, phenobarbitone is thought to enhance GABA-mediated postsynaptic inhibition as part of its anticonvulsant activity both experimentally and in patients (Engel 1989). The use of benzodiazepines, for instance clonazepam, has also been associated with the development of depression (Browne 1983). The development of depression is generally seen during the first few weeks of treatment as the dose is being increased, or following subsequent increases after a period of fixed dose administration. A past history of psychiatric disturbance also appears to be more common in those developing depressive symptoms on vigabatrin.

Aggression. The development of aggression in a study of mentally handicapped patients is described elsewhere in this review. Aggressive behaviour is also reported by Robinson et al (1990) in 9 out of 119 patients with refractory epilepsy treated with vigabatrin. Seven of these patients had a history of aggression and varying degrees of brain damage.

Cognitive effects. There is currently no published evidence that vigabatrin has any deleterious effects on indices of cognitive function. McGuire et al (1991) examined 15 patients with chronic treatment-resistant epilepsy at baseline and after one month of open treatment with 2 g per day of vigabatrin, comparing them to 15 patients on standard antiepileptics and matched for age, sex and IQ. Use of critical flicker fusion, reaction time, digit symbol substitution and arithmetic tests found no treatment-related deterioration in attention, central cognitive processing or perceptuomotor performance.

Side effects leading to withdrawal from vigabatrin

Of the 305 patients entering the studies described in Tables 11.1 and 11.2, a total of 16 were withdrawn from vigabatrin treatment because of adverse side effects. Table 11.5 lists the most frequent side effects implicated in these patients. A comparison with the frequency of all reported side effects (Table 11.4) indicates that the most frequently experienced problems are not too severe whereas the effects warranting cessation of treatment occur more rarely. Where adverse effects have led to withdrawal it has been observed that these effects have subsided over approximately two weeks (Gram et al 1985, Ring et al 1990).

Adverse effects associated with long-term use

The most common adverse effects, somnolence and fatigue, are seen relatively early in the course of treatment and if they do not necessitate withdrawal they tend to remit with continued exposure to the drug (Matilainen et al 1988, Pedersen et al 1985, Rimmer & Richens 1984, Sivenius et al 1987). Weight gain starting soon after initiation of therapy may continue for up to six months (Tartara et al 1989). No new side effects have been reported to emerge on long-term treatment that are not seen in the short term.

Neuropathological examinations

In the course of preclinical animal toxicology studies of vigabatrin it was observed that high doses were associated with the development of dose-dependent central nervous system myelin vacuolation in mice, rats and dogs (Butler et al 1987, Graham 1989, Hauw et al 1988). These changes were reversible on reducing or stopping treatment (Graham 1989, Butler 1989, Arezzo et al 1989). The mechanism of these effects has been investigated by John et al (1987), who examined the hypothesis that increased GABA concentrations were responsible for vacuolation. They compared the effects of vigabatrin and of ethanolamine-O-sulphate, another GABA-T inhibitor, on rat brains. On the latter drug there was a small degree of vacuolation, but the effects were much greater after vigabatrin, suggesting that increased GABA alone could not explain the phenomenon. Studies in a range of animals have demonstrated that vacuolation is a species-specific effect. In monkeys administration of vigabatrin at a dose of 300 mg/kg per day for six months did not lead to any difference in brain pathology from that seen in untreated controls (Graham 1989).

   In dogs the development of histopathological vacuolation was associated with increased central latency of somatosensory evoked potentials (SEPs)

(Arezzo et al 1989). A number of evoked potential studies have been performed in humans to look for electrophysiological evidence of vacuolation in clinical use (Cosi et al 1988, Hammond & Wilder 1985a, Cosi et al 1989, Mervaala et al 1989). These studies have failed to demonstrate any abnormality of visual, brainstem auditory or somatosensory evoked potentials during administration of 2–4 g per day for up to 42 months. It was concluded by Liegeois-Chauval et al (1989) that the absence of any such change in evoked potentials in humans, despite the clear increase in SEPs in dogs, implied that vigabatrin does not cause microvacuolation in man. Support for this conclusion comes from studies of the histological examination of brain tissue obtained from patients treated with vigabatrin (Butler 1989, Hauw et al 1988, Pedersen et al 1987). Currently brains have been obtained from 11 post-mortem cases. These patients had received vigabatrin at doses of 1–4 g per day for a mean of 29 (and a maximum of 69) months. Comparison with 10 control autopsy cases revealed no differences. Additionally surgical brain specimens from 51 patients treated with vigabatrin for a mean of 32.5 months showed no relevant differences from 20 untreated control cases (Merrell Dow, personal communication).

Use in children

Two groups have described the use of vigabatrin as add-on therapy in children. In an open uncontrolled study of 135 children aged between 2 months and 12 years, suffering from a range of seizure types, altogether 38% achieved a greater than 50% reduction in seizure frequency (Livingston et al 1989). A single-blind placebo-controlled study of 61 children with intractable epilepsy reported similar efficacy (Luna et al 1989). These rates are lower than those reported in open or double-blind adult studies. One explanation for this discrepancy may be that the adult test populations contained a higher proportion of patients with partial epilepsy, which has been demonstrated to be particularly responsive to vigabatrin. Livingston et al (1989) initially used a dose range between 40 and 80 mg/kg per day, but increased doses if indicated. The final mean dose used was 87 mg/kg per day. In the study by Luna et al (1989) the dose range was 50–150 mg/kg per day. Doses greater than 100 mg/kg per day were not associated with any further increase in efficacy in either study. Luna et al (1989) did not observe any significant deterioration in seizure frequency in 22 responders followed beyond the 16 week single-blind phase for a further 2–11 months (mean 8 months).

   Like adults, children with complex partial seizures responded best to vigabatrin (Livingston et al 1989). Although some children with severe generalized epilepsy improved significantly, most with myoclonic epilepsy and Lennox–Gastaut syndrome failed to improve, or deteriorated. An open study examining the effects of vigabatrin on 45 children aged 2 months to 10 years suffering from treatment-resistant infantile spasms found that 30 children experienced a reduction in spasms of at least 50%. The children responding most positively in this group were those with a seizure history of less than one year, and the 8 children with tuberose sclerosis. Seven of the latter group achieved complete control of their spasms (Chiron et al 1990).

The most common adverse effects in the childhood studies were agitation or aggression. They were generally reversible on reducing or withdrawing medication, although in 2 out of their 135 patients Livingston et al (1989) note that symptoms persisted after vigabatrin was stopped. Thus agitation is seen more often in children than in adults and may be particularly common in children with mental retardation (Luna et al 1989). In 6 children taking very high doses of vigabatrin (250–600 mg/kg per day) a moderate decrease in haemoglobin concentration (2.5 g per 100 ml on average) was reported (Livingston et al 1989). These changes reversed after reducing the dose. In the other study in children, in which a lower maximum dose of about 150 mg/kg per day was used, no changes in haemoglobin were seen (Luna et al 1989).

Use in patients with mental impairment

Matilainen et al (1988) have studied the effect of vigabatrin in a group of 36 mentally handicapped patients with drug-refractory epilepsy in an open add-on study for seven months. A 50% reduction in seizure frequency was observed in 43% of those with partial seizures and in 33% (2 patients) of those with primary generalized epilepsy. The benefit was maintained throughout the seven-month follow-up period. Vigabatrin was more effective in patients with mild to moderate mental handicap and less so in those with severe mental retardation and multiple seizure types. The side effects observed were reported to be mild and most commonly drowsiness, seen in 21%, and aggressiveness, seen in 8% (3 patients).

SUMMARY AND CONCLUSIONS

Seven double-blind, placebo-controlled trials (six cross-over and one parallel) have confirmed the efficacy of vigabatrin in adult patients with intractable epilepsy and this experience is reinforced by several single-blind and open studies. The drug is particularly useful for partial seizures with or without secondary generalization, but patients with primary generalized seizures may benefit to a lesser extent. No benefit has been reported in myoclonus or petit mal but experience in these areas is limited. In intractable adult populations (i.e. mainly complex partial seizures with or without secondary generalization), approximately 50% of the patients achieve at least a 50% fall in seizure frequency following the addition of vigabatrin to one or two, sometimes more, standard antiepileptic drugs. A few patients may demonstrate complete seizure control. In long-term follow-up studies most patients maintain their initial benefit and if tolerance occurs at all it seems to be slight.

The acute and short-term side effects are similar to those of standard antiepileptic drugs. Drowsiness and fatigue are common and may regress with continued use or reduction of the dose. There is increasing recognition of occasional serious side effects, i.e. psychosis, depression or behavioural disturbance, to which some patients may be predisposed for constitutional or other reasons, such as a past history of mental illness. These will also usually regress on withdrawal of the drug, but may occasionally require specific treatment. No new long-term side effects have so far been reported even up to five years of treatment. Psychiatric side effects may be delayed and weight gain can be insidious. No microvacuolation in myelin has so far been seen in postmortem or surgically resected specimens from patients treated with the drug. Obviously vigilance for long-term clinical or pathological effects must be maintained.

Limited experience in children suggests a similar spectrum of antiepileptic action to that in adults with additional benefit in infantile spasms. Behavioural side effects, especially excitement or agitation, have been prominent. The presence of mental retardation, whether in adults or children, may slightly reduce the degree of efficacy and increase the risk of behavioural side effects.

Our practice is to introduce the drug carefully in adults in a dose of 0.5 g twice daily, increasing by 0.5-g increments depending on clinical progress up to a maximum of 3–4 g daily. As there is no correlation between plasma levels of vigabatrin and clinical efficacy such measurements are not usually undertaken. As the drug is not protein bound or metabolized and is not an enzyme inducer, the potential for drug interaction is limited. Only a slight but unexplained fall in phenytoin levels has been consistently reported. As with other antiepileptic drugs, vigabatrin should always be withdrawn slowly, since earlier theoretical assumptions that it could be withdrawn abruptly have not been borne out in clinical practice.

The introduction of vigabatrin into clinical practice may prove to be a milestone in the treatment of epilepsy, not only because it is the first novel antiepileptic drug since valproate in the 1970s, but because it appears to be the first successful rational approach to the treatment of epilepsy. So far experience is limited to chronic epileptic patients, a notoriously difficult group of patients to treat, and a very demanding test for any new drug. The stage is now set to evaluate the drug as monotherapy in newly diagnosed patients in comparison with other standard antiepileptic drugs. This will provide a clearer picture of the overall role of this promising new drug in the treatment of epilepsy.

REFERENCES

Arezzo J C, Schroeder C E, Litwak M S, Steward D L 1989 Effects of vigabatrin on evoked potentials in dogs. Br J Clin Pharmacol 27 (Suppl 1): 53S–60S

Beart P M, Scatton B, Lloyd K G 1985 Subchronic administration of GABAergic agonists elevates [³H]GABA binding and produces tolerance in striatal dopamine catabolism. Brain Res 335: 169–173

Ben-Menachem E 1989 Pharmacokinetic effects of vigabatrin on cerebrospinal fluid amino acids in humans. Epilepsia 30 (Suppl 3): S12–S14

Ben-Menachem E, Treiman D M 1989 Effect of gamma-vinyl GABA on interictal spikes and sharp waves in patients with intractable complex partial seizures. Epilepsia 30: 79–83

Ben-Menachem E, Persson L I, Schechter P J et al 1989 The effect of different vigabatrin treatment regimens on CSF biochemistry and seizure control in epileptic patients. Br J Clin Pharmacol 27 (Suppl 1): 79S–85S

Betts T, Thomas L 1990 Vigabatrin and behaviour disturbances. Lancet 335: 605–606

Brodie M J, McKee P J W 1990 Vigabatrin and psychosis. Lancet 335: 1279

Browne T R 1983 Benzodiazepines. In: Browne T R, Feldman R G (eds) Epilepsy: diagnosis and management. Little Brown, Boston, pp 235–246

Browne T R, Mattson R H, Penry J K et al 1987 Vigabatrin for complex partial seizures: multicenter single-blind study with long-term follow-up. Neurology 37: 184–189

Browne T R, Mattson R H, Penry J K et al 1989 A multicentre study of vigabatrin for drug-resistant epilepsy. Br J Clin Pharmacol 27 (Suppl 1): 95S–100S

Butler W H 1989 The neuropathology of vigabatrin. Epilepsia 30 (Suppl 3): S15–S17

Butler W P, Ford G P, Newberne J W 1987 A study of the effects of vigabatrin on the central nervous system and retina of Sprague Dawley and Lister-Hooded rats. Toxicol Pathol 15: 143–148

Chadwick D, Crawford P 1986 Clinical, biochemical and pharmacological factors in seizures. In: Trimble M R, Reynolds E H (eds) What is epilepsy? Churchill Livingstone, Edinburgh, pp 53–66

Chiron C, Dulac O, Luna D et al 1990 Vigabatrin in infantile spasms. Lancet 335: 363–364

Cocito L, Maffini M, Perfumo P et al 1989 Vigabatrin in complex partial seizures: a long-term study. Epilepsy Res 3: 160–166

Cosi V, Callieco R, Galimberti C A et al 1988 Effect of vigabatrin (gamma-vinyl-GABA) on visual, brainstem auditory and somatosensory evoked potentials in epileptic patients. Eur Neurol 28: 42–46

Cosi V, Callieco R, Galimberti C A et al 1989 Effects of vigabatrin on evoked potentials in epileptic patients. Br J Clin Pharmacol 27 (Suppl 1): 61S–68S

Dam M 1989 Long-term evaluation of vigabatrin (gamma vinyl GABA) in epilepsy. Epilepsia 30 (Suppl 3): S26–S30

Dam M 1990 Vigabatrin and behaviour disturbances. Lancet 335: 605

Editorial 1989 Vigabatrin. Lancet i: 532–533

Engel J Jr 1989 Seizures and epilepsy. Davis, Philadelphia, pp 411–412

Gale K 1989 GABA in epilepsy: the pharmacologic basis. Epilepsia 30 (Suppl 3): S1–S11

Graham D 1989 Neuropathology of vigabatrin. Br J Clin Pharmacol 27 (Suppl 1): 43S–45S

Gram L, Blatt Lyon B, Dam M 1983 Gamma-vinyl-GABA: a single-blind trial in patients with epilepsy. Acta Neurol Scand 68: 34–39

Gram L, Klosterskov P, Dam M 1985 Gamma-vinyl GABA: a double-blind placebo-controlled trial in partial epilepsy. Ann Neurol 17: 262–266

Gram L, Larsson O M, Johnsen A, Schousboe A 1989 Experimental studies of the influence of vigabatrin on the GABA system. Br J Clin Pharmacol 27 (Suppl 1): 13S–17S

Haegele K D, Huebert N D, Ebel M et al 1988 Pharmacokinetics of vigabatrin: implications of creatinine clearance. Clin Pharmacol Ther 44: 558–565

Halonen T, Lehtinen M, Pitkanen A et al 1988 Inhibitory and excitatory amino acids in CSF of patients suffering from complex partial seizures during chronic treatment with gamma-vinyl GABA (vigabatrin). Epilepsy Res 2: 246–252

Hammond E J, Wilder B J 1985a Effect of gamma-vinyl GABA on human pattern evoked visual potentials. Neurology 35: 1801–1803

Hammond E J, Wilder B J 1985b Effects of gamma-vinyl-GABA on the human electroencephalogram. Neuropharmacology 24: 975–984

Hauw J-J, Trottier S, Boutry J-M et al 1988 The neuropathology of vigabatrin. Br J Clin Pract Suppl 61: 10–13

John R A, Rimmer E M, Williams J et al 1987 Micro-vacuolation in rat brains after long term administration of GABA-transaminase inhibitors. Comparison of effects of ethanolamine-O-sulphate and vigabatrin. Biochem Pharmacol 36: 1467–1473

Jung M J, Lippert B, Metcalf B W et al 1977 Gamma-vinyl GABA (4-amino-hex-5-enoic acid), a new selective irreversible inhibitor of GABA-T: effects on brain GABA metabolism in mice. J Neurochem 29: 797–802

Lancet Editorial. Vigabatrin. Lancet i: 532–533

Larsson O M, Gram L, Schousboe I, Schousboe A 1986 Differential effect of gamma-vinyl GABA and valproate on GABA-transaminase from cultured neurones and astrocytes. Neuropharmacol 25: 617–625

Liegeois-Chauvel C, Marquis P, Gisselbrecht D et al 1989 Effects of long-term vigabatrin on somatosensory-evoked potentials in epileptic patients. Epilepsia 30 (Suppl 3): S23–S25

Lippert B, Metcalf B W, Jung M J, Casara P 1977 4-Amino-hex-5-enoic acid: a selective catalytic inhibitor of 4-aminobutyric-acid aminotransferase in mammalian brain. Eur J Biochem 74: 441–445

Livingston J H, Beaumont D, Arzimanoglou A, Aicardi J 1989 Vigabatrin in the treatment of epilepsy in children. Br J Clin Pharmacol 27 (Suppl 1): 109S–112S

Loiseau P, Hardenberg J P, Pestre M et al 1986 Double-blind placebo-controlled study of vigabatrin (gamma-vinyl GABA) in drug-resistant epilepsy. Epilepsia 27: 115–120

Löscher W, Jackel R, Muller F 1989 Anticonvulsant and proconvulsant effects of inhibitors of GABA degradation in the amygdala-kindling model. Eur J Pharmacol 163: 1–14

Luna D, Dulac O, Pajot N, Beaumont D 1989 Vigabatrin in the treatment of childhood epilepsies: a single-blind placebo-controlled study. Epilepsia 30: 430–437

Matilainen R, Pitkanen A, Ruutiainen T et al 1988 Effect of vigabatrin on epilepsy in mentally retarded patients: a 7-month follow-up study. Neurology 38: 743–747

McGeer P L, McGeer E G 1989 Amino acid neurotransmitters. In: Siegel G, Agranoff B, Albers R W, Molinoff P (eds) Basic neurochemistry. Raven Press, New York, pp 311–332

McGuire A M, Duncan J S, Trimble M R 1991 Effects of vigabatrin on cognitive function and mood, when used as add-on therapy in patients with intractable epilepsy. Epilepsia (in press)

Meldrum B 1984 Amino acid neurotransmitters and new approaches to anticonvulsant drug action. Epilepsia 25 (Suppl 2): S140–S149

Mervaala E, Partanen J, Nousiainen U et al 1989 Electrophysiological effects of gamma-vinyl GABA and carbamazepine. Epilepsia 30: 189–193

Michelucci R, Tassinari C A 1989 Response to vigabatrin in relation to seizure type. Br J Clin Pharmacol 27 (Suppl 1): 119S–124S

Miller J A, Richter J A 1986 Effects of GABAergic drugs in vivo on high-affinity choline uptake in vitro in mouse hippocampal synaptosomes. J Neurochem 47: 1916–1918

Olsen R W 1982 Drug interactions at the GABA receptor–ionophore complex. Ann Rev Pharmacol Toxicol 22: 245–277

Pedersen B, Hojgaard K, Dam M 1987 Vigabatrin: no microvacuoles in a human brain. Epilepsy Res 1: 74–76

Pedersen S A, Klosterskov P, Gram L, Dam M 1985 Long-term study of gamma-vinyl GABA in the treatment of epilepsy. Acta Neurol Scand 72: 295–298

Pitkanen A, Matilainen R, Ruutiainen T et al 1988 Effect of vigabatrin (gamma-vinyl GABA) on amino acid levels in CSF of epileptic patients. J Neurol Neurosurg Psychiatry 51: 1395–1400

Remy C, Beaumont D 1989 Efficacy and safety of vigabatrin in the long-term treatment of refractory epilepsy. Br J Clin Pharmacol 27 (Suppl 1): 125S–129S

Remy C, Favel P, Tell G et al 1986 Etude en double aveugle contre placebo en permutations croisees du vigabatrin dans l'epilepsie de l'adulte resistant a la therapeutique. Boll Lega It Epil 54/55: 241–243

Reynolds E H 1990 Vigabatrin: rational treatment for chronic epilepsy. Br Med J 300: 277–278

Reynolds E H, Ring H A, Farr I N et al 1991 Open, double blind and long term study of vigabatrin in chronic epilepsy. Epilepsia (in press)

Richens A 1989 Potential antiepileptic drugs: vigabatrin. In: Levy R H, Dreifuss F E, Mattson R H et al (eds) Antiepileptic drugs. Raven Press, New York, pp 937–946

Riekkinen P J, Ylinen A, Halonen T et al 1989a Cerebrospinal fluid GABA and seizure control with vigabatrin. Br J Clin Pharmacol 27 (Suppl 1): 87S–94S

Riekkinen P J, Pitkanen A, Ylinen A et al 1989b Specificity of vigabatrin for the GABAergic system in human epilepsy. Epilepsia 30 (Suppl 3): S18–S22

Rimmer E M, Richens A 1984 Double-blind study of gamma-vinyl GABA in patients with refractory epilepsy. Lancet ii 189–190

Rimmer E M, Richens A 1989 Interaction between vigabatrin and phenytoin. Br J Clin Pharmacol 27 (Suppl 1): 27S–33S

Ring H A, Reynolds E H 1990 Vigabatrin and behaviour disturbance. Lancet 335: 970

Ring H A, Heller A J, Farr I N, Reynolds E H 1990 Vigabatrin: rational treatment for chronic epilepsy. J Neurol Neurosurg Psychiatry 53: 1051–1055

Robertson M M, Trimble M R, Townsend H R A 1987 Phenomenology of depression in epilepsy. Epilepsia 28: 364–372

Robinson M K, Richens A, Oxley R 1990 Vigabatrin and behaviour disturbances. Lancet 336: 504

Sander J W A S, Trevisol-Bittencourt P C, Hart Y M, Shorvon S D 1990 Evaluation of vigabatrin as an add-on drug in the management of severe epilepsy. J Neurol Neurosurg Psychiatry 53: 1008–1010

Sander J W A S, Hart Y M, Trimble M R, Shorvon S D 1991 Vigabatrin and psychosis. J Neurol Neurosurg Psychiatry (in press)

Schechter P J 1986 Vigabatrin. In: Meldrum B S, Porter R J (eds) Current problems in epilepsy: new anticonvulsant drugs, Vol 4. Libby, London, pp 265–275

Schechter P J 1989 Clinical pharmacology of vigabatrin. Br J Clin Pharmacol 27 (Suppl 1): 19S–22S

Schechter P J, Hanke N F, Grove J et al 1984 Biochemical and clinical effects of gamma-vinyl-GABA in patients with epilepsy. Neurology 34: 182–186

Sivenius M R J, Ylinen A, Murros K et al 1987 Double-blind dose reduction study of vigabatrin in complex partial epilepsy. Epilepsia 28: 688–692

Tartara A, Manni R, Galimberti C A et al 1986 Vigabatrin in the treatment of epilepsy: a double-blind, placebo-controlled study. Epilepsia 27: 717–723

Tartara A, Manni R, Galimberti C A et al 1989 Vigabatrin in the treatment of epilepsy: a long-term follow-up study. J Neurol Neurosurg Psychiatry 52: 467–471

Tassinari C O, Michelucci R, Ambrosetto G, Salvi F 1987 Double-blind study of vigabatrin in the treatment of drug-resistant epilepsy. Arch Neurol 44: 907–910

Van Wieringen A, Binnie C D, De Boer P T E et al 1987 Electroencephalographic findings in antiepileptic drug trials: a review and report of 6 studies. Epilepsy Res 1: 3–15

12

Lamotrigine

A. Richens

INTRODUCTION

Sometimes in medicine the trail leading to a new discovery is a tortuous one and the researcher, on looking back down the pathway that he has taken, may be tempted to say that if he were to start again he would not start from where he did. Such is the history of lamotrigine. This chapter reviews the background and summarizes the current position with regard to its clinical use. Previous reviews have been published by Miller et al (1986a), Gram (1989) and Yuen (1991).

In the 1960s it was realized that the antiepileptic drugs in use at that time, predominantly phenobarbitone and phenytoin, could lower serum folate levels and occasionally cause macrocytosis. Following their observations that folic acid supplements could worsen seizures, Reynolds et al (1966) put forward the hypothesis that antiepileptic drugs might reduce seizures by an antifolate effect. Although controlled studies have failed to support this hypothesis, researchers at the Wellcome Research Laboratories looked among a number of antifolate compounds for a new antiepileptic drug. A series of phenyltriazine compounds were investigated and anticonvulsant activity was demonstrated in animal models, but this did not appear to correlate with their antifolate activity. One of these compounds, lamotrigine, was selected for development. Further pharmacological studies suggest that its mode of action is by interfering with glutamate transmission.

CHEMISTRY

Lamotrigine is the approved name for 3,5-diamino-6-(2,3-dichlorophenyl)-1,2,4-triazine. Its structure is shown in Figure 12.1. It has been given the proprietary name Lamictal in the UK. It is a chemically stable white powder with a molecular weight of 256.09 and a pK_a of 5.5. It has a solubility in water of <1 mg/ml and in ethanol of approximately 1 mg/ml. A high-performance liquid chromatographic method has been developed for measuring lamotrigine in body fluids (Cohen et al 1987).

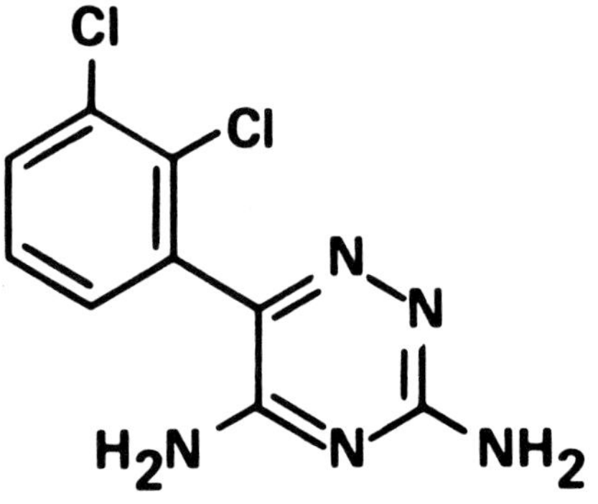

Fig. 12.1   Chemical structure of lamotrigine

PRECLINICAL STUDIES (a review can be found in Miller et al 1986a)

Antiseizure activity in animal models

In maximal electroshock tests in rodents, a dose-dependent abolition of hind limb extension by single doses of lamotrigine has been demonstrated (Lamb et al 1985, Miller et al 1986b). Oral ED_{50} values for mice are shown in Table 12.1. In this test, lamotrigine showed a potency similar to phenytoin and diazepam, but greater than carbamazepine or phenobarbitone. Sodium valproate was weak in this test and ethosuximide was inactive.

The duration of action of lamotrigine was long in both rats and mice and no tolerance to the anticonvulsant action of the drug was observed on oral administration of lamotrigine for up to 28 days in both species. The drug was active by all routes tested, namely oral, subcutaneous, intraperitoneal and intravenous; the peak ED_{50} values were of a similar order with each route.

In maximal seizures induced in mice by intravenous infusion of pentylenetetrazole or bolus injections of picrotoxin or bicuculline, lamotrigine abolished or reduced the incidence of hind limb extension, with ED_{50} values being similar to those found in electroshock testing. In chemically induced threshold tests, lamotrigine, like phenytoin, failed to increase

Table 12.1   Oral ED_{50} values (mg/kg) for abolition of hind limb extension in maximum electroshock testing in mice (from Lamb et al 1985)

Drug	ED_{50} at peak activity	ED_{50} at 24 h post-drug
Lamotrigine	2.6–3.8	10.1
Carbamazepine	6.9–8.5	352
Phenobarbitone	9.1–11.4	64.7
Phenytoin	3.5–5.2	35.9
Diazepam	3.2–5.5	119
Sodium valproate	332–461	Not tested
Troxidone	750–609	Not tested
Ethosuximide	Inactive	

clonus latency and at high doses both drugs lowered clonus latency, suggesting a proconvulsant action at these doses.

In electrically evoked afterdischarges in the rat and dog, the duration of the response was reduced in a dose-dependent manner with ED_{50} values of 11.7 and 4.5 mg/kg, respectively, following intravenous lamotrigine (Miller & Wheatley 1985). Visually evoked afterdischarges in the rat were inhibited by lamotrigine, an effect which resembles diazepam and ethosuximide but contrasts with phenytoin and carbamazepine. Similar results have been found with further studies in the marmoset (Wheatley & Miller 1989).

In electrically induced cortical kindling in rats, lamotrigine increased the number of negative responses (absence of behavioural or EEG responses to electrical stimulation) in a dose-related manner (Leach et al 1983). At high doses of 18 mg/kg the number and duration of kindled responses was reduced although lamotrigine failed to block kindling development completely.

Toxicity

Acute toxicological studies in rodents have shown a 40–100-fold separation between the oral anticonvulsant ED_{50} and LD_{50} (Miller et al 1986a). Subacute oral toxicity studies in rats and marmosets at dose levels of up to 50 mg/kg per day, and 3, 6 and 12-month chronic toxicity studies in rats and cynomolgus monkeys in doses of up to 25 mg per day, demonstrated no effects which precluded its oral administration to man. Carcinogenicity, reproductive toxicity and mutagenicity tests have demonstrated no toxic actions.

Behavioural toxicological studies (Miller et al 1986b) have shown that lamotrigine has a behavioural depressant effect, including decreased locomotor activity, ataxia and reflex impairment, but only in doses considerably higher than those required to produce an anticonvulsant action. In mice there was a 35-fold separation between the anticonvulsant ED_{50} value and the dose required to induce ataxia. The separation for phenytoin was 11-fold.

Pharmacology

Initial studies of the anticonvulsant spectrum of lamotrigine indicated that it resembled phenytoin. As there is some evidence for a presynaptic site of action for the latter drug, Leach et al (1986) studied the effect of lamotrigine and phenytoin on the release of endogenous amino acids in rat cerebral cortex slices in vitro. Amino acid release was stimulated by veratrine or high potassium concentrations. Lamotrigine inhibited veratrine-induced release of glutamate and aspartate, with ED_{50} values of 21 μM, but was less potent in inhibiting GABA release, with an ED_{50} of 44 μM. However, lamotrigine had no effect on potassium-evoked release at concentrations up to 300 μM. Veratrine is known to cause transmitter release by opening up presynaptic voltage-sensitive sodium channels, while high potassium concentrations evoke release simply by reversing the potassium electrochemical gradient across the membrane. The results observed with lamotrigine therefore indicated that this drug is acting like phenytoin at presynaptic sodium channels. As this occurred in concentrations which are achieved in rat brain after administration of anticonvulsant doses of lamotrigine, inhibition of the release of excitatory amino acids was considered to be a likely mechanism of lamotrigine's anticonvulsant effect.

Lamotrigine weakly displaces [^{3}H]diazepam from its binding sites, but has no effect on the binding of a wide range of radiolabelled ligands (Miller et al 1986a).

Drug metabolism and pharmacokinetics

Parsons & Miles (1984) studied the disposition of lamotrigine in several animal species. It was found to be well absorbed and widely distributed in the body tissues. It is eliminated largely in the urine but the elimination half-life varies widely between species (2–5 hours in the beagle dog and up to 52 hours in the cynomolgus monkey). The kinetics are independent of the dose and duration of administration in the rat and monkey.

In the rat, an N-oxide and glucuronide conjugate are formed but the predominant substance in the urine is the parent compound. In the cynomolgus monkey, extensive metabolism to a glucuronide conjugate occurs and smaller amounts of the unmetabolized drug is found in the urine.

The influence of chronic oral administration of lamotrigine on the hepatic microsomal metabolizing activity of various substrates has been examined in rats and marmosets. Slight inducing effects were seen with subtherapeutic doses in the marmoset only (Miller et al 1986a).

CLINICAL STUDIES

Pharmacokinetics

Single and multiple-dose studies in healthy human volunteers have shown that lamotrigine is well absorbed, with the peak plasma concentration occurring at 2–3 hours (Cohen et al 1987). A linear relationship was found between the dose administered and both the maximum plasma concentration and area under the plasma concentration–time curve. Absolute bioavailability was not measured but urine collections over 144 hours showed that at least 70% of the dose must have been absorbed.

The drug was excreted mainly (about 90%) in the form of a 2N-glucuronic acid conjugate, which is advantageous because the glucuronidation mechanism has a large capacity and is little affected by age. The possibility that patients with unconjugated hyperbilirubinaemia (Gilbert's syndrome) might conjugate lamotrigine less readily, with the result that the drug might accumulate, was examined by Posner et al (1989). Some impairment of lamotrigine elimination was found in that the clearance was 32% lower and the elimination half-life was 37% higher but this was thought not to be of clinical significance.

The plasma protein binding of lamotrigine is about 55%, measured by in vitro techniques and by the saliva to plasma concentration ratio in vivo. Therapeutic concentrations of phenytoin, phenobarbitone and valproate do not influence its binding (Miller et al 1986a).

The plasma elimination half-life following single doses was 24.1 ± 5.7 hours and was not significantly changed by repeated doses. A half-life of this length predicted that once or twice-daily dosing would be possible. The single-dose kinetics were found to predict the behaviour of the drug after multiple doses, suggesting that autoinduction or saturation of metabolism does not occur.

Studies in epileptic patients, however, have shown that the background antiepileptic therapy that the patient is receiving alters the elimination rate of lamotrigine. In patients on hepatic enzyme-inducing drugs (i.e. carbamazepine, phenytoin, phenobarbitone and primidone) the elimination half-life is shortened. Binnie et al (1986) found values of 7.8–33.3 hours (mean 15 hours, $n=9$) and Jawad et al (1987) found values of 6.4–32.2 hours (mean 14.3 hours, $n=12$). This presumably reflects an induction of the glucuronidation mechanism, an effect which is recognized with enzyme inducers.

On the other hand, patients on valproate have longer half-lives than healthy volunteers. Binnie et al (1986) included four patients on valproate alone in their study; they had a half-life of 30.5–88.8 hours (mean 59 hours).

When valproate is combined with enzyme inducers intermediate half-lives are seen. Jawad et al (1987) found mean ($\pm$ SD) values of 29.6 ± 10 hours in 10 patients on combined therapy compared with 14.3 ± 6.9 hours in 12 patients on inducers alone.

It was clear from these pharmacokinetic studies that the dosage of lamotrigine would have to be tailored to the background therapy when definitive clinical trials were started. The recommended maintenance doses were 200 mg daily in those patients on enzyme-inducing drugs without valproate, 100 mg daily in those on a combination and 75 mg daily in those on valproate alone. This ensured that the plasma lamotrigine levels were roughly the same in the three groups.

These interactions will complicate the use of lamotrigine in clinical practice because the incidence of adverse reactions, including skin rashes, is related to the plasma concentration achieved.

Efficacy

Single-dose studies

Single-dose techniques have been little used in the preliminary assessment of potential antiepileptic drugs in man. With lamotrigine, however, two groups performed such studies at a time when insufficient animal toxicology data were available to justify multiple doses in man. In open studies, Binnie et al (1986) found a reduction in the photosensitivity range in six photosensitive patients given single 120–240 mg doses of lamotrigine. In two patients, the photic response was completely abolished. In a further five patients with frequent interictal spike or sharp wave abnormalities, lamotrigine reduced the frequency of these phenomena.

Jawad et al (1986) also studied patients with interictal spike abnormalities. In a double-blind study in which 240 mg of lamotrigine, 20 mg of diazepam or a matching placebo were given orally to 6 patients, the spike frequency was reduced to about 60% of the baseline level by lamotrigine, this effect being significantly different from placebo although slightly less than with diazepam.

The data from both of these groups indicate that peak effects occur 1.5–6.5 hours after oral administration, and some effect was still present (on photosensitivity) at 24 hours. The positive results of these trials encouraged further evaluation of the compound.

One-week studies

In an open study primarily designed to investigate the single and multiple-dose pharmacokinetics of lamotrigine, Jawad et al (1987) found a significant reduction in the frequency of complex partial seizures in 11 patients with refractory epilepsy given lamotrigine for one week. The mean $\pm$ SE seizure count was reduced from 8.7 ± 1.3 in the baseline week to 4.1 ± 0.8 in the treatment week, in which the patients were given a daily dose designed to achieve a peak plasma concentration of 1.5 mg/l at the end of three days dosing and 3 mg/l after seven days dosing. The doses were calculated from a single-dose kinetic study performed in each patient. Secondarily generalized tonic–clonic seizures were also reduced (from 4.3 ± 1.5 to 2.4 ± 0.6 per week, $n = 14$) but this difference was not statistically significant.

Binnie et al (1987) also performed a one-week trial, but used a double-blind cross-over technique in which either lamotrigine or placebo was added on to existing therapy in a group of ten patients with therapy-resistant seizures. The dose of lamotrigine was tailored according to an elimination half-life calculated over 26 hours after the first (200 mg) dose. The seizure type in these patients was not uniform and therefore an analysis of seizure frequency could be undertaken only on the basis of total seizures regardless of type. Median seizure count fell from 5.0 in the baseline period to 2.5 during lamotrigine administration, but this reduction did not reach statistical significance ($p = 0.055$). Six patients experienced a seizure reduction of 50% or more.

These two trials were not primarily designed to examine the efficacy of lamotrigine, but nevertheless, despite the short duration of treatment, they gave encouraging signs of an antiseizure effect. Definitive efficacy studies were therefore set up.

Definitive clinical trials

The initial approach was to use the cross-over technique in limited numbers of patients in four centres: the Welsh Epilepsy Unit, Cardiff, UK (Jawad et al 1989), the Instituut voor Epilepsiebestrijding, Heemstede, Holland (Binnie et al 1989), the Chalfont Centre for Epilepsy, Chalfont St Giles, UK (Sander et al 1990a) and the University Hospital, Bordeaux, France (Loiseau et al 1990). The first three trials had the same design, while the Bordeaux study used shorter treatment periods (8 weeks compared with 12 weeks). All included patients with therapy-resistant seizures, which were mainly partial with or without secondary generalization. Lamotrigine 50–400 mg per day or a matching placebo was added to existing therapy in a double-blind randomized cross-over manner. The dosage administered allowed for drug interactions, higher starting doses being used for patients on enzyme-inducing drugs only, and lower doses for those on valproate.

Two further cross-over trials have been completed since the European trials have been analysed, and at the time of writing a draft unpublished report of each was available to the Wellcome Foundation (Wellcome 1991a, 1991b). Both were multicentre, one in the USA and the other in Australia. The design of both of the trials resembled the European studies. The outcome of each of these six trials is summarized for total seizure counts in Table 12.2. All seizure types have been added together but the most common during the trials were partial seizures, predominantly complex. In all of the trials except that at Chalfont, a significant reduction in seizures during the lamotrigine treatment phase was seen. The other findings in each of the studies is summarized below.

Cardiff trial. In this trial the dose of lamotrigine was tailored to produce trough plasma concentrations of 1.5–2.5 mg/l, and this required between 75 mg and 400 mg daily. All the patients were receiving enzyme-inducing drugs and only one received valproate also. Two 12-week treatment periods were used. Seventeen of the 21 patients who completed this trial had partial

Table 12.2 Changes in total seizure count in six double-blind cross-over trials in patients suffering mainly from partial seizures with or without secondary generalization

Study centre	Number of patients	% with >50% reduction in seizures	Mean % reduction	Confidence intervals		p
Cardiff	21	67	60	42	73	0.001
Heemstede	30	7	16	5	25	0.01
Chalfont	18	11	8	−20	29	NS
Bordeaux	23	30	27	2	46	0.05
US multicentre	88	20	25	14	35	0.001
Australian multicentre	41	22	24	11	35	0.001

seizures, and of these, 16 had fewer during the lamotrigine phase, and 12 had a greater than 50% reduction ($p<0.002$). Eight of 15 patients with secondarily generalized tonic–clonic seizures benefited, of whom 7 had a greater than 50% reduction ($p<0.05$). The overall response rate in this trial was greater than in any of the other five trials; this may be partly explained by the fact that they were all outpatients and may have had less intractable epilepsy than those patients entered into some of the other trials.

Heemstede trial. Dosing in this trial was designed to achieve peak plasma lamotrigine concentrations of 3 mg/l and the required dose varied between 50 mg and 400 mg daily. Nine of the 30 patients completing the trial were receiving valproate in addition to enzyme-inducing antiepileptic drugs, and higher plasma lamotrigine concentrations than those on enzyme inducers only (2.3 ± 0.5 mg/l and 1.5 ± 0.4 mg/l, respectively) despite receiving a smaller mean dose of lamotrigine (114 ± 38 mg daily compared with 242 ± 81 mg daily). Twenty of the 30 patients had fewer partial seizures on lamotrigine ($p<0.01$) but only 2 showed a greater than 50% improvement. Insufficient patients had tonic–clonic seizures during the trial for a subanalysis to be made.

Chalfont trial. Trough plasma lamotrigine concentrations of 0.5–3 mg/l were aimed at in this study and the final daily doses required were between 100 mg and 300 mg daily. Twelve of the 18 patients completing the trial were on valproate in addition to enzyme inducers. No significant reduction in seizures was found except that, in the last four weeks of the lamotrigine treatment period, there was a significant fall in the frequency of generalized seizures when compared with placebo and baseline.

Bordeaux trial. The dosage strategy in this trial was aimed at achieving plasma concentrations of 1.5–2.5 mg/l. Doses of 150–300 mg were given, five of the 23 patients being on valproate. Partial seizures were reduced in 14 of the 23 patients, with 8 benefiting by more than 50% ($p<0.05$). An insufficient number of patients experienced generalized seizures for an analysis to be made of this type.

Meta-analysis of the four European trials. The numbers of patients included in each of these trials was relatively small and therefore the power of the individual studies was low. Furthermore, only a proportion of the patients had secondarily generalized seizures and therefore the effectiveness of lamotrigine was not well assessed in this seizure type. As the studies were of a similar design a meta-analysis of the four trials was undertaken with the statistical advice of Dr Tony Johnson at the Medical Research Council Biostatistical Department (Yuen 1991). Of the 92 patients involved, 64 (70%) experienced fewer total seizures while on lamotrigine compared with placebo. Twenty-five (27%) had a greater than 50% reduction ($p<0.001$). The median seizure reduction (Fig. 12.2) was 27%, with a confidence interval of 19–34%. The meta-analysis also showed a significant reduction in partial seizures ($n=92$) and in generalized tonic–clonic seizures ($n=45$).

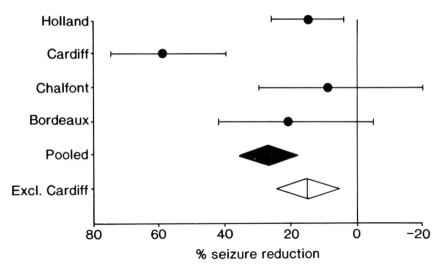

Fig. 12.2 Meta-analysis of the four European double-blind cross-over trials giving the median reduction in total seizures and 95% confidence intervals. (Reproduced with permission from Yuen 1991.)

US multicentre trial. This involved seven centres (Detroit, Miami, Houston, Richmond, Chapel Hill, West Haven and Dallas). Ninety-eight patients with refractory partial seizures were recruited, of which 88 completed the trial. It was designed as a placebo-controlled cross-over study with the treatments added to existing therapy and each treatment was given for a nine-week maintenance period, excluding dose ascension and tapering. Mean trough plasma lamotrigine levels ranged from 1.64 to 2.94 mg/l, with doses of 150–400 mg daily. The frequency of total partial seizures was reduced in 57 (65%) of the patients, 18 (20%) having a 50% or more seizure reduction. The median reduction across all centres was 25% ($p < 0.001$). Simple and complex partial seizures responded in a similar way. Only 29 patients had secondarily generalized seizures and no significant difference emerged between lamotrigine and placebo in this seizure type.

Australian multicentre trial. Four centres recruited a total of 41 patients into this study (Sydney, Adelaide and two in Melbourne). A placebo-controlled cross-over, add-on design was used with treatment phases of 12 weeks' duration. Lamotrigine doses of 100–300 mg per day were given with the aim of producing plasma concentrations of 1.5–2.5 mg/l. All 41 patients completed the trial and 26 (63%) showed an improvement on lamotrigine treatment. Nine patients (22%) experienced a 50% or greater reduction in total seizure count, the mean reduction being 24%. Partial seizures were significantly improved by lamotrigine treatment (mean reduction of 30%) but the reduction in generalized tonic–clonic seizures (46%) did not quite reach statistical significance ($0.05 < p < 0.10$). Only 19 of the patients experienced seizures of this latter type during the trial.

Other physiological actions

Van Wieringen et al (1989) studied the effects of lamotrigine on the EEG power spectrum in normal human volunteers. Two single doses of lamotrigine were used: 120 mg and 240 mg at an interval of one week. A placebo control was used as well and an active control comprising phenytoin 500 mg and 1000 mg each given in two equally divided doses 2.5 hours apart. The latter dose gave low therapeutic levels of phenytoin during the 7 hours in which testing was done. Plasma lamotrigine concentrations were a little over 2 mg/l. Both drugs produced marked effects on the power spectra, some of which were dose related. The effects of the two drugs were similar in some respects but in others differences appeared, e.g. the centre of gravity of the spectrum was increased by lamotrigine but decreased by phenytoin.

Cortical and brainstem evoked responses were measured in this study. An increased latency in wave 1 in the brainstem auditory evoked response was found with phenytoin, and considered to be an effect of the drug in delaying nerve conduction. This was not found with lamotrigine, suggesting that this drug might be less neurotoxic than phenytoin.

Cohen et al (1985) studied the effects of lamotrigine compared to phenytoin and diazepam on various measures of CNS activity in healthy volunteers: adaptive tracking, eye movements, body sway and visual analogue scales. Lamotrigine was given in single doses of 120 and 240 mg, phenytoin 500 and 1000 mg and diazepam 10 mg. A placebo control was used and the trial was double-blind, randomized cross-over in design. Plasma levels of phenytoin at 4 hours were 11.5 ± 2.2 mg/l and lamotrigine 2.7 ± 0.4 mg/l. Lamotrigine produced no important side effects but diazepam caused sedation and phenytoin unsteadiness. Subjective effects increased by analogue rating scales occurred with phenytoin and diazepam. Whereas both phenytoin and diazepam improved adaptive tracking, increased body sway and impaired eye movements, lamotrigine produced only a possible slight increase in body sway. The effects of phenytoin and diazepam correlated with saliva concentrations of the drugs. It was concluded that lamotrigine might have a more favourable CNS side effect profile than phenytoin.

Adverse events in clinical trials

In a seven-day pharmacokinetic study in healthy volunteers, no clinically important side effects or changes in CNS or cardiovascular system variables, haematology, biochemistry or urinalysis were observed with lamotrigine (Cohen et al 1987).

CNS effects in patients

In the four European double-blind studies several adverse events were more commonly seen during lamotrigine treatment than during placebo: asthenia, diplopia, headache, somnolence, ataxia, dizziness, nausea and nervousness. However, the differences between the two treatment periods were not signficant for any of these symptoms; ataxia and headache were close to significant.

In the US multicentre study ataxia and nystagmus were noted during lamotrigine treatment but not significantly more so than during placebo.

Open studies are unsatisfactory for determining the incidence of adverse effects caused by a new drug because a high incidence of CNS symptoms is seen randomly and in association with placebo. A placebo control is therefore essential in order to evaluate what is really due to the drug and what is coincidental. In the open long-term tolerability study reported by Sander et al (1990b) the commonest adverse events were diplopia, headache and ataxia – three symptoms which are common in cohorts of epileptic patients.

Skin rashes

Type IV allergic skin rashes related to the administration of lamotrigine have been reported in all clinical trials. Typically they occur in the second week of administration and present as erythema multiforme or maculopapular rashes. In a few cases there has been oral involvement but none has satisfied the definition of Stevens–Johnson syndrome. A fever, lymphadenopathy and eosinophilia have occasionally been seen. There is no evidence of a phototoxic mechanism.

In-house data (Wellcome 1990a) in which experience in 2620 patients and volunteers has been reviewed indicate that the incidence in double-blind placebo-controlled trials is 10.3% with the active drug compared to 5.4% in the placebo-treated group. Withdrawal of lamotrigine was necessary in 1.9% of those on the active treatment compared with 0.2% on placebo. In open studies involving 1446 patients, withdrawal of lamotrigine was necessary in 4.3% (but the rashes were not necessarily caused by lamotrigine).

Much higher rash rates have been found in volunteers and in patients not on hepatic enzyme-inducing therapy. In these subjects high initial plasma lamotrigine concentrations have been measured. This suggests that the rash rate is dependent upon the starting dose and plasma level, as has been reported with carbamazepine and phenytoin (Chadwick et al 1984). This indicates that low starting doses should be used especially where it is used as monotherapy or added to a non-enzyme-inducing drug such as valproate (in fact, this drug inhibits lamotrigine metabolism; see below). A starting dose of 50 mg per day should not be exceeded in these patients.

Laboratory monitoring

In the European double-blind studies, a reduction in blood white cell count

(WCC) was observed. This is a frequent finding in epileptic patients (32% had low WCC while on placebo) but it occurred more frequently during lamotrigine therapy. However, the decrease was not sustained, nor did it occur at any particular time during treatment. No change in WCC was noted in the US multicentre trial. An in-house analysis of databases from 40 clinical trials, involving 972 patients, gave no indication that lamotrigine lowers WCC (Wellcome 1990b). No other haematological abnormalities have occurred in lamotrigine trials.

Pooled data from the six double-blind trials ($n = 221$) shows no change in liver function tests (Wellcome 1989). The US multicentre study, however, showed a significant *reduction* in alanine transaminase – an effect not mirrored in any other study – and is probably a chance finding.

γ-Glutamyl transpeptidase levels are frequently higher than normal in patients on enzyme-inducing drugs. When lamotrigine is added to existing treatment the proportion of patients with abnormal values increases slightly (Wellcome 1990b) but with a very slow time-course, making it unlikely that it is due to enzyme induction. No other measure of liver function was altered. An in-house study has shown that lamotrigine lacks significant hepatic enzyme-inducing properties when given in doses of 200 mg daily to healthy volunteers for two weeks (Wellcome 1991c).

Drug interactions

Plasma concentrations of the standard antiepileptic drugs have not been altered by addition of lamotrigine in any of the double-blind cross-over studies. Multiple doses of paracetamol have been shown to facilitate lamotrigine clearance in volunteers by an unknown mechanism (Depot et al 1990). The effects of enzyme-inducing antiepileptic drugs and sodium valproate on lamotrigine dispositions have been described earlier in this review.

SUMMARY AND CONCLUSION

Lamotrigine is a novel antiepileptic drug which probably acts by reducing the release of excitatory amino acids from presynaptic terminals. Its beneficial effect in refractory simple and complex partial seizures is proven when added on to existing therapy, although the benefit is modest (about a 25–30% reduction in mean seizure frequency). Whether it will be more effective in less severe seizures remains to be demonstrated. The power of published trials to demonstrate an effect in secondarily generalized seizures has been weaker but the balance of evidence points to a reduction in this seizure type of about 10%. No trials have so far been completed in primary generalized seizure disorders. Its spectrum of adverse effects appears at this stage to be as good as or better than existing drugs, but skin rashes are a nuisance, especially with high starting doses. Furthermore, the dose needs to be adjusted to the background therapy because lamotrigine's metabolism is stimulated by enzyme-inducing antiepileptic drugs and inhibited by valproate. At the time of writing, marketing approval had been granted in the Irish Republic but applications have been filed in various other countries. More extensive investigation will be required to define the exact position of lamotrigine in treating epilepsy.

REFERENCES

Binnie C D, van Emde Boas W, Kasteleijn-Nolste-Trenite D G A et al 1986 Acute effects of lamotrigine (BW430C) in persons with epilepsy. Epilepsia 27: 248–254
Binnie C D, Beintema D J, Debets R M C et al 1987 Seven day administration of lamotrigine in epilepsy: placebo-controlled add-on trial. Epilepsy Res 1: 202–208
Binnie C D, Debets R M C, Engelsman M et al 1989 Double-blind cross-over trial of lamotrigine (Lamictal) as add-on therapy in intractable epilepsy. Epilepsy Res 4: 222–229
Chadwick D, Shaw M D M, Foly P et al 1984 Serum anticonvulsant concentrations and the risk of drug induced skin eruptions. J Neurol Neurosurg Psychiatry 47: 642–644
Cohen A F, Ashby L, Crowley D et al 1985 Lamotrigine (BW430C), a potential anticonvulsant: effects on the central nervous system in comparison with phenytoin and diazepam. Br J Clin Pharmacol 20: 619–629
Cohen A F, Land G S, Breimer D D et al 1987 Lamotrigine, a new anticonvulsant: pharmacokinetics in normal humans. Clin Pharmacol Ther 42: 535–541
Depot M, Powell J R, Messenheimer J A et al 1990 Kinetic effects of multiple oral doses of acetaminophen on a single oral dose of lamotrigine. Clin Pharmacol Ther 48: 346–355
Gram L 1989 Potential antiepileptic drugs: lamotrigine. In: Levy R, Mattson R, Meldrum B et al (eds) Antiepileptic drugs, 3rd edn. Raven Press, New York, pp 947–953
Jawad S, Oxley J, Yuen W C et al 1986 The effect of lamotrigine, a novel anticonvulsant, on interictal spikes in patients with epilepsy. Br J Clin Pharmacol 22: 191–193
Jawad S, Yuen W C, Peck A W et al 1987 Lamotrigine: single-dose pharmacokinetics and initial 1 week experience in refractory epilepsy. Epilepsy Res 1: 194–201
Jawad S, Richens A, Goodwin G et al 1989 Controlled trial of lamotrigine (Lamictal) for refractory partial seizures. Epilepsia 30: 356–363
Lamb R J, Leach M J, Miller A A et al 1985 Anticonvulsant profile in mice of lamotrigine, a novel anticonvulsant. Br J Pharmacol 85: 235
Leach M J, Miller A A, O'Donnell R A et al 1983 Reduced cortical glutamine concentration in electrically kindled rats. J Neurochem 41: 1492–1494
Leach M J, Marden C M, Miller A A 1986 Pharmacological studies on lamotrigine, a novel potential antiepileptic drug: II. Neurochemical studies on the mechanism of action. Epilepsia 27: 490–497
Loiseau P, Yuen A W C, Duche B et al 1990 A randomized double-blind placebo-controlled cross-over add-on trial of lamotrigine in patients with treatment-resistant partial seizures. Epilepsy Res 7: 136–145
Miller A A, Wheatley P L 1985 Anticonvulsant action of lamotrigine, phenytoin and phenobarbitone on electrically-induced after discharge. Br J Pharmacol 85: 366
Miller A A, Sawyer D A, Roth B et al 1986a Lamotrigine. In: Meldrum B S, Porter R J (eds) New anticonvulsant drugs. Libbey, London, pp 165–177
Miller A A, Wheatley P L, Sawyer D A et al 1986b Pharmacological studies on lamotrigine, a novel potential antiepileptic drug: I. Anticonvulsant profile in mice and rats. Epilepsia 27: 483–489
Parsons D M, Miles D W 1984 Metabolic studies with BW430C. Epilepsia 25: 655
Posner J, Cohen A F, Land G et al 1989 The pharmacokinetics of lamotrigine (BW430C) in healthy subjects with uncomplicated hyperbilirubinaemia (Gilbert's syndrome). Br J Clin Pharmacol 28: 117–120
Reynolds E H, Milner G, Matthews D M et al 1966 Anticonvulsant therapy, megaloblastic haemopoiesis and folic acid metabolism. Q J Med 35: 521–537

Sander J W A S, Patsalos P N, Oxley J R et al 1990a A randomised double-blind placebo-controlled add-on trial of lamotrigine in patients with severe epilepsy. Epilepsy Res 6: 221–226

Sander J W A S, Trevisol-Bittencourt P C, Hart Y M et al 1990b The efficacy and long-term tolerability of lamotrigine in the treatment of severe epilepsy. Epilepsy Res 7: 226–229

van Wieringen A, Binnie C D, Meijer J W A et al 1989 Comparison of the effects of lamotrigine and phenytoin on the EEG power spectrum and cortical and brain stem-evoked responses of normal human volunteers. Pharmacoelectroencephalography 21: 157–169

Wellcome 1989 Company Document. BLZG/89/022. Wellcome Foundation Ltd, UK

Wellcome 1990a Company Document. BLZG/90/011. Wellcome Foundation Ltd, UK

Wellcome 1990b Company Document. BLZG/90/012. Wellcome Foundation Ltd, UK

Wellcome 1991a Company Document. BLZG/90/008. Wellcome Foundation Ltd, UK

Wellcome 1991b Company Document. BLZG/90/008. Wellcome Foundation Ltd, UK

Wellcome 1991c Company Document. BLVS/90/27. Wellcome Foundation Ltd, UK

Wheatley P L, Miller A A 1989 Effects of lamotrigine on electrically induced after-discharge duration in anaesthetised rat, dog, and marmoset. Epilepsia 30: 34–40

Yuen A W C 1991 Lamotrigine. In: Pisani F, Perucca E, Avanzini G, Richens A (eds) New antiepileptic drugs. Elsevier, Amsterdam (in press)

13

Gabapentin

D. Chadwick

INTRODUCTION

Gabapentin is a chemically novel compound related in structure to the neurotransmitter γ-aminobutyric acid (GABA) that has been developed by Warner-Lambert. Gabapentin was synthesized as a GABA-mimetic that could freely cross the blood–brain barrier. Despite its structural relationship to GABA and its anticonvulsant activity, gabapentin does not appear to act pharmacologically as a GABA-mimetic.

CHEMISTRY

Gabapentin (CI-945), 1-(aminomethyl)cyclohexaneacetic acid (Fig. 13.1), has a molecular weight of 171.34, is freely soluble in water ($>10\%$ at pH 7.4), and does not exist in enantiomeric forms (Bartoszyk et al 1986).

In the crystalline form it is stable at room temperature, but a slow formation of the lactam occurs in aqueous solutions. Gabapentin may be assayed in plasma and urine by sensitive high-performance liquid chromatography with pre-column labelling for ultraviolet detection (Hengy & Kolle 1985).

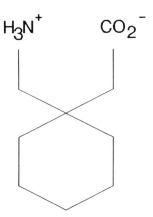

Fig. 13.1   Structure of gabapentin.

TOXICOLOGY

Gabapentin is well tolerated with no deaths in acute animal studies at doses up to 8000 mg per day in rats and up to 5000 mg per day in mice. Chronic studies show similar good tolerance with doses up to 1500 mg per day in rats, up to 2000 mg per day in dogs and up to 500 mg per day in monkeys. Minor increases in liver enzymes and increased organ weights seen at the highest doses all reversed promptly after cessation of therapy. Gabapentin is not mutagenic in bacterial and mammalian assays and is not teratogenic in three animal species (Bartoszyk et al 1986).

Toxicology data from two-year bioassay studies conducted in rats and mice have recently become available (personal communication). These studies show an increase in acinar cell carcinomas of the pancreas in male Wistar rats only. The tumours were not seen in female rats or mice of either sex. In the study, designed to evaluate carcinogenicity, male and female rats were given gabapentin at 250, 1000 and 2000 mg/kg daily for two years. Mean plasma concentrations at these doses were 24.2, 51.2 and 84.6 μg/ml, respectively. For reference, plasma concentrations from ongoing clinical studies commonly range from 2 μg/ml up to peak concentrations of 15 μg/ml.

The clinical relevance of these data is uncertain but probably does not warrant interruption of clinical trials in refractory patients.

PHARMACOLOGICAL PROPERTIES

Animal models of epilepsy

Gabapentin has been tested in a wide variety of animal models of epilepsy (Bartoszyk et al 1986). Table 13.1 summarizes the protective effect of gabapentin in various chemically and electrically induced acute seizure models in mice or rats in comparison with sodium valproate.

Gabapentin was tested in male DBA/2J mice genetically susceptible to sound-induced seizures (Bartoszyk et al 1983). Gabapentin, given orally 60 minutes prior to the test, protected against wild running and/or chronic convulsions with an ED_{50} of 16 mg/kg, and against tonic extensions with an ED_{50} of 3 mg/kg. Gabapentin was also effective in protecting gerbils selectively bred to show reflex epilepsy in response to environmental change with an ED_{50} of 10 mg/kg.

Gabapentin did not show efficacy in a third genetic model using a strain of Wistar rats that show the EEG and clinical symptoms of absence seizures. Gabapentin dose-dependently aggravated the spike and wave bursts at doses of 25 and 100 mg/kg in these studies.

Gabapentin (1–20 mg/kg) showed only weak anticonvulsant activity in baboons with photosensitive epilepsy. No neurological side effects were observed, but seizures were facilitated at very high doses (240 mg/kg).

When excitatory amino acids were used as convulsants, gabapentin

Table 13.1 Anticonvulsant activity of gabapentin; ED_{50} values in mg/kg orally (95% confidence interval)

Convulsant/test	Model	Gabapentin[a]	Valproate[b]
Semicarbazide	Inh. GABA synth.	5 (3–11)	76 (52–114)
Isoniazid	Inh. GABA synth.	20 (9–31)	325 (277–372)
3-Mercaptoproprionate	Inh. GABA synth.	31 (15–75)	71 (49–97)
Bicuculline	GABA recep. antag.	32 (13–53)	Not tested
Picrotoxin	Cl^- channel block	57 (36–89)	131 (99–163)
Strychnine	Glycine antagonist	34 (1–69)	252 (167–308)
MES	Tonic–clonic	9.4	236.6
PTZ maximal	Tonic–clonic	52 (30–75)	155 (130–181)
PTZ minimal	Absence	147 (62–1596)	83 (50–114)

[a] Gabapentin given 60–120 minutes prior to convulsant.
[b] Valproate given 30–60 minutes prior to convulsant.

(30–420 mg/kg intraperitoneally) given 90 minutes prior to the convulsants, markedly prolonged the latency of onset of convulsions and death in the N-methyl-D-aspartic acid (NMDA) model, but did not affect either time to onset or severity of convulsions in the kainic acid or quisqualate models (Bartoszyk 1983).

Gabapentin at doses of 45–100 mg/kg intraperitoneally showed anticonvulsant activity in a kindled rat model. It reduced behavioural seizures to a greater extent than afterdischarge following electrical hippocampal stimulation – a property it shares with phenytoin (Lothman, unpublished data).

Electrophysiology

The electrophysiological effects of gabapentin on spinal cord neurones cultured in vitro have been examined (Taylor et al 1988). Gabapentin did not change postsynaptic GABA or glutamate responses, did not depress spontaneous neuronal activity, and did not block high-frequency sustained repetitive action potentials at concentrations up to 30 μg/ml. This contrasts with phenytoin, carbamazepine and valproate, which interact with voltage-sensitive sodium channels and block sustained firing at low concentrations.

Gabapentin (3 mg/kg intraperitoneally) did decrease GABAergic inhibition in an experiment where paired pulse orthodromic stimulation of rat hippocampal pyramidal cells is used to evaluate GABAergic mechanisms. The first pulse activates inhibitory interneurones, which inhibit or attenuate the response to a second pulse given within an interstimulus range of 200 ms. The results obtained with gabapentin were comparable to those seen with baclofen and anticonvulsant doses of phenytoin.

Glycine has been shown to potentiate NMDA-mediated responses in vitro (Johnson & Ascher 1987). Antagonists at this strychnine-insensitive glycine site have been shown to possess anticonvulsant effects (Kemp et al 1988, Singh et al 1990).

In thalamic and hippocampal in vitro slice preparations gabapentin (100–200 μM) antagonized NMDA, but not kainate-induced depolarizations. Mechanistic studies in cultured striatal neurones have shown that gabapentin (10–200 μM) antagonism of NMDA-induced currents in the presence of glycine (1 μM) is reversible by increasing the glycine concentration or by the addition of D-serine (an agonist at the glycine modulatory site). These results are consistent with gabapentin antagonizing the action of glycine at the glycine modulatory site on the NMDA receptor complex (Sprosen et al, personal communication) despite the finding that gabapentin does not appear to inhibit strychnine-insensitive glycine binding (see below).

Biochemical pharmacology

In the search for a mode of action for gabapentin and to test its direct GABA-mimetic activity, a wide range of receptor-binding and other in vitro studies have been undertaken (Schmidt 1989). Gabapentin does not bind to GABA receptors (A or B), or to benzodiazepine, or muscarinic receptors, and it does not block sodium channels. Initial data suggested that gabapentin does not interfere with GABA metabolism. No increase in brain GABA levels in whole brain or in synaptosomal fractions was observed, nor any effect on GABA turnover or uptake (Schmidt 1989).

However, gabapentin (23 mg/kg intraperitoneally) does increase aminoxyacetic acid-induced accumulation of GABA throughout rat brain, suggesting an effect on GABA synthesis (Löscher et al 1991). The precise mechanism of this effect remains unclear. The time-course of this effect in the substantia nigra parallels gabapentin's antiepileptic effect. This region may be important for antiepileptic drug (AED) effects (Gale 1988).

Gabapentin's anticonvulsant activity when given before pentylenetetrazol is dose-dependently antagonized by D-serine, a glycine receptor antagonist (Oles et al 1990).

Studies using purified synaptic membranes prepared from rat cortex have revealed the presence of high-affinity binding sites ($K_D = 100$ nM) for [^{3}H]gabapentin. The binding site still remains to be fully characterized but preliminary experiments show it to be sensitive to a range of gabapentin analogues that also possess anticonvulsant activity, but no interaction with any putative neurotransmitters or neuromodulators has yet been demonstrated.

The binding site, which seems to be regionally distributed throughout the brain, appears to be independent of sodium and does not appear to be associated with either the GABA uptake site or the benzodiazepine receptor associated with the GABA$_A$ receptor. Experiments designed to determine the nature of the binding site are in progress (Hill, personal communication).

CLINICAL PHARMACOKINETICS

In healthy volunteers, gabapentin is rapidly absorbed after oral administration. Maximum plasma levels occur 2–3 hours post-administration and the elimination half-life ranges from 5 to 7 hours (Vollmer et al 1989). Gabapentin is not bound to plasma proteins and is not metabolized (Vollmer et al 1986). It is excreted unchanged in urine with renal clearance approximately equalling total clearance (120–130 ml/min). The renal clearance and elimination half-life are not altered by increasing dose, although oral bioavailability is reduced at higher doses. Gabapentin may be titrated to full therapeutic doses in two to three days with good tolerance. The pharmacokinetics of gabapentin are not altered following multiple dosing (Tuerck et al 1989) and the bioavailability of gabapentin is not affected by food. The pharmacokinetics of gabapentin were not altered in patients with epilepsy who were receiving phenytoin monotherapy (Anhut et al 1988).

Gabapentin levels in a single-specimen human brain are 80% of serum levels, confirming animal tissue distribution studies (Ojemann et al 1988).

As part of a placebo-controlled double-blind study, patients suffering from intractable complex partial seizures with or without secondary generalization were followed with lumbar punctures at baseline and after three months of gabapentin treatment (900 mg per day or 1200 mg per day) (Ben-Menachem et al 1990). Cerebrospinal fluid (CSF) was analysed for concentrations of gabapentin, free and total GABA. Preliminary results indicate that GABA concentrations were not affected by gabapentin treatment. At steady state, CSF/plasma ratios of gabapentin ranged from 0.056 to 0.34. No linear relationship was observed between plasma and CSF gabapentin levels in these patients.

CLINICAL EFFICACY

Human exposure

By 1st February 1990 over 2200 people had been exposed to gabapentin. Of these, 264 healthy volunteers received the drug in pharmacokinetic studies and 158 patients had taken gabapentin as monotherapy for indications other than epilepsy (spasticity and as migraine prophylaxis). Over 1800 patients with refractory epilepsy received gabapentin in open-label or double-blind, placebo-controlled studies. The number of patients who have been treated long-term is extensive, with over 460 patients receiving gabapentin for longer than one year, 119 for longer than two years, 39 for longer than three years and 32 for longer than four years.

Double-blind cross-over study

Early indications of the efficacy of gabapentin as an anticonvulsant came from a 25-patient dose-ranging, cross-over study (Crawford et al 1987). Following an eight-week baseline period and two-week titration phase, patients were randomized to 300 mg, 600 mg or 900 mg per day of gabapentin as add-on therapy for eight weeks at each dosage in a three-way cross-over design. Stable dosages of pre-existing antiepileptic drug (AED) therapy were maintained throughout the study. In addition to routine monthly monitoring of seizure frequency, side effects and serum AED levels, a psychometric test battery was also performed during baseline and each treatment phase.

The 15 male and 10 female patients had a mean age of 33 years (range 18–53) and a median duration of epilepsy of 18.5 years (range 6–40). Eighteen had partial seizures (with and without secondary generalization) and 7 patients had primary generalized seizures. Four patients were excluded from the efficacy analysis, 3 patients due to questionable compliance or the addition of AEDs during the study and one patient withdrew during the titration phase due to absence status.

The median frequency of all seizures was reduced from 3.3 to 2.1 per week (45%) on 900 mg per day of gabapentin compared to baseline ($p < 0.001$, Wilcoxon signed rank test). There was a dose-related antiepileptic effect, with the 900-mg dose significantly better than 600 mg ($p < 0.05$) and 300 mg ($p < 0.01$). Similar trends towards improvement with an increasing dose of gabapentin were seen for both partial seizures and tonic–clonic seizures, although gabapentin appeared to be more effective in the reduction of tonic–clonic seizures.

No trends were observed in any of the psychometric tests, indicating that no impairment of performance was noted with gabapentin therapy in the tests used.

Of the 25 patients who entered the study, 8 (32%) patients reported one or more adverse events on 300 mg per day; 15 (44%) on 600 mg per day and 11 (44%) on 900 mg per day. The most common adverse events were drowsiness and tiredness. None led to withdrawal from the study, except for the patient who reported absence status during the titration period. This patient frequently reported such episodes and they had occurred previously when he had been challenged with new AEDs.

OPEN-LABEL, DOSE-TITRATION STUDY

Seventy patients with refractory partial and generalized epilepsies were recruited to an open-label study where, following a 12-week baseline, gabapentin was added to the standard AEDs in doses beginning with 300 mg per day (Bauer et al 1989). The dose of gabapentin was individually titrated to a maximum of 1800 mg per day. Treatment continued for a period of at least two months at the optimal dose, with standard AED treatment remaining constant throughout the study.

Eighteen patients were excluded from the efficacy sample: 13 due to poor documentation or protocol violations and 5 due to early withdrawals related to adverse events.

The median reduction in seizure frequency during treatment with gabapentin compared to baseline was 27% for all seizures, 32% for partial seizures, 36% for tonic–clonic seizures and 49% for absence seizures. Where response is defined as a 50% or greater reduction in seizure frequency, 29% of patients with all seizure types combined ($n = 52$) were responders compared to 31% of patients reporting partial seizures ($n = 29$), 35% of patients with tonic–clonic seizures ($n = 20$) and 50% of patients with absence seizures ($n = 10$).

Thirty-six of the 70 patients who received gabapentin reported a total of 60 adverse events. The most common events were fatigue (20%) and dizziness (12.9%). Five patients withdrew from treatment due to adverse events.

DOUBLE-BLIND, PARALLEL GROUP STUDIES

A multicentre, placebo-controlled, double-blind, parallel-group study was undertaken in patients with drug-resistant partial epilepsy reporting at least one partial seizure per week despite optimal therapy with one or two standard AEDs (Andrews et al 1990). Following a three-month baseline, patients were randomized to either gabapentin or placebo. Patients received 600 mg per day of gabapentin or matching placebo during a two-week titration period and then entered a three-month evaluation period at the full 1200 mg per day dose or placebo. Seizure frequency, adverse events, biochemistry, haematology and plasma levels of gabapentin and standard AEDs were monitored throughout the study.

One hundred and twenty-seven patients were randomized: 61 to gabapentin and 66 to placebo. Both groups were well matched at baseline with respect to age, duration of epilepsy, sex and baseline seizure frequency per 28 days.

Of the 127 patients recruited, 113 (61 placebo and 53 gabapentin) were included in the efficacy sample. Fourteen were excluded due to having less than one seizure per week during baseline, less than 58 days diary available during baseline or treatment or because they stopped study medication for more than 14 days.

The evaluation of efficacy showed that 25% of gabapentin patients showed a reduction of at least 50% in partial seizures compared to 9.8% of placebo patients ($p = 0.043$, Fisher's exact test). Figure 13.2 shows the distribution of responders in 25 percentile groups for all partial seizures.

Efficacy was also determined by calculating response ratios (RR). $RR = (T - B)/(T + B)$, where B is the seizure frequency per 28 days during baseline and T is the seizure frequency per 28 days during treatment. The response ratio makes the response distribution more normal as it lies in the range -1 to $+1$. Percentage changes in seizure frequency range from -100% to $+$infinity. The mean adjusted response ratio for gabapentin (-0.192) was significantly better than with placebo (-0.060, $p = 0.0056$). The median percentage change from baseline in partial seizure frequency

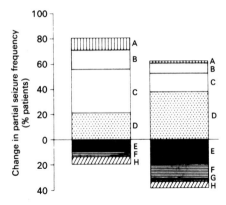

Fig. 13.2 Distribution of patients by percentage change in partial seizure frequency compared with baseline for gabapentin (left) and placebo (right). Positive deflection represents decreased seizure frequency A = over -75%; B = -50 to -75%; C = -25 to -50%; D = 0 to -24%; E = $+1$ to 25%; F = $+26$ to 50%; G = 51 to 74%; and H = over $+75\%$. (Reproduced with permission from Andrews et al 1990.)

was greater in the gabapentin group (-29.2%) than in the placebo group (-12.5%).

Of the 61 patients who received gabapentin and the 66 who received placebo, 38 (62%) reported adverse events on gabapentin compared to 27 (41%) on placebo. The most frequent reports on gabapentin were somnolence (15%), fatigue (13%), dizziness (7%) and weight increase (5%). In the placebo group, headache (9%), was the most commonly reported adverse event, followed by dizziness (5%) and somnolence (5%). Even the most common symptoms such as somnolence and fatigue were mostly rated as mild to moderate, did not appear to be disabling and, in the gabapentin group, mostly resolved during the double-blind phase. Eleven patients – 7 on gabapentin and 4 on placebo – withdrew from the study due to adverse events. There were no significant trends for any abnormalities in the haematological or biochemical parameter in either treatment group.

A similarly designed study of patients with complex partial epilepsy has recently been reported (Bauer, personal communication). A statistically significant reduction ($p = 0.031$, Fisher's exact test) of seizure frequency of more than 50% was seen in 23% of 96 patients treated with gabapentin 900 mg per day compared to 10% of 99 placebo patients. Fifty patients were randomized to gabapentin 1200 mg per day.

The mean response ratio and equivalent percentage change in seizure frequency for the double-blind period were: gabapentin 900 mg per day -0.154, 16.4% reduction; gabapentin 1200 mg per day (50 patients) -0.185, 15.9% reduction; and placebo -0.028, 4.9% increase. Again, the difference between the gabapentin 900 mg per day and placebo groups were statistically significant ($p = 0.0046$, ANOVA).

LONG-TERM GABAPENTIN TREATMENT

Following completion of a double-blind, cross-over study of 1200 mg per day gabapentin as add-on therapy (Andrews et al 1990), patients who had received gabapentin in the blinded phase and who had benefited could elect to continue therapy, whilst those who received placebo could commence open-label add-on gabapentin (1200 mg per day).

Thirty-one patients who had received double-blind gabapentin elected to continue open-label gabapentin, of whom 27 continued for a further three to six months and 21 continued for a further nine months. Compared to baseline, median percentage seizure reduction was -33% for the three to six-month period, -38% for six to nine months, and -41% for nine to 12 months. Six patients discontinued gabapentin during open-label because of loss of efficacy and 3 because of adverse events possibly (diplopia and increased seizure frequency) and probably not (breast carcinoma) related to gabapentin.

Fifty-seven patients who received placebo during double-blind elected to receive open-label gabapentin. Forty-five completed three months' therapy. Thirty-three completed six months' therapy, 25 completed nine months' therapy, 19 completed 12 months' therapy. After three months median seizure reduction was 41%; 43% after six months, 20% after nine months and 40% after 12 months. Twelve patients stopped treatment because of lack of efficacy, 9 because of adverse events possibly related to treatment.

DRUG INTERACTIONS

Gabapentin was shown not to induce hepatic enzymes in a controlled study comparing the effect of gabapentin and phenytoin on antipyrine kinetics in healthy volunteers (Allen et al 1987). Phenytoin, a known hepatic enzyme inducer, significantly increased antipyrine clearance, and significantly decreased antipyrine area under the curve (AUC).

Considering gabapentin is not metabolized, does not induce hepatic enzymes and is not protein bound, pharmacokinetic interactions with other drugs are unlikely. To date, no interactions have been observed between gabapentin and the standard AEDs (carbamazepine, sodium valproate, phenytoin and phenobarbitone) in clinical studies (Crawford et al 1987, Bauer et al 1989, Andrews et al 1990).

A formal interaction study of gabapentin with phenytoin in patients with epilepsy demonstrated that co-administered gabapentin does not influence plasma levels of phenytoin and vice versa (Anhut et al 1988).

CONCLUSIONS

These studies indicate an antiepileptic effect for gabapentin in partial and generalized tonic–clonic seizures which may be comparable with that for conventional antiepileptic drugs and which appears to be maintained over 12 months. Adverse events with this drug are relatively few and relatively mild. The drug may therefore be a valuable introduction, being potentially better tolerated than some existing antiepileptic drugs. However, the recent findings of potential carcinogenicity in the male Wistar rats will require further elucidation before the use of the drug can become widespread.

REFERENCES

Allen E, Jarad B, Wroe S, Richens A 1987 Does the anticonvulsant gabapentin lack enzyme inducing properties? Abstracts 17th Epilepsy International Congress, Jerusalem.
Andrews J, Chadwick D, Bates D et al 1990 Gabapentin in partial epilepsy. Lancet 335: 1114–1117
Anhut H, Leppik I, Schmidt B, Thomann P 1988 Drug interaction study of the new anticonvulsant gabapentin with phenytoin in epileptic patients. Naunyn-Schmiedebergs Arch Pharmacol 337/Suppl R127
Bartoszyk G D 1983 Gabapentin and convulsions provoked by excitatory amino acids. Naunyn-Schmiedebergs Arch Pharmacol 324/Suppl R24
Bartoszyk G D, Fritschi E, Herrmann M, Satzinger G 1983 Indications for an involvement of the gaba-system in the mechanism of action of gabapentin. Naunyn-Schmiedebergs Arch Pharmacol 322/Suppl R94
Bartoszyk G D, Meyerson N, Reimann W et al 1986 In: Meldrum B S, Porter R J (eds) Current problems in epilepsy 4. New anticonvulsant drugs. Libbey, London, pp 147–163
Bauer G, Bechinger D, Castell M et al 1989 Gabapentin in the treatment of drug-resistant epileptic patients. Adv Epileptol 17: 219
Ben-Menachem E, Hender T, Persson L I 1990 Seizure frequency and CSF gabapentin, GABA, and monoamine metabolite concentrations after 3 months' treatment with 900 mg or 1200 mg gabapentin daily in patients with intractable complex partial seizures. Neurology 40 (Suppl 1): 158
Crawford P, Ghadiali E, Lane R et al 1987 Gabapentin as an antiepileptic drug in man. Neurol Neurosurg Psychiatry 50: 682–686
Gale K 1988 Progression and generalisation of seizure discharge: anatomical and neurochemical substrates. Epilepsia 29 (Suppl 2): S15–S34
Hengy H, Kolle E 1985 Determination of gabapentin in plasma and urine by high-performance liquid chromatography and pre-column labelling for ultraviolet detection. J Chromatogr 341: 473–478
Johnson J W, Ascher P 1987 Glycine potentiates the NMDA response in cultured mouse brain neurons. Nature 325: 529–531
Kemp J A, Foster A C, Leeson P D et al 1988 7-Chlorokynurenic acid is a selective antagonist at the glycine modulatory site of the N-methyl-D-aspartate receptor complex. Proc Natl Acac Sci USA 85: 6547–6550
Loscher W, Honack D, Taylor C P 1991 Gabapentin increases GABA turnover in several regions of rat brain, including substantia nigra. Brain Res (in press)
Oles R J, Singh L, Hughes J, Woodruff G N 1990 The anticonvulsant action of gabapentin involves the glycine/NMDA receptor. Abst Soc Neurosci St Louis 16: 763
Ojemann L M, Friel P N, Ojemann G A 1988 Gabapentin concentrations in human brain. Epilepsia 29: 694
Schmidt B 1989 Potential antiepileptic drugs: gabapentin. In: Levy R (ed) Antiepileptic drugs, 3rd edn. Raven Press, New York, pp 925–935
Singh L, Oles R J, Tricklebank M D 1990 Modulation of seizure susceptibility in the mouse by the strychnine-insensitive glycine recognition site at the NMDA receptor/ion channel complex. Br J Pharmacol 99: 285–288
Taylor C P, Rock D M, Weinkauf R J, Ganong A H 1988 In vitro and in vivo electrophysiological effects of the anticonvulsant gabapentin. Soc Neurosci Abst 14/2: 866
Tuerck D, Vollmer K, Bockbrader H, Sedman A 1989 Dose-linearity of the new

anticonvulsant gabapentin after multiple oral doses. Eur J Clin Pharmacol 36/Suppl A310
Vollmer K, von Hodenberg A, Kolle E 1986 Pharmacokinetics and metabolism of gabapentin in rat, dog and man. Drug Res 36: 830–839
Vollmer K, Anhut H, Thomann P et al 1989 Pharmacokinetic model and absolute bioavailability of the new anticonvulsant gabapentin. Adv Epileptol 17: 209

14

Behavioural therapy of epilepsy

P. Fenwick

INTRODUCTION

New models of seizure genesis are moving away from the static image of a damaged area of brain spontaneously and randomly generating seizure discharges, to a more dynamic view. This new view recognizes that the damaged area of brain from which seizures arise is central to seizure genesis, but that activity in surrounding brain areas may be of equal importance. It is now being suggested that the cortical spike discharge which was initially thought to be excitatory might be inhibitory. Recent work both from UCLA and Erlangen, using magnetoencephalographic techniques, has shown that the focal cortical spike itself is a compound wave, and correlates with large populations of cells which are excited in deep brain structures. Animal work also suggests that there may be seizure suppressor zones and activity from these areas can significantly modify and influence firing rates in epileptic foci, and thus the probability of seizure occurrence.

This new dynamic view has led to the recognition that surrounding brain activity can significantly alter the likelihood of seizure occurrence, and that there are close links between brain activity, the psychic life of the individual, and the genesis of seizure activity.

These observations raise the possibility that behavioural methods which seek to modify the activity in populations of cells surrounding the focus could contribute to the control of seizure activity.

FOCAL SEIZURE GENESIS

Lockard's (1980a) animal model of focal epilepsy defines two populations of epileptogenic cells: group 1 neurones, which are partially damaged neurones at the centre of the focus which always fire in an epileptic, bursting mode, and group 2 neurones, partially damaged neurones surrounding the focus, which can fire in both the bursting, epileptic mode, and in a normal mode. The activity of the group 1 cells is not modified to any significant extent by surrounding brain activity; that of the group 2 cells can be so modified.

When a seizure occurs, the continually discharging group 1 cells recruit group 2 cells into the seizure discharge, to form a focal seizure. If group

2 cells recruit surrounding normal brain cells, the focal seizure spreads to become secondarily generalized. There are two points in the evolution of a seizure when ongoing brain activity can affect the likelihood of the seizure developing. The first is between group 1 and group 2 neurones, and the second between group 2 and normal brain neurones.

Lockard (1980b) has also shown, in her monkey model, that psychosocial processes can modify both spike frequency and seizure frequency.

GENERALIZED SPIKE–WAVE SEIZURES

Musgrave & Gloor (1980) and Avoli & Gloor (1982) have suggested that the reticular formation may directly affect generalized spike–wave seizures. Reticular activity, like cortical activity, varies as a function of behaviour, and thus behaviour could also be expected to affect the occurrence of generalized seizures.

EVOKED SEIZURES

The precipitation of seizures by specific external stimuli has been called 'reflex epilepsy' (Gowers 1891). 'Evoked seizures' was the term preferred by Symonds (1959) and will be used here.

Evoked seizures are said to occur in about 5% of people with epilepsy (Symonds 1959). Fenwick (1981b) has suggested in those epileptics attending the Maudsley Hospital that the rate may be nearer 25%. Reading, eating, stimulation of the skin, movement, sounds and smells can all trigger seizures (Merliss 1974, Fenwick 1981b), probably because peripheral stimulation raises the level of activity within a damaged area of the cortex, by rhythmic driving of the cells, and so allows seizure discharges to spread within this area. An alteration in the level of excitation in the area of damaged cortex may also *prevent* seizure activity from arising and spreading.

PSYCHOGENIC EPILEPTIC SEIZURES

Fenwick (1981a) proposed a classification of seizures generated by an action of mind. These he called 'psychogenic epileptic seizures', indicating that they arose as a consequence of mental activity. Primary psychogenic epileptic seizures are produced by a deliberate mental attempt to induce a seizure. Secondary psychogenic seizures (also called the 'thinking epilepsies') occur when the subject is thinking, calculating or 'feeling', but not trying to induce a seizure (Ingvar & Nyman 1962, Fenwick 1981b, Fenwick & Brown 1989, Merliss 1974, Ch'en et al 1965, Forster et al 1975, Forster 1977a, Cirignotta et al 1980).

In a recent survey of 76 patients attending the Maudsley Epilepsy Clinic, 22.4% admitted that they had on occasion deliberately induced a seizure; 15.6% admitted encouraging seizures when upset; 28.6% could describe how they did this. Thus between a quarter and a third of patients attending a psychiatric epilepsy clinic can generate their own epileptic seizures at will. Dahl et al (1985) report that 16% of their children 'can elicit seizure on demand'. In a further survey of 36 patients attending a general hospital epilepsy clinic, Finkler and Fenwick found only 3% admitted having induced or encouraged a seizure. Thus seizure induction is commoner in patients attending psychiatric clinics.

Patients are known to report having more seizures in certain situations. In the Maudsley survey, over 50% of the patients had seizures when they were tense, depressed or tired, compared with only a third in the general hospital group. Over 30% of the Maudsley group had seizures when they were angry, excited or bored, and only 4% when they were happy. In the general hospital group, a quarter had seizures when excited, angry or bored, and 3% when happy. Tempkin & Davis (1984) studied the effect of major life events, and of more minor stresses and strains on the likelihood of patients having seizures, and confirmed that high stress levels were associated with more frequent seizures – and that happiness is a powerful anticonvulsant. Dahl et al (1985) also reported that 66% of their children 'can identify low-risk situation for seizure occurrence'.

SEIZURE INHIBITION

Seizure inhibition, like seizure generation, has both primary and secondary components. Primary seizure inhibition is the direct inhibition of seizures by an act of will; secondary seizure inhibition is the inhibition of seizures by an action and mind or behaviour which interferes with seizure generation, but is not deliberately intended to do so (Brown & Fenwick 1989).

Primary inhibition

The use of external stimulation to inhibit seizure occurrence is reported by Efron (1956), Forster et al (1969), Forster (1977b) and de Weerdt & van Rign (1975). Most patients will admit to using a mental mechanism to try to inhibit their seizures. In the Maudsley Hospital study, in answer to the question 'Do you sometimes make yourself have fewer seizures?', 33.8% said yes. To the question 'Can you sometimes stop your seizures from happening?' 36.4% said yes, and to the question 'Can you stop your seizures from spreading?' 27.3% said yes. In the general hospital study, only 6% said they could sometimes stop their seizures.

A 42-year-old woman with a right temporal focus on EEG had had feelings of déjà vu since the age of 6, which had at times been associated with feelings of guilt. Her therapy, in part, consisted of helping her deal with her guilt, which she described as the *most powerful* anticonvulsant that she had ever been given.

In this patient the group 1 neurones were probably situated in the hippocampus and amygdala, and these areas were activated when she felt guilty.

Indirect primary inhibition

Indirect primary inhibition of seizures occurs when the patient carries out a set of physical or mental actions intended to stop the seizure occurring or generalizing.

Reticular formation activity changes the excitability of the brain in a global fashion. Many non-specific inhibitory strategies use this mechanism (Mostofsky & Balaschack 1977). The alerting of the patient alters the level of cortical arousal in a non-specific way. Patients whose seizures have focal onsets will commonly either say 'no' to themselves, or try to attend to something different at the onset of the aura.

Deliberate alerting in boring situations has been known to produce a reduction in petit mal seizures (Jung 1962, Ounsted et al 1966).

Pritchard et al (1985) found that about 10% (7 of 71) of their patients with complex partial seizures could reduce their seizure frequency using varied, highly idiosyncratic strategies. These patients had attained higher educational status, better social and vocational adjustment, and better psychological adjustment than those who could not. They were also more likely to have right hemisphere EEG abnormalities. None of 18 patients with simple partial seizures were able to reduce seizure frequency. Dahl et al (1985) reported that in a group of 18 children about 40% were 'at some time able to counteract seizure'.

Secondary inhibition

Secondary inhibition occurs when a patient unintentionally reduces seizure frequency, for example by maintenance of interest or alertness. There is now some evidence that if psychological variables are targeted in treatment programmes seizure frequency decreases (Davis et al 1984).

Although these strategies do not work for everybody, it does seem that certain types of activity tend to enhance the possibility of seizure occurrence, while others tend to prevent it. The final common pathway for all such activity in those patients who have focal seizures is the alteration in activity of group 2 neurones.

PSYCHOLOGICAL METHODS FOR TREATMENT OF EPILEPSY

Mostofsky & Balaschak (1977) and Mostofsky (1981) have written major reviews of early studies in this area, so this section will concentrate on more recent work. The classification system used by Mostofsky and Balaschak defines three areas: reward management, self-control and psychophysiological treatments. Many of the cases reported in the literature are single-case studies, without proper controls, and there is likely to be more than one therapeutic factor in a conditioning programme. Methodological points were first raised by Mostofsky & Balaschak (1977), and later by Krafft & Poling (1982).

Reward management

Overt reward

Reward programmes aim to reinforce seizure-free periods positively by an increase in privileges, or tokens allowing the purchase of privileges (Flannery & Cautela 1973, Balaschak 1976, Zlutnick et al 1975, Iwata & Lorentzson 1976, Cataldo et al 1979).

Cinciripini et al (1980) used both restraint and reward to reduce seizure frequencies significantly in a 7-year-old child with petit mal seizures, both spontaneous and self-precipitated (by putting his hand in front of a light). Differential reinforcement consisted of praise for using his hands appropriately, or keeping them flat on the table. Rapid improvement was well maintained at an eight-month follow-up.

Covert reward

The patient imagines situations in which seizures may occur, and then fantasizes the non-occurrence of seizures and the positive gains that would follow. These fantasy sessions are usually part of a relaxation programme, so the mechanism involved may be covert desensitization rather than covert reward. However, no study has yet tried to disentangle these two aspects (Cautela 1971, Daniels 1975).

Denial of reward

Overinvolvement and overprotection by the patient's caregiver may inadvertently reinforce behaviours leading to seizures, and become a powerful method of controlling the patient's relationships. Dahl et al (1985) found that 50% of children in her study 'reported mainly positive consequences associated with seizures'. Denial of reward is a direct attempt to break this cycle. Gardner (1967) reports the abolition of seizures in a 10-year-old girl when the parents were instructed to ignore their daughter's attacks (?pseudo-seizures or true seizures) (see also Daniels 1975).

Punishment programme

Penalty programme. This involves intervention after a seizure by either withdrawal of privileges or 'time-out' (Adams et al 1973, Iwata & Lorentszon 1976).

Punishment programmes. A seizure is followed immediately with an unpleasant stimulus such as a foul odour, electric shocks, shouting, or hitting the patient (Adams et al 1973, Wright 1973, Zlutnick 1972, Zlutnick et al 1975, Bandler 1957).

Relief avoidance. This is similar to overt punishment, except that the punishment is discrete and continuous until there is an improvement in either seizure behaviour or EEG activity (Ounsted et al 1966, Stevens 1962, Dorcas & Schaffer 1945).

Self-control strategies

These allow the patient, by cognitive processes, to gain control of his seizure activity.

Self-control

Most patients use cognitive strategies to inhibit seizures, both by avoiding circumstances likely to cause seizures, and attempting to terminate seizures (Fenwick & Brown 1988, Brown & Fenwick 1988, Fenwick 1988) (also see above).

Relaxation and desensitization

The patient is taught progressive deep muscular relaxation (Wolpe 1969). He can then reproduce the feelings of relaxation when a seizure seems imminent. Wells et al (1978), treating patients with psychomotor seizures, reported that training generalized well from a hospital to a home situation, with a reduction of seizures.

Rousseau et al (1985), taking into account previous methodological criticisms, studied 15 patients suffering mainly from partial complex seizures, with and without secondary generalization. Each group had baseline assessment followed by two periods of treatment. Group 1 had two periods of progressive relaxation therapy; group 2 had a period of sham treatment, consisting of two 20-minute periods of relaxing 'as best they could', and later a period of progressive relaxation therapy. An overall significant decrease in seizure frequency for the treatment conditions was found. However, there was also a significant decrease in 2 of the 4 patients given sham treatment. This could suggest that non-specific factors played a part, or that the sham condition was a weaker form of therapy.

An extension of this method is relaxation and covert densensitization. The patient carries out a protocol of relaxation and, while relaxed, imagines the occurrence of a seizure and the consequent anxiety. Densitization to seizure occurrence may result in a reduction in seizure frequency (Brown & Fenwick 1989, Ince 1976, Cabral & Scott 1976, Muthen 1978, Mostofsky 1975, Standage 1972, Parrino 1971). Melin & Dahl (1981) looked at the effect of contingent relaxation on 4 single subjects with different seizure types. All patients showed a significant fall in seizures. In two cases they tried a short period of reversal, telling subjects not to relax on seizure occurrence. This may have increased seizures. Seizure reduction was maintained at six months follow-up. Psychomotor seizures and auras responded more than grand mal seizures.

Dahl et al, in a study of 18 children, found that they were all able to predict the likelihood of a seizure. Three could elicit them on demand, and 12 could identify low-risk situations. They were split up into three groups of six: an active treatment group, who were taught to recognize seizure onset and given a method of relaxation to counteract this; an attentional control group, who were given the same amount of attention by the psychologist; and a control group who received no specific treatment. The study showed that the children could discover pre-seizure cues, and that using a relaxation technique as a counter-measure significantly reduced seizure frequency. Non-specific attention did not have this effect.

In 1987 Dahl et al, in a more sophisticated controlled study, looked at three groups of 6 adults with refractory epileptic seizures, including a non-treatment waiting-list control group. Patients in the first group were taught to carry out muscle relaxation every day, particularly in situations of high risk for seizures. The second, attentional control group received supportive therapy for an equal number of sessions. Patients in the relaxation group were able to determine the early onset of their seizures and abort them with the relaxation procedure used as a counter-measure; they showed a significant seizure reduction. However, not all seizures could be stopped this way, and the authors could find no clear predictors as to which seizures could be stopped. Patients reported increased confidence and greater control over their epilepsy. The attention group, surprisingly, showed an increase in seizures, probably due to focusing on seizure behaviour.

Dahl et al (1988) showed that it is not enough to identify pre-seizure behaviour; there must be an active intervention to stop seizures spreading and reduce seizure frequency. Three children with severe refractory epileptic seizures were taught to identify the onset of paroxysmal EEG activity and/or sensations preceding seizures. This had no effect on seizure frequency. However, when they were taught an intervention technique consisting of an adapted counter-measure, e.g. the moving of an arm in the direction opposite to that caused by seizure onset, both seizure frequency and paroxysmal EEG activity were significantly reduced.

Brown (personal communication) has taught children in his epilepsy centre to identify seizure onset and then to carry out the 'opposite' (whatever they identify as opposite) behaviour. He reports that two 20-minute sessions with the neuropsychologist are all that is required to produce a significant reduction in seizure frequency.

Flooding, by exposing the patient to the situation in which a seizure is likely to be evoked, has been used by Pinto (1972) in one patient, with some success.

Psychotherapy

Individual or group psychotherapy aims to help the patient understand himself and the relationship of his seizures to life events. Better life adjustment leads to greater relaxation and a sense of fulfilment, both powerful anticonvulsants, and occasionally to the reduction of covert seizure induction, and to enhanced strategies of self-control (Gottschalk 1953, Williams et al 1978). However, Correa (1987) attempted unsuccessfully to change the locus of control and seizure frequency in 13 children with epilepsy.

Tan & Bruni (1986) compared cognitive/behaviour therapy and supportive counselling with a waiting-list and no-treatment control, in alleviating psychosocial problems and reducing seizure frequency of 27 patients. The first group received a total of eight 2-hour sessions of group cognitive/behaviour therapy each week. The supportive counselling group had a similar number of sessions, aimed at clarification of feelings; no specific control behaviours were taught. There were no significant differences for seizure frequency, or patients' complaints. However, a global rating of psychological adjustment was improved for the two therapy groups. The authors comment that overall group cognitive/behaviour therapy does not reduce psychosocial difficulties or seizures.

Rosenbaum & Palmon (1984) suggested that the emotional sequelae of epilepsy are a joint function of the severity of the epilepsy and the individual's self-control skills. The patients were divided into two groups: high resourceful and low resourceful. They found that in the low/medium categories of seizure frequency high-resourceful subjects were significantly less depressed and anxious and coped better with their disability. However, in the high-frequency range of seizures, high and low-resourceful epileptics showed equally low levels of emotional adjustment. These data suggest that patients with less severe epilepsy are influenced by their ability to cope with personal and social circumstances.

Feldman & Paul (1976) reported significant seizure reduction in 5 patients whose treatment included watching videotapes of their seizures. Although the authors claim that the improvement was due to 'the conscious awareness of the association between the specific emotional stimulus and the seizure', several other psychological mechanisms could have been involved (Mostofsky & Balaschak 1977).

Psychophysiological

Epileptic seizures can be conditioned (habituation and extinction) in a classical Pavlovian paradigm (Forster 1972). Abnormal cortical discharges evoked by a specific stimulus are habituated by continual exposure to the stimulus. This has been tried in the visual, auditory and sensory modalities, with some success (Booker et al 1965, Forster & Campos 1964, Forster et al 1964, 1965, Forster 1977). However, the conditioning of seizures is a fragile process and can be obliterated by one grand mal seizure.

Biofeedback

There is insufficient space to review biofeedback in detail. The following is an outline for the reader.

Anticonvulsant rhythms

Sterman (1973) was the first to investigate successfully the anticonvulsant properties of the 12–16-Hz sensorimotor rhythm in man, by using biofeedback training. Other authors have reported varying degrees of success (Siefert & Lubar 1975, Lubar & Bhaler 1976, Lubar 1977, Finlay et al 1975, Tansey 1985).

Some studies reported no success, and attributed any reduction in seizure frequency to non-specific factors (Finlay 1977, Kuhlman & Allison 1977, Sterman 1977, Quy et al 1979), although Kuhlman (1978), using yoked and random feedback controls, was able to show that biofeedback training for a 9–14-Hz SMR was effective in 60% of the subjects tested. However, the experiment still left unanswered the specificity of the SMR (Review, Fenwick 1981b).

Sterman & Shouse (1980) investigated the difference between fast activity and SMR feedback and concluded that SMR feedback training may be non-specific and that other EEG frequencies are effective.

Lantz & Sterman (1988) found that following feedback training cognitive and motor functioning improved only in those subjects who showed the greatest seizure reduction, and this was confined to those who had undergone active feedback, and was not seen in subjects whose seizures had fallen during the control conditions. Improvement in MMPI scores was not specific to feedback.

Current opinion now supports the view that the SMR change may contain components specific to the reduction of epileptic seizures.

Non-specific EEG biofeedback

Non-specific biofeedback is the deliberate enhancement or reduction of background cerebral rhythms, and has been used successfully. Cabral & Scott (1976) used conventional occipital rhythm biofeedback; Whyler et al (1976) used biofeedback to increase fast low-voltage activity and suppress slow wave activity surrounding the epileptic focus. Kaplan (1975) and Kuhlman & Allison (1977) used augmentation of Mu activity. Lubar et al (1981) found a reduction in seizure frequency associated with increased fast activity. Suppression of slow activity produced a levelling off of seizure reduction – further evidence of the non-specific nature of EEG operant feedback.

Feedback of other physiological parameters

Fried et al (1984) argued that patients who showed a high end-tidal carbon dioxide level were likely to have more seizures. They used training in breathing to reduce end-tidal carbon dioxide. Respiratory pattern, end-tidal carbon dioxide levels and respiratory rate were normalized in the patient group. Their EEG power spectrum 'normalized', and their seizure frequency was significantly reduced, though whether these changes were due to a placebo effect or to the active treatment is not yet known. However, this suggests that biofeedback methods could lead to seizure reduction by modification of physiological variables other than the EEG.

SUMMARY

Epileptic seizures do not occur in a behavioural vacuum. There is abundant evidence of the close interrelation between seizure activity and behaviour, and it is not surprising that seizure control is significantly influenced by altering the attitude and behaviour of the epileptic patient. In the focal epilepsies, information about the nature and characteristics of the aura and the spread of the seizure allows accurate location of the seizure focus, and determines the relationship between the individual and his epilepsy, and how he may both trigger and inhibit seizures.

A complete treatment of epilepsy involves not just the giving of drugs. It includes teaching the patient that his seizures are not part of a random process, but are intimately related to how he feels, what he is doing, what he is thinking, and showing him how these can all be used in the control of his epilepsy.

REFERENCES

Adams K M, Klinge V, Keiser T W 1973 The extinction of a self-injurious behaviour in an epileptic child. Behav Res Ther 11: 351–356
Avoli M, Gloor P 1982 Role of the thalamus in generalised penicillin epilepsy: observations on decorticate cats. Exp Neurol 77: 386–402
Balaschak B A 1976 Teacher-implemented behaviour modification in a case of organically based epilepsy. J Consult Clin Psychol 44: 218–223
Bandler B, Kaufman I, Dykens J et al 1957 Seizures and the menstrual cycle. Am J Psychol 113: 704–798
Booker H E, Forster F M, Klove H 1965 Extinction factors in startle (acoustico-motor) seizures. Neurology 15: 1095–1103
Brown S, Fenwick P 1989 Evoked and psychogenic epileptic seizures II. Inhibition. Acta Neurol Scand 80: 541–547
Cabral R J, Scott D F 1976 Effects of two desensitization techniques, biofeedback and relaxation, on intractable epilepsy: follow-up study. J Neurol Neurosurg Psychiatry 39: 504–507
Cataldo M F, Russo C C, Freeman J M 1979 A behaviour analysis approach to high rate myoclonic seizures. J Autism Dev Disord 9: 413–427
Cautela J R 1971 Covert extinction. Behav Ther 2: 192–200
Ch'en H, Ch'in C, Ch'u C 1965 Chess epilepsy and card epilepsy. Chin Med J 84: 470–474
Cinciripini P M, Epstein L H, Kotanchik N L 1980 Behavioural intervention for

self-stimulatory, attending and seizure behaviour in a cerebral palsied child. J Behav
Ther Exp Psychiatry 11: 313–316

Cirignotta F, Cicogna P, Lugaresi E 1980 Epileptic seizures during card games and
draughts. Epilepsia 21: 137–140

Correa S 1987 Locus of control in children with epilepsy. Psychol Rep 60: 9–10

Dahl J, Brorson L 1983 The behaviour analysis of epilepsy: in theory and practice.
Scand J Behav Ther 12: 195–209

Dahl J, Melin L, Brorson L, Schollin J 1985 Effects of a broad-spectrum behaviour
modification treatment programme on children with refractory epileptic seizures. Epilepsia
26: 303–309

Dahl J, Melin L, Lund L 1987 Effects of a contingent relaxation treatment programme
on adults with refractory epileptic seizures. Epilepsia 28: 125–137

Dahl J, Melin L, Leissner P 1988 Effects of a behavioural intervention on epileptic
seizure behaviour and paroxysmal activity: a systematic replication of three cases of children
with intractable epilepsy. Epilepsia 29: 172–183

Daniels L K 1975 The treatment of grand mal epilepsy by covert and operant conditioning
techniques: a case study. Psychosomatics 16: 65–67

Davis G R, Armstrong H E, Donovan D M, Tempkin N R 1984 Cognitive-behavioural
treatment of depressed affect among epileptics: preliminary findings. J Clin Psychol
40: 930–935

de Weerdt C J, van Rijn A J 1975 Conditioning therapy in reading epilepsy.
Electroencephalogr Clin Neurophysiol 39: 417–420

Dorcas R M, Schaffer G W 1945 Textbook of abnormal psychology, 3rd edn. Williams
and Wilkins, Baltimore

Efron R 1956 The effect of olfactory stimuli in arresting uncinate fits. Brain 79: 267–281

Feldman R G, Paul N L 1976 Identity of emotional triggers in epilepsy. J Nerv Ment
Dis 162: 345

Fenwick P 1981b Precipitation and inhibition of seizures. In: Reynolds E, Trimble
M (eds) Epilepsy and psychiatry. Churchill Livingstone, Edinburgh

Fenwick P 1988 The significance of a seizure. In: Trimble M R, Reynolds E H (eds)
Bridge between neurology and psychiatry. Churchill Livingstone, Edinburgh

Fenwick P, Brown S 1989 Evoked and psychogenic epileptic seizures 1. Precipitation.
Acta Neurol Scand 80: 535–540

Finlay W W 1977 Operant conditioning of the EEG in two patients with epilepsy:
methodological and clinical considerations. Pavlov J Biol Sci 12: 93–111

Finlay W W, Smith H A, Etherton M D 1975 Reduction of seizures and normalisation
of the EEG in a severe epileptic following sensorimotor biofeedback training:
preliminary study. Biol Psychol 2: 189–203

Flannery R B Jr, Cautela J R 1973 Seizures: controlling the uncontrollable. J Rehabil
39: 34–36

Forster F M 1972 Classification and conditioning treatment of the reflex epilepsies.
Int J Neurol 9: 73–86

Forster F M 1977a Epilepsy evoked by higher cognitive functions: decision-making
epilepsy. In: Reflex epilepsy, behaviour therapy and conditioned reflexes. Thomas,
Springfield, pp 124–134

Forster F M 1977b Behavioral therapy of reflex epilepsy: maintenance or reinforcement
of therapy. In: Reflex epilepsy, behaviour therapy and conditioned reflexes. Thomas,
Springfield, pp 242–255, 318

Forster F M, Campos G B 1964 Conditioning factors in stroboscopic-induced seizures.
Epilepsia 5: 156–165

Forster F M, Ptacek L J, Peterson W G et al 1964 Stroboscopic-induced seizure
discharges: modification by extinction techniques. Arch Neurol 11: 603–608

Forster F M, Ptacek L J, Peterson W G 1965 Auditory clicks in extinction of
stroboscope-induced seizures. Epilepsia 6: 217–225

Forster F M, Paulsen W, Baughman F 1969 Clinical therapeutic conditioning in
reading epilepsy. Neurology 19: 71–77

Forster F M, Richards J F, Panitch H S 1975 Reflex epilepsy evoked by decision
making. Arch Neurol 32: 54–56

Fried R, Rubin S R, Carlton R M, Fox M C 1984 Behavioural control of intractable
idiopathic seizures: 1. Self regulation of end-tidal CO_2. Psychosomatic Med 46: 315–331

Gardner J E 1967 Behaviour therapy treatment approach to a psychogenic seizure case. Consult Psychol 31: 209–212

Gottschalk L A 1953 Effects of intensive psychotherapy on epileptic children. Arch Neurol Psychiatry 70: 361–384

Gowers W 1901 Epilepsy and other chronic convulsive disorders: their causes, symptoms and treatment. Churchill, London, p 29

Ince L P 1976 The use of relaxation training and a conditioned stimulus in the elimination of epileptic seizures in a child: a case study. J Behav Ther Exp Psychiatry 7: 39–42

Ingvar D H, Nyman G E 1962 A new psychological trigger mechanism in a case of epilepsy. Neurology 12: 282

Iwata B A, Lorentzson A M 1976 Operant control of seizure-like behaviour in an institutionalised retarded adult. Behav Ther 7: 247–251

Jung R 1962 Blocking of petit mal attacks by sensory arousal and inhibition of attacks by an active change in attention during the epileptic aura. Epilepsia 3: 435

Kaplan B J 1975 Biofeedback in epilepsy: equivocal relationship of reinforced EEG frequency to seizure reduction. Epilepsia 16: 477–485

Krafft K M, Poling A D 1982 Behavioural treatments of epilepsy: methodological characteristics and problems of published studies. Appl Res Ment Retard 3: 151–162

Kuhlman W N 1978 EEG feedback training of epileptic patients: clinical and electroencephalographic analysis. Electroencephalogr Clin Neurophysiol 45: 699–710

Kuhlman W M, Allison T 1977 EEG feedback training in the treatment of epilepsy: some questions and answers. Pavlov J Biol Sci 12: 112–122

Lantz D, Sterman M B 1988 Neuropsychological assessment of subjects with uncontrolled epilepsy: effects of EEG feedback training. Epilepsia 29: 163–171

Lockard J S 1980 A primate model of clinical epilepsy: mechanisms of action through quantification of therapeutic effects. In: Lockard J S, Ward A A (eds) Epilepsy: a window to brain mechanisms. Raven Press, New York

Lubar J F 1977 Electroencephalographic methodology and the management of epilepsy. Pavlov J Biol Sci 12: 147–185

Lubar J F, Bhaler J F 1976 Behavioural management of epileptic seizures following EEG biofeedback training of the sensori-motor rhythm. Biofeedback Self Regul 1: 77–104

Lubar J F, Shabsin H S, Natelson S E et al 1981 EEG operant conditioning in intractable epileptics. Arch Neurol 38: 700–704

Melin L, Dahl J 1981 Effects of contingent relaxation on epileptic seizures. J Psychiatr Treatment Eval 3: 201–207

Merlis J K 1974 Reflex epilepsy. In: Handbook of Clinical Neurology, Vol 15: The epilepsies. pp 440–456

Mostofsky D I 1975 Teaching the nervous system. New York Univ Educational Quarterly, Spring: 8–13

Mostofsky D I 1981 Recurrent paroxysmal disorders of the central nervous system. In: Turner S (ed) Handbook of Clinical Behaviour Therapy. Ch 16

Mostofsky D I, Balaschak B A 1977 Psychobiological control of seizures. Psychol Bull 84: 723–759

Musgrave J, Gloor P 1980 The role of the corpus callosum in bilateral interhemisphereic synchory of spike and wave discharge in feline penicillin epilepsy. Epilepsia 21: 369–378

Muthen J 1978 Psychological treatment of epileptic seizures. Thesis, Institute of Applied Psychology, Uppsala University, Sweden

Ounsted C, Lee D, Hut S J 1966 Electroencephalographic and clinical changes in an epileptic child during repeated photic stimulation. Electroencephalogr Clin Neurophysiol 21: 388–391

Parrino J J 1971 Reduction of seizures by desensitization. J Behav Ther Exp Psychiatry 2: 215–218

Pinto R 1972 A case of movement epilepsy with agarophobia, treated successfully by flooding. Br J Psychiatry 121: 287–288

Pritchard P, Holmstrom V, Giacinto J 1985 Self-abatement of complex partial seizures. Ann Neurol 18: 265–267

Quy R J, Hut S J, Foresst S 1979 Sensorimotor rhythm feedback training in epilepsy. Biol Psychol 9: 129–149

Rosenbaum M, Palmon N 1984 Helplessness and resourcefulness in coping with epilepsy. J Consult Clin Psychol 52: 244–253

Rousseau A, Herman B, Whitman S 1985 Effects of progressive relaxation on epilepsy: analysis of a series of cases. Psychol Rep 57: 1203–1212

Siefert A R, Lubar J F 1975 Reduction of epileptic seizures through EEG biofeedback training. Biol Psychol 3: 156–184

Standage K F 1972 Treatment of epilepsy by reciprocal inhibition of anxiety. Guys Hosp Rep 121: 217

Sterman M B 1973 Neurophysiological and clinical studies of sensori-motor EEG biofeedback training: some effects of epilepsy. In: Birk L (ed) Biofeedback: behaviour medicine. Grune and Stratton, Boston, pp 507–526

Sterman M B 1977 Effects of sensorimotor EEG feedback training on sleep and clinical manifestation of epilepsy. In: Beatty J, Legewie H (eds) Biofeedback and behaviour. Plenum Press, New York, pp 167–200

Sterman M B, Shouse M N 1980 Quantitative analysis of training, sleep EEG and clinical response to EEG operant conditioning in epileptics. Electroencephalogr Clin Neurophysiol 49: 558–576

Sterman M B, Macdonald L R, Stone R K 1974 Biofeedback training of the sensorimotor EEG rhythm in man: effects on epilepsy. Epilepsia 15: 395–416

Stevens J R 1962 Endogenous conditioning to abnormal cerebral electrical transience in man. Science 137: 974–976

Symonds C 1959 Excitation and inhibition in epilepsy. Brain 82: 133–146

Tan S, Bruni J 1986 Cognitive-behaviour therapy with adult patients with epilepsy: a controlled outcome study. Epilepsia 27: 225–233

Tansey M A 1985 The response of a case of petit mal epilepsy to EEG sensorimotor rhythm biofeedback training. Int J Psychophysiol 3: 81–84

Tempkin N, Davis G 1984 Stress as a risk factor for seizures among adults with epilepsy. Epilepsia 25: 450–456

Wells K, Turner S, Bellack A, Hersen M 1978 Effects of cue-controlled relaxation on psychomotor seizures. Behav Res Ther 16: 51–54

Whyler A R, Lockard J S, Ward A A, Finch C A 1976 Condition EEG desynchronisation and seizure occurrence in patients. Electroencephalogr Clin Neurophysiol 41: 501–512

Williams D T, Spiegel H, Mostofsky D I 1978 Neurogenic and hysterical seizures in children and adolescents: differential diagnostic and therapeutic considerations. Am J Psychiatry 135: 82–86

Wolpe J 1969 The practice of behaviour therapy. Pergamon Press, New York

Wright L 1973 Aversive conditioning of self-induced seizures. Behav Ther 4: 712–713

Zlutnick S I 1972 The control of seizures by the modification of pre-seizure behaviour: the punishment of behavioural chain components (Doctoral dissertation, Utah State College). Dissertation Abstracts International 33, 6B (Univ Microfilms No. 72–31, 182)

Zlutnick S I, Mayville W J, Moffat S 1975 Behavioural control of seizure disorders: the interruption of chained behaviour. In: Katz R C, Zlutnick S I (eds) Behaviour therapy and health care: principles and applications. Pergamon Press, New York

Index